Midwifery
at a Glance

This title is also available as an e-book.
For more details, please see
www.wiley.com/buy/9781118874455

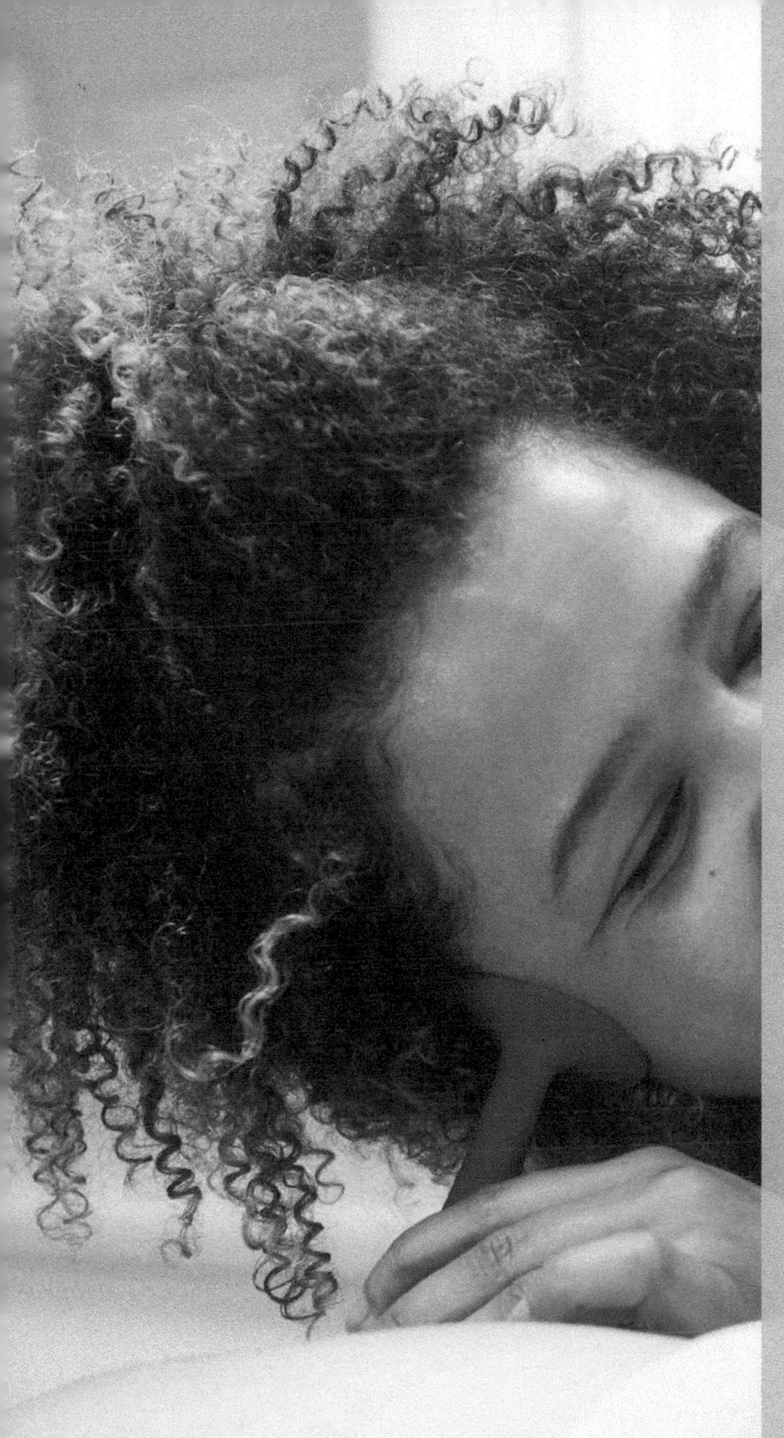

Midwifery at a Glance

Edited by

Eleanor Forrest
Glasgow Caledonian University
Glasgow, UK

Series Editor: Ian Peate OBE, FRCN

WILEY Blackwell

This edition first published 2019

Registered Offices
John Wiley & Sons, Inc., 111 River Street, Hoboken, NJ 07030, USA
John Wiley & Sons Ltd,. The Atrium, Southern Gate, Chichester,
West Sussex, PO19 8SQ, UK

Editorial Office
9600 Garsington Road, Oxford, OX4 2DQ, UK

For details of our global editorial offices, customer services, and more information about Wiley products visit us at www.wiley.com.

Wiley also publishes its books in a variety of electronic formats and by print-on-demand. Some content that appears in standard print versions of this book may not be available in other formats.

Library of Congress Cataloging-in-Publication Data

Names: Forrest, Eleanor, editor. Title: Midwifery at a glance / edited by Eleanor Forrest.
Description: Hoboken, NJ : Wiley-Blackwell, 2018. | Series: At a glance series |
Includes bibliographical references and index. |
Identifiers: LCCN 2018034897 (print) | LCCN 2018035390 (ebook) | ISBN
9781118873618 (Adobe PDF) | ISBN 9781118873601 (ePub) |
ISBN 9781118874455 (pbk.)
Subjects: | MESH: Midwifery—methods | Postnatal Care—methods |
Prenatal Care—methods | Pregnancy—physiology | Handbooks
Classification: LCC RG950 (ebook) | LCC RG950 (print) | NLM WQ 165 | DDC
618.2—dc23
LC record available at https://lccn.loc.gov/2018034897

Cover image: © SolStock/Getty Images
Cover design by Wiley

Set in Minion Pro 9.5/11.5 by Aptara
Printed and bound by CPI Group (UK) Ltd, Croydon CR0 4YY

10 9 8 7 6 5 4 3 2 1

Contents

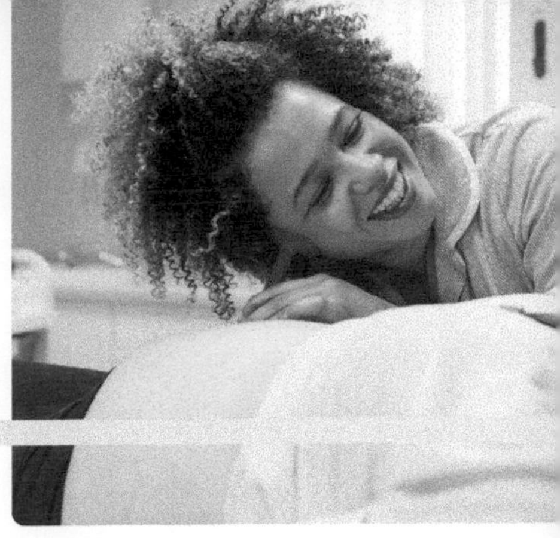

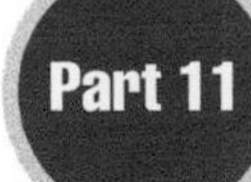

Midwifery skills 171

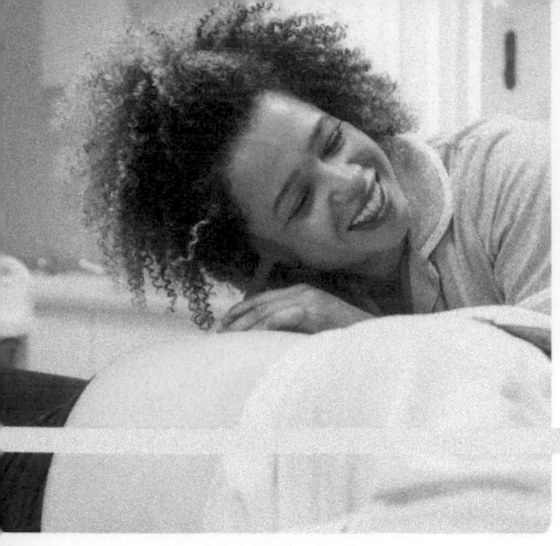

Contributors

Lynda Bateman
University of Hull
Hull, England

Sarah Bennett-Day
University of Suffolk
Suffolk, England

Nicola Bradley
NHS Greater Glasgow & Clyde
Glasgow, Scotland

Jo Butler
University of Suffolk
Suffolk, England

Sam Chenery-Morris
University of Suffolk
Suffolk, England

Laura Coltart
NHS Greater Glasgow & Clyde
Glasgow, Scotland

Fenella Cowie
NHS Tayside
Perth, Scotland

Catriona Hendry
Glasgow Caledonian University
Glasgow, Scotland

Cindy Horan
Queen Elizabeth University Hospital Maternity Unit
Glasgow, Scotland

Lyz Howie
University of the West of Scotland
Paisley, Scotland

Anne Lennie
Princess Royal Maternity Hospital
Glasgow, Scotland

Helene Marshall
NES Scotland
Edinburgh, Scotland

Marion McPhillips
Family Nurse Partnership National Unit
Edinburgh, Scotland

Ola Ogbuehi
University of Hull
Hull, England

Heather Passmore
University of Suffolk
Suffolk, England

Lorna Pender
Gender Based Violence Resource Unit
Glasgow, Scotland

Angela Poat
University of Hull
Hull, England

Liz Teiger
Glasgow Caledonian University
Glasgow, Scotland

Jane Tyler
University of Hull
Hull, England

About the companion website

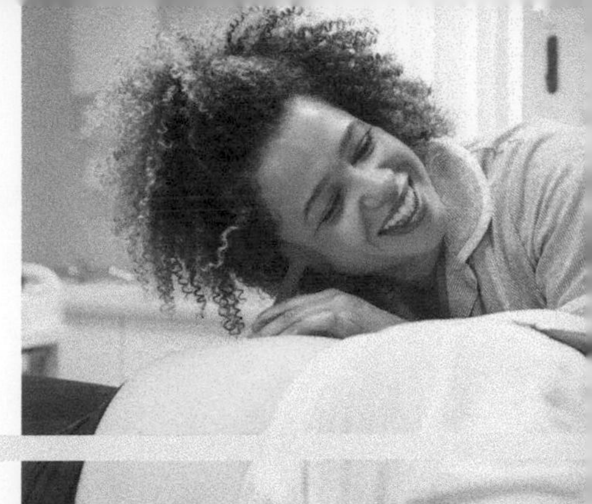

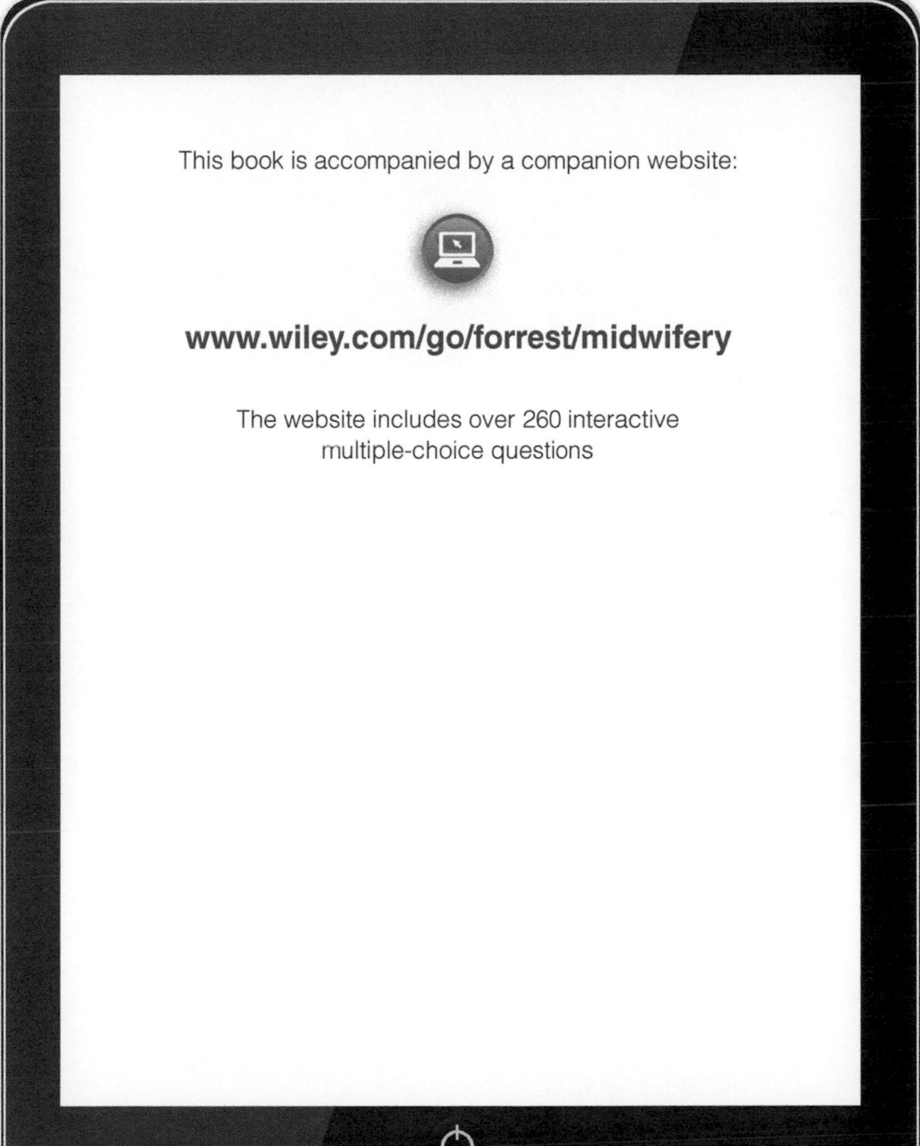

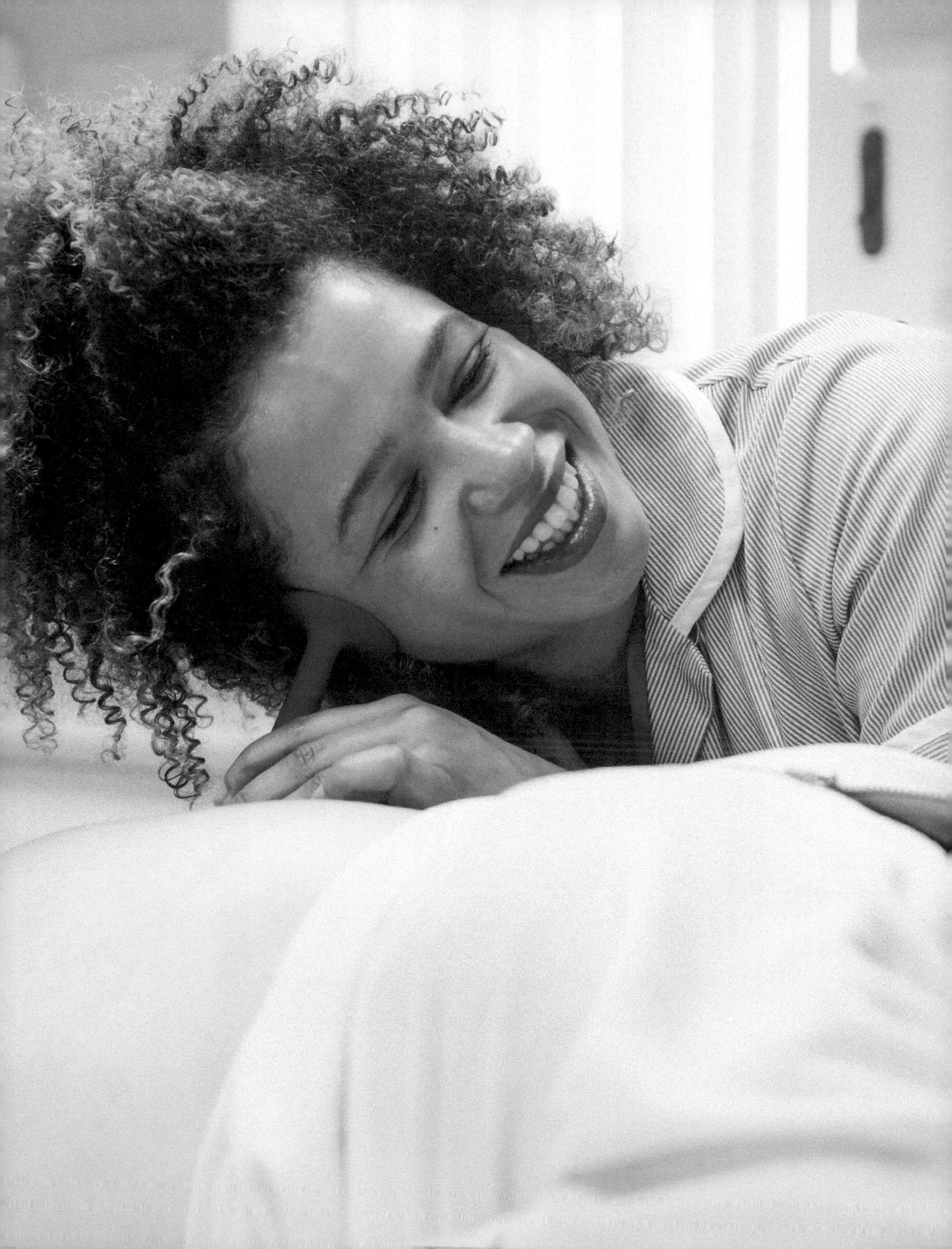

Introduction

Chapters

Historical overview of midwifery

Table 1.1 Major historical events in midwifery during the 20th and 21st centuries.

Date	Development	Recommendations/Effects
1902	Midwives Act	Central Midwives Board (CMB) in England and Wales formed to provide a roll of certified midwives – included those registered with the London Obstetrical Society and bona fide midwives 3-month training for entrants to midwifery; examinations conducted and certificates issued Local supervision of midwives established to ensure high quality care
1915		Legal regulation of midwifery in Scotland. Provision of antenatal care; compulsory notification of birth
1916		Training doubled to 6 months for direct entrants; 4-month training for nurse entrants
1918	Amendment to Midwives Act	Local authority responsible for paying doctor's fee and mileage; statutory provision of a midwife's stationery; CMB powers to suspend and remove midwives from the roll
1922		Legal regulation of midwifery in Northern Ireland
1926	Amendment to Midwives Act	12-month training for direct entrants: 6-month training for nurse entrants Midwife Teachers Certificate established
1936	Midwives Act	Adequate salaried domiciliary midwifery service; working conditions improved Improved provision of antenatal care Qualifications for Supervisor of Midwives prescribed. End of bona fide midwives
1938		Training doubled to 2 years for direct entrants; 1 year for SRNs Training divided into two parts; length of part 1 determined by previous experience of applicant; part 2 – 6 months for all pupils
1941		Midwives Institute became the College of Midwives, gaining Royal Charter in 1947
1943	Rushcliffe Report	Identification of midwifery as a distinct profession from nurisng and salary scale greater in recognition of responsibility of the work. Recommended caseload of 66 confinements a year without a pupil; 90 a year with a pupil; 96-hour fortnight for hospital midwives-
1952	CEMD commenced	Confidential Enquiry into Maternal Deaths (CEMD) – enquiries around maternal deaths and triennial report produced to save lives of women and babies, reduce complications and improve quality of maternity care
1968		Single period midwifery training – parts 1 and 2 phased out
1970	Peel Report	Recommended 100% availability of beds for hospital confinement Consequent effect of this was majority of care provided within hospital with a more medicalised approach; increased use of technology including induction of labour, use of cardiotocography, intrauterine pressure monitoring-1978 – first IVF baby born
1972	Briggs Report	Midwives would be expected to complete nurse training prior to 1 year post-registration midwifery; led to Nurses, Midwives and Health Visitors Act 1979
1979	Demise of CMB	Formation of United Kingdom Central Council for Nurses, Midwives and Health Visitors, with four National Boards (e.g. English National Board)
1980	Short Report	Actions to reduce high perinatal and neonatal mortality rates
1981		3-year training for direct entrants: 18-month training for nurse entrants Changes implemented in line with European Directives 1980
1992	Winterton Report	Midwives the key professionals to care for the majority of women with normal pregnancies and births; obstetricians to look after the few women who have complicated pregnancies. No evidence to suggest that home birth is unsafe for healthy women and every woman should know of their right to choose a home birth
1993	DH Changing Childbirth Report	Followed findings of Winterton Report, and established 3 'Cs': Choice (of type of care), Control (of what is happening by participating in decisions) and Continuity (knowing a small group of professionals who will care throughout her maternity experience) as dominating principles for women during pregnancy and birth (chaired by Baroness Cumberldge)
1996		Health authorities assume responsibility for supervision of midwives
2002	NMC formed	Regulatory funtion of United Kingdom Central Council for Nurses, Midwives and Health Visitors replaced by Nursing and Midwifery Council (NMC)
2007	Maternity Matters	High quality, safe and accessible maternity service through a new national choice guarantee, together with improved access to services and continuity of midwifery care and support
2010	Midwifery 2020	Vision of the midwife as lead professional for women with normal pregnancies and to work as the key co-ordinator with the multidisciplinary team for women with complex needs. Development of a greater public health role and provision of innovative, evidence-based, cost effective, high quality care for women, responsive to change-
2011	MINT Report	Evaluation of contribution and impact of midwife teachers on care provided by students and newly qualified midwives and demonstration of fitness for practice-
2012	MBRRACE	Mothers and Babies Reducing Risk through Audits and Confidential Enquiries replaces CEMD
2015	Kirkup Report	Recommended removal of supervision of midwifery from NMC regulatory framework
2016	Better Births	*Better Births: Improving Outcomes of Maternity Services in England – A Five Year Forward View of Maternity Care* (chaired by Baroness Cumberldge)

Midwifery at a Glance, First Edition. Edited by Eleanor Forrest © 2019 John Wiley & Sons, Ltd. Published 2019 by John Wiley & Sons, Ltd.
Companion website: www.wiley.com/go/forrest/midwifery

Midwifery is one of the oldest occupations in the world, if considered simply as the presence of a woman accompanying another woman during her childbearing event, with knowledge passed from one generation to another. The term midwife is understood to mean 'with woman' but older terms have existed such as 'howdie' in Scotland. Midwives' status in the community rose and fell over the centuries, influenced by medical men and concern over their mysterious powers. Soranus of Ephesus (2nd century AD) is credited with writing the first textbook on midwifery, which described desirable characteristics of a good midwife to be 'literate, with her wits about her, good memory, loving work, respectable, not unduly handicapped as regards her senses, sound of limb, robust, long slim fingers and short nails, soft hands, free from superstition and of sympathetic disposition.' The contemporary concept of a 'good midwife' is related to the complementary areas of theoretical knowledge and skilled competence underpinned by lifelong learning, communication skills, and personal qualities including emotional intelligence, with a midwife's professionalism being central to women's empowerment during childbirth. However, often women became midwives by default of attending a birth with a midwife and then being asked to attend others.

The first school to train midwives was founded in Edinburgh in 1726, followed by Glasgow in 1739, with others following in England. However, training was mainly under the auspices of the Faculty of Physicians and Surgeons. The 18th century also saw the rise of male midwives among controversy regarding their role in attending women. Smellie (c. 1750) provided anatomical knowledge that contributed to understanding the mechanism of normal labour, while Chamberlen (c. 1733) used forceps to aid delivery of a live baby rather than just to extract the often dead fetus. During the 19th century, educated middle class women tried to improve the status of midwifery as a profession through the eradication of caricatures such as the uneducated, drunken Sarah Gamp portrayed by Charles Dickens. The Ladies Obstetrical College (1846) was formed by these educated women, offering theoretical and practical training, but was disbanded due to puerperal fever. The London Obstetrical Society Examining Board (1872) required candidates for midwifery to be aged between 21 and 30 years and have proof of attending a minimum of 25 cases; however only six took the exam.

Rosalind Paget and Zepherina Veitch were influential women in the establishment of the Midwives Institute (1881; to become the Royal College of Midwives (RCM)), which campaigned for the registration of midwives, culminating in the Midwives Act 1902 (England and Wales) which specified the education and training, registration and certification, supervision and control of midwifery practice. Therefore it was not until the 20th century that legislation existed to regulate midwifery practice. The roll of qualified midwives maintained by the Central Midwives Board (CMB), included women who already possessed a recognised qualification in midwifery and women of good character who had already practiced as a midwife for at least 1 year (bona fide midwives). Legislation laid down several aspects of midwifery practice and rules concerning equipment, clothing and standards of hygiene that were considered essential, which continued until the 1970s.

Improvements in midwifery practice focused on strategies to reduce maternal and perinatal mortality rates, aided by social and environmental and technological advances, combined with changes in working practices and education and training for midwives. Pressure groups such as the Association of Radical Midwives (ARM) and the National Childbirth Trust (NCT), together with the RCM as a professional and trade union-affiliated organisation, through various reports and campaigns, have influenced both the provision of care and status of the midwife as professionals (Table 1.1).

Changes in the regulatory body (CMB to UK Central Council (UKCC) to Nursing Midwifery Council (NMC)) over the years have seen modifications to the *Midwives Rules and Standards* (NMC, 2012) and *The Code* (NMC, 2015) to less specified activity with greater use of professional knowledge and competence. Supervision of midwives increased after 1996, with their role and function being prescribed within the *Midwives Rules and Standards*; however recent investigations into the practice of midwifery supervision (such as Morecombe Bay and Guernsey) have led to the demise of this within the regulatory function of the NMC (Chapter 5).

In 1986, Project 2000 recommended a 3-year curriculum, with midwifery being seen as a branch of nursing. This was fiercely rejected by the profession and a year later the RCM advocated a 3-year curriculum for midwifery in the UK with direct entrant midwifery, which was supported by the English National Board in 1988. Whilst two hospitals continued some direct entrant training (Edgware and Derby), in 1989 seven 'midwifery schools' commenced 3-year direct entrant midwifery training, and by 1994 there were 35 three-year pre-registration programmes, at both degree and diploma level, linked to higher education institutions. The formation of the UKCC in 1989 had led to removal of the requirements for specified hours of medical practitioner input into the midwifery curriculum and examination. By 2009, the NMC, within their standards for pre-registration midwifery education, stipulated that midwifery should became an all degree profession.

Midwifery remains an important occupation and is highly valued by women. However, constant tension between personal qualities, as aligned to the NHS values and the six 'C's of Care (Chapter 2), and professional competencies of midwives and other occupations have all had an impact on the status of midwifery and the autonomy and control of midwives. Changes in relation to the skill mix in maternity services and in midwifery supervision and the future of the *Midwives Rules and Standards* have set the scene for the potential of professional control remaining an important issue in the future of midwifery practice.

2 NHS values

Box 2.1 The NHS principles.

- To provide a comprehensive service to all
- Care is based on clinical need, not ability to pay
- Aspires to the highest standards of excellence and professionalism
- The patient is at the heart of everything the NHS does
- To work across organisational boundaries and in partnership with other organisations in the interests of patients, local communities and wider population
- Committed to providing best value for taxpayers' money and most effective, fair and sustainable use of finite resources
- To be accountable to the public, communities and patients it serves

Box 2.2 NHS Scotland – 10 essential shared capabilities supporting person-centred approaches.

- Working in partnership
- Respecting diversity
- Practising ethically
- Challenging inequality
- Promoting recovery, wellbeing and self-management
- Identifying people's needs and strengths
- Providing person-centred care
- Making a difference
- Promoting safety and risk enablement
- Personal development and learning

Box 2.3 Recent inquiry and review summaries into the NHS. Source: http://www.midstaffspublicinquiry.com, https://www.england.nhs.uk/2013/12/sir-bruce-keogh-7ds/, https://www.gov.uk/government/publications/berwick-review-into-patient-safety. Licensed under Open Governement License v3.0.

Francis Inquiry February 2013

- A public inquiry into the failings at Mid Staffordshire NHS foundation Trust made 290 recommendations for improvement. At the heart of these was a need to develop: a culture of openness and transparency; a system of accountability for all; a system for promoting clinical leadership and emphasis on always putting patients first (www.midstaffspublicinquiry.com)

Keogh Review July 2013

- A review of 14 hospital trusts with a persistently high mortality rate of which 11 hospitals were put into special measures. 8 key ambitions set out for improving care and this has informed the Care Quality Commission in developing its process of inspecting all trusts throughout England (www.nhs.uk/NHSEngland/bruce-keogh-review)

Berwick Review August 2013

- In response to the Francis inquiry this review explored how 'zero harm' could be made a reality in the NHS. 10 recommendations made with core themes around transparency, continual learning, leadership, regulation and seeking patient and carer opinions (www.gov.uk/government/publications/berwick-review-into-patient-safety)

Box 2.4 Chief nurse's 6 'C's of care. Source: NHS. Licensed under Open Gov License v3.0.

- Care
- Compassion
- Commitment
- Courage
- Communication
- Competence

CNO and DH CN (2012) Compassion in Practice. Commissioning Board. Leeds https://www.england.nhs.uk/wp-content/uploads/2012/12/compassion-in-practice.pdf

Box 2.5 NMC 4 'P's for professional standards.

- Prioritise people
- Practise effectively
- Preserve safety
- Promote professionalism and trust

Box 2.6 Remit of the National Institute for Health and Care Excellence. Source: https://www.nice.org.uk.

NICE provides national guidance and advice to improve health and social care. It achieves this by:

- Producing evidence-based guidance and advice for health, public health and social care practitioners
- Developing legally binding quality standards for those providing and commissioning health, public health and social care services
- Providing a range of informational services for commissioners, practitioners and managers across the spectrum of health and social care (www.nice.org.uk)

Figure 2.1 NHS Outcomes Framework 2016/17 showing relevance to midwifery.

Domain 1: Preventing people from dying prematurely	
Indicators: potential years of life lost; children & young people; neonatal mortality & stillbirths	Improvement areas: reducing premature mortality in people with mental illness; suicide & mortality from injury of undetermined intent; reducing mortality in children/infant mortality

↓

Domain 4: Ensuring that people have a positive experience of care	
Indicators: patient experience of patient care–GP services/NHS dental/hospital care/friends & family test	Improvement areas: improving people's experience of outpatient services; responsiveness to in-patient needs; access to GP and NHS dental services; women's experiences of maternity services

↓

Domain 5: Treating & caring for people in a safe environment & protecting them from avoidable harm	
Indicators: deaths attributable to problems in healthcare; severe harm attributable to harm in healthcare	Improvement areas: reducing the incidence of avoidable harm; incidence of venous thromboembolism (VTE), healthcare-associated infection (HCAI), methicillin-resistant *S. aureus* (MRSA) *C. difficile*; newly acquired category 2, 3 & 4 pressure ulcers; improving safety of maternity services; admission of full term babies to neonatal care

The NHS was founded in 1947 to improve health and wellbeing within a common set of principles. The NHS Constitution was first published in 2009 by the Department of Health as part of a 10-year plan to provide the highest quality of care and service for patients in England. Updated in 2015, it explicitly states the principles (Box 2.1), values and pledges that patients, the public and staff can expect from the NHS and what the NHS expects from them in return.

NHS Scotland has published the 10 Essential Shared Capabilities supporting person-centred approaches to care (Box 2.2) that has themes comparable to the NHS Constitution. Following the failings at the Mid Staffordshire NHS Foundation Trust, it is vital that everyone involved in the NHS learns from the findings of the subsequent Francis Inquiry and Keogh and Berwick Reviews (Box 2.3). The NHS values describe how everyone using or working within the NHS should be treated and the updated constitution reflects that the NHS's most important value is for patients to be at the heart of everything the NHS does.

Six values

The six NHS values are respect and dignity; compassion; working together for patients; improving lives; everyone counts; and commitment to quality of care. These apply to all recipients and providers of care and describe the aspiration to facilitate co-operative working at all levels of the NHS.

Applied to midwifery practice these values can be considered as:

1 **Respect and dignity** – every person is valued as an individual and respect is given to their aspirations and commitments in life, and their priorities, needs, abilities and limits should be understood, irrespective of whether they are a mother/baby, family member or staff. Care should be provided with honesty and integrity and listening to the views of others, for example when formulating a birth plan, to enhance provision of safe and effective care.

2 **Compassion** – midwives should respond with humanity and kindness to each mother's need, pain or distress and find things that will provide comfort and relieve suffering to mothers and their families but also their colleagues, for example during labour and in times of bereavement.

3 **Working together for patients** – mothers, babies and their family come first in everything a midwife does. Collaboration with the multidisciplinary team and networking plus seeking the views of service users will contribute to effective care delivery.

4 **Improving lives** – the public health role of the midwife and health promotion can affect the mother's health. Midwives can innovate and improve care to improve health and wellbeing plus the mother's experience of the NHS, for example establishing teams to support vulnerable women.

5 **Everyone counts** – midwives should maximise resources for the benefit of the whole community of mothers, babies and their families, whatever their social or educational background, their race, religion or culture; for example all women should have equal access to antenatal classes.

6 **Commitment to quality of care** – midwives must provide safe and effective care. The right care, in the right way at the right time is dependent upon midwives' knowledge and skills, communication and competence and ability to work with others. Midwives should offer evidence-based care, for example using National Institute for Health and Care Excellence (NICE) guidance and participate in clinical audits.

Six 'C's

In 2012 the Chief Nursing Officer for England launched a vision for nurses and midwives entitled Compassion in Practice, to provide for basic human needs with care and compassion; all patients can expect to receive such care within the NHS. This applies to midwives as well as nursing. The 6 'C's – care, compassion, commitment, courage, communication and competence – are the core elements of the vision (Box 2.4). Care is the core business of midwives, which improves the lives of mothers, babies and their families. Mothers expect care to be right for them, consistently, throughout every stage of their childbearing process. Compassion is how care is given through relationships based on empathy, respect and dignity – it can also be described as emotional intelligence, and is central to how people perceive their care.

The 6 'C's reaffirm the qualities and standards that the public can expect from midwives, and those in the profession are aware that no matter how midwifery changes, the six values remain at the core. If midwives work in accordance with the 4 'P's of professional practice (Box 2.5) as defined by the Nursing and Midwifery Council (NMC) in *The Code* (NMC, 2015), their practice will be congruent with the NHS principles and values. This will enable practitioners to maintain their professional knowledge and competence to perform safely but also report when care does not fulfil these standards.

Quality is defined as excellence in patient safety, clinical effectiveness and patient experience and is an organising principle of the NHS. Clinically effective care delivery is supported through the remit of NICE (Box 2.6) and numerous guidelines support midwives and their colleagues in the delivery of high-quality care, for example intrapartum care and antenatal and postnatal mental health. An effective healthcare system should: (i) prevent people from dying prematurely, (ii) improve the quality of life for people living with long-term health conditions, and (iii) aid recovery for those with ill health. The NHS Outcomes Framework identifies five overall principles, three of which relate to midwifery care (domains 1, 4 and 5) (Figure 2.1).

The NHS values require the development of a culture where it is the 'norm' to Observe others, Praise good practice, Challenge poor practice and Escalate concerns readily (OPCE). Adherence to this will improve outcomes and satisfaction for mothers and their families.

3 Ethics

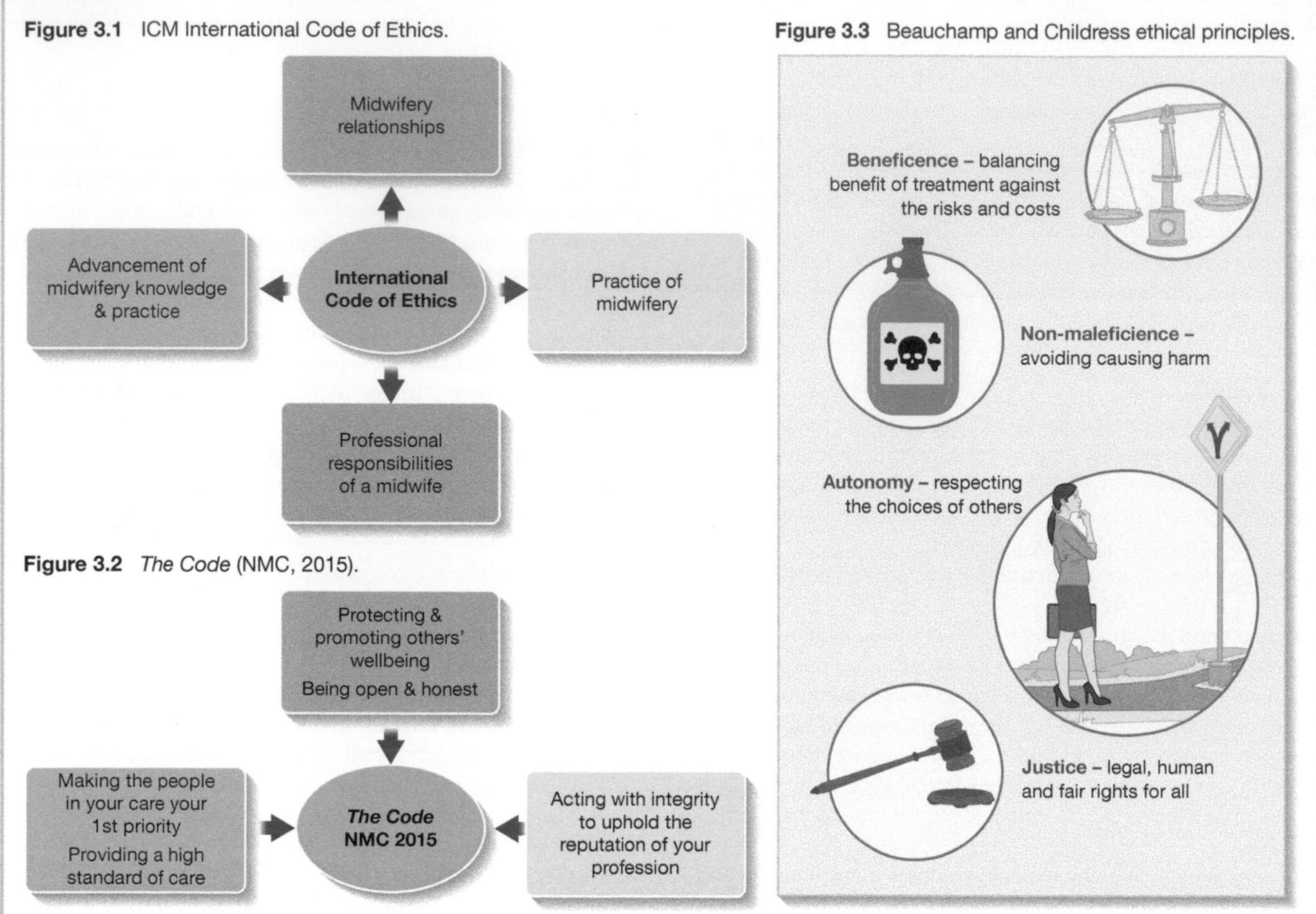

Figure 3.1 ICM International Code of Ethics.

Figure 3.2 *The Code* (NMC, 2015).

Figure 3.3 Beauchamp and Childress ethical principles.

Ethics are pervasive in midwifery practice. Ethics is a term used to cover fundamental principles of what is right and wrong and what people should or ought to do. Ethical principles can be explored at the micro or macro level or from a personal, professional and societal viewpoint.

Micro and macro

Micro-level ethics promotes good interactions between women and midwives, based on mutual respect and trust. It offers all women equitable care and promotes truly individualised information so each woman can make the right choice according to her needs, religious beliefs and values. Macro-level ethics looks at policies, technologies and practices across the reproductive health span. These include issues of sexual consent, the rights of women to choose contraception, abortion or to be sterilised, or where to give birth to their baby.

Personal, professional and theoretical

Everyone has a right to their own ethical values and beliefs. Beliefs come from our parents, upbringing, schooling, education, religious figures and the media. Most people have views on what they believe to be morally right or wrong on issues such as life or death and reproductive choices.

As midwives our personal beliefs need to be set aside when offering professional midwifery care and information to pregnant women or new mothers. Across the globe each country will have their own professional code of ethics which generally follow those produced by the International Confederation of Midwives (ICM) based around four concepts (Figure 3.1). In the UK, the Nursing and Midwifery Council publishes *The Code* (NMC, 2015) which includes the ethical principles nurses and midwives must understand and adhere to (Figure 3.2). These include: making the people in your care your first priority, protecting and promoting others' wellbeing, providing a high standard of care, being open and honest and acting with integrity to uphold the reputation of your profession. Key terms like gaining informed consent and maintaining professional barriers and confidentiality are explained in further detail. How you offer informed consent to any treatment or intervention in midwifery, from screening tests to suturing, matters. What you say and how you say it either enables or acts as a barrier to empowering the individual women to make autonomous decisions about what is acceptable to her. Doing or saying what we think is right is not acceptable, we need to give women the evidence, carefully describing the risks and benefits so they can make their own decisions whether to accept or decline care options.

There are only two areas of professional practice where your views as a person matter. The term used is contentious objection and the two practices are: providing abortion care and technological procedures to achieve a pregnancy. However, if the woman needs emergency treatment in either case, the midwife has a duty to provide this, regardless of their personal views.

Theoretically, one of the most prevalent ethical frameworks used in healthcare was devised by Beauchamp and Childress (Figure 3.3). Their four principles were originally non-hierarchical, meaning each principle had equal weight, but now the principle of respect for autonomy is seen as paramount.

Autonomy

The word originates from the Greek for self-govern. It is often applied to midwifery practice but in ethics it means the individual is capable to decide for themselves what matter in their life. The moral obligation of a midwife regarding autonomy of another person is to respect their choices. In order for women to make informed choices the midwife imparts information that must be factual and complete. The midwife's role is not to bombard individual women with information but to have conversations in language they understand so they can choose which care and which tests they want and where to have their baby. Not giving enough information is not acceptable, it assumes you are treating the woman as a child (paternalism) and disengages the woman and her family actively in her care decisions. Legally, information is required prior to consent, whether this is to take a blood pressure measurement, an ultrasound scan or examination. If a woman lacks autonomy, her competence or capacity to consent to care may be undertaken by another person in her best interest. This is unusual in midwifery.

Beneficence

In order to act for the benefit of others, all the evidence must be considered. As a midwife it is your obligation to maintain contemporaneous research knowledge. As a practitioner you will know smoking in pregnancy is harmful to the woman and her developing fetus. You have a responsibility to offer smoking cessation advice (beneficence) but the woman has the right to decide whether to take this advice or not (autonomy). Her right to autonomy must be upheld, but you still have a duty to promote wellbeing. Open and honest interaction between you and the woman regarding her choices and informing her of the benefits of smoking cessation are required. The woman cannot choose to quit if she does not know the benefits of cessation for her and the baby.

Non-maleficience

Avoiding harm to others seems simple enough, yet there are many interventions in midwifery that may cause harm which should be considered. For example, a vaginal examination may be offered, especially in labour. This may be uncomfortable and an invasion of the woman's personal body, yet the information gained from performing a vaginal examination may be needed to offer her care options. So the benefit of undertaking this exam may outweigh the harm it causes. However, some women may experience significant harm from having this exam, so the concept of non-maleficience is not always straightforward. A woman may decline blood products due to her religious beliefs; although the blood may do no physical harm, her moral beliefs would be harmed in accepting it. All midwifery interventions require consideration for potential harm for individuals.

Justice

This is concerned with the distribution of healthcare, to make sure that everyone has access to a fair system. As midwives you have an obligation to treat all women equally.

4 Role of the midwife

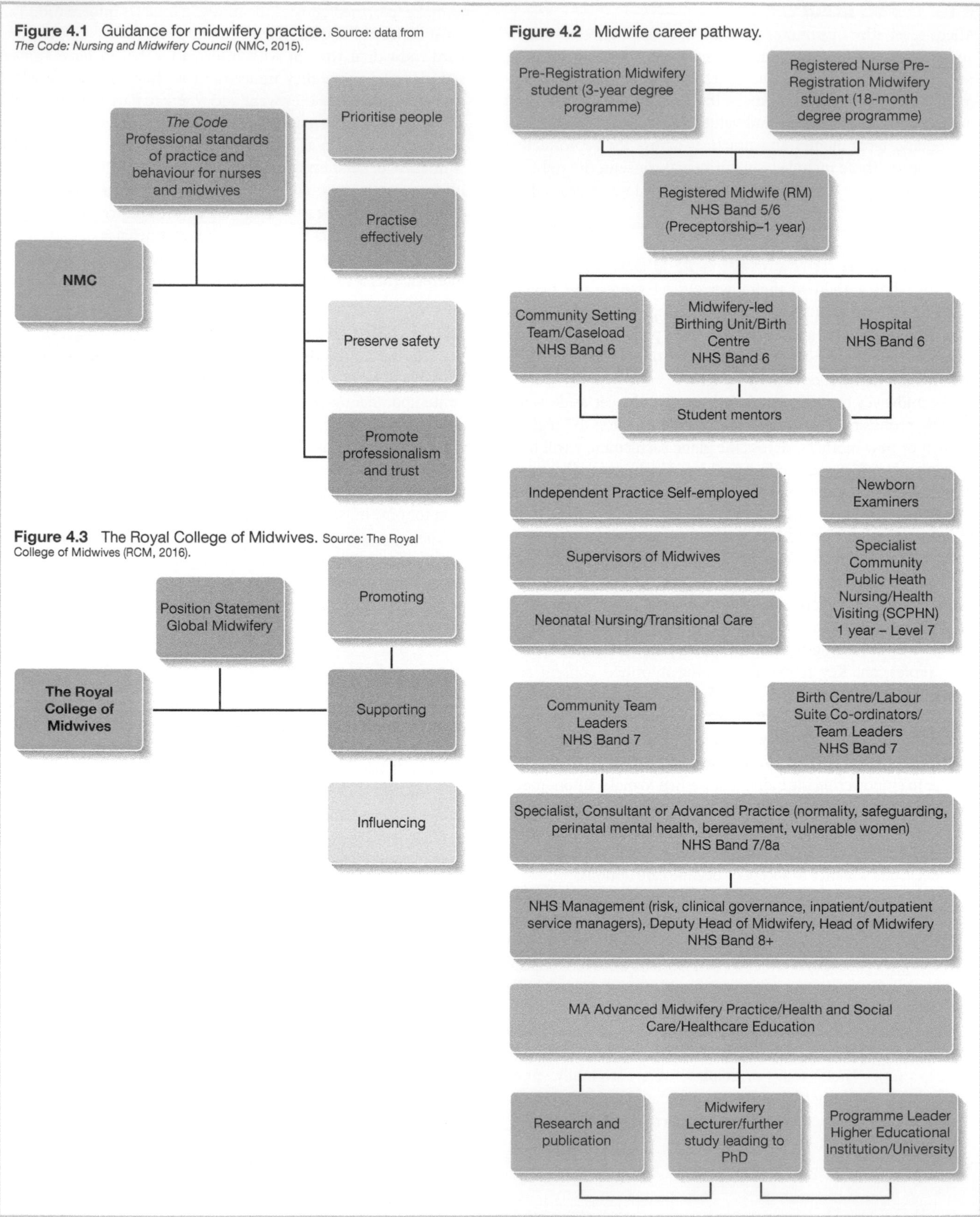

Figure 4.1 Guidance for midwifery practice. Source: data from *The Code: Nursing and Midwifery Council* (NMC, 2015).

Figure 4.2 Midwife career pathway.

Figure 4.3 The Royal College of Midwives. Source: The Royal College of Midwives (RCM, 2016).

Midwifery at a Glance, First Edition. Edited by Eleanor Forrest © 2019 John Wiley & Sons, Ltd. Published 2019 by John Wiley & Sons, Ltd.
Companion website: [illegible]

Definition

The International Confederation of Midwives (ICM) represents the midwifery profession worldwide. For the title 'midwife' to be used; a person must demonstrate competency in the practice of midwifery through the acquisition of specific skills, leading to qualification by a recognised midwifery education programme.

> *'The midwife is recognised as a responsible and accountable professional who works in partnership with women to give the necessary support, care and advice during pregnancy, labour and the postpartum period, to conduct births on the midwife's own responsibility and to provide care for the newborn and the infant. This care includes preventative measures, the promotion of normal birth, the detection of complications in mother and child, the accessing of medical care or other appropriate assistance and the carrying out of emergency measures' (ICM, 2011).*

Midwives are also professionals who engage with women and their families. This is an insightful time and an opportunity to make a lasting, positive impact. The midwife is in a prime position to assume a wider public health role, including preconception care, health counselling and education for the woman, her partner and other children. As the midwife's role is complex, the midwife continuously must adapt to the needs of the woman and her family. Women want a midwife to be with them through all aspects of their care. The midwife must be the expert in normality and health promotion and the co-ordinator when care falls outside her remit; knowing when to refer to other professionals such as obstetricians, general practitioners, health visitors, social workers and specialist services (such as mental health).

Scope of practice

The majority of midwives (96%) in the UK work within the NHS, with the remainder working in a self-employed capacity as independent practitioners, often as part of a small team. However, all qualified midwives must be registered with and are regulated by the Nursing and Midwifery Council (NMC). Midwives have a direct responsibility to the women in their care and for actions taken when providing care – professional accountability. Fundamental to practising as a midwife is the commitment to upholding the professional standards set out by the NMC (2015), published in *The Code* (Figure 4.1). To maintain registration and continue to practice in the UK, a midwife, as of April 2016, must 'revalidate' with the NMC every 3 years. The NMC exists to protect the public and ensure that only those registered to practice midwifery can provide care in the UK. In serious cases, a midwife may have her registration suspended or revoked. Revalidation ensures not only that the public are safe from practitioners who have failed to meet the required standards of professionalism and competence, but maintains a culture of continued professional development and life-long learning for midwives, upholding a high, deeply respected public profile.

A midwife may work in a wide variety of settings, from community centres, to women's homes, stand-alone midwife-led birthing centres, co-located birthing units and hospitals. Her sphere of practice may include preconception care; she is the first point of contact for a woman upon conception, and for health promotion, education and support through the antenatal period, as well as clinical assessment and documentation. She is the primary care giver for a woman experiencing a normal pregnancy and documentation would include direct referral for ultrasound scans, all screening tests and referral to other practitioners, such as obstetricians. A midwife is the lead professional at a home birth or within a midwifery-led birthing centre/unit and a co-ordinator of care when a woman requires input from the medical team. Midwives provide immediate care to the newborn baby and must be competent in managing emergency situations. Midwives support women in the earliest days of parenting, ensuring this transition is a positive and life-affirming one, advising and offering support and education on breastfeeding, basic care and hygiene principles. The postpartum is an emotional and testing time for a new family, the midwife will care for a woman and her baby within the hospital environment and at home, typically for up to 10 days but this may be extended in some areas to 28 days postpartum. Midwives may look to progress in their career, entering varying levels of management, education and research (Figure 4.2).

In general, the midwifery model of care is social rather than medical and is underpinned by a philosophy of normality and the natural ability for the woman to give birth to her baby with minimum intervention, enhancing her wellbeing and feelings of empowerment, placing the woman at the centre of care. The midwife must then be competent in the planning, organisation and delivery of an individualised care plan, made with the woman at her first booking appointment and reviewed with the woman throughout her pregnancy. In this model, continuity is important. This may refer to continuity of carer or of care. A small team of midwives, based within a community setting, where their workload is organised by geographical location and where the midwifery team acts as the lead professional, may offer the greatest balance in ensuring the woman has such continuity of care, a deeper relationship with the midwives caring for her and the highest quality of care and satisfaction, maximising the chances of the best outcomes. The Royal College of Midwives is a professional organisation (Figure 4.3) and trade union that supports midwives in practice, providing legal and statutory information, guidance and support and works to promote the profession on an international level. The midwife has a unique place in society, working on a very personal level with women and their families, and much of the role cannot be quantified or measured because the midwife is as important emotionally to the individual woman as she is physically.

5 Drug exemptions

Figure 5.1 Illegal drugs.

CLASS A – morphine, diamorphine, heroin, ectasy, Lysergic Acid Diethylamine (LSD)

CLASS B – barbiturates, speed, cannabis, mephedrone, codeine

CLASS C – ketamine, gammahydroxybutrate (GHB), anabolic steriods, benzodiazepines

Box 5.1 Prescription only medicines (POMs).

- Diclofenac
- Hydrocortisone acetate
- Miconazole
- Nystatin
- Phytomenadione

Box 5.2 Exemptions from restriction on administration.

This list is subject to commercial availability and may change over time

- Adrenaline
- Anti D Immunoglobulin
- Carboprost
- Cyclizine lactate
- Diamorphine
- Ergometrine maleate
- Gelofusine
- Hartmann's solution
- Hepatitis B vaccine
- Hepatitis B immunoglobulin
- Lidocaine
- Lidocaine hydrochloride
- Morphine
- Naloxone hydrochloride
- Phytomenadione
- Prochloperazine
- Sodium chloride 0.9%

Midwives at the point of registration and on notifying their intention to practice may supply and/or administer on their own initiative any of the substances that are indicated in medicines legislation under midwives' exemptions, provided this is during their professional practice. They may do this without a prescription, patient-specific directive or patient group directive (PGD) from a medical practitioner provided the requirements of any conditions attached to the exemptions are met. The two main acts of parliament controlling the administration and use of medicines are the Medicines Act 1968 and the Misuse of Drugs Act 1971. There are, however, exemptions from the general rules provided specifically for midwives in the Prescription Only Medicine (Human Use) Order 1997, the Medicines (Sale or Supply) (Miscellaneous Provisions) Regulations 1980 and the Medicines (Pharmacy and General Sale – Exemption) Order 1980. In July 2011, new legislation came into force that amended the list of medicines which midwives are able to supply and administer in their professional practice. These specific amendments can be found on the Nursing and Midwifery Council (NMC) website.

Under the Medicines Act 1968, medicines classified as pharmacy (P) medicines may be sold or supplied only through registered pharmacies by or under the supervision of a pharmacist (section 52). Prescription only medicines (POMs) are subject to an additional requirement: they may only be sold or supplied through pharmacies against a prescription from an appropriate practitioner (section 58). General sale list (GSL) medicines may be sold through retail outlets other than pharmacies as they do not need to be sold or supplied under the supervision of a pharmacist (sections 51 and 53).

Under the Misuse of Drugs Act 1971 dangerous or otherwise harmful drugs are divided into Class A, B and C (Figure 5.1) according to the perceived degree of harm. Class A drugs are those considered the most harmful when misused. Class B drugs, although still dangerous, are classified as less harmful then Class A drugs. Class C are the least dangerous but still illegal.

Exemptions vary for prescribing, which requires the involvement of a pharmacist in the sale or supply of the medicine, and PGDs, where the midwife must comply with specific legal criteria and needs the PGD to be signed by a doctor or dentist and a pharmacist and authorised by an appropriate body.

Exemption from restrictions on sale or supply

Under the 'sale or supply' exemptions for midwives, a registered midwife, in the course of her professional practice, may supply but not offer for sale:

- All medicinal products on the general sales list and all pharmacy medicines
- POMs containing *only* the substances in Box 5.1.

Exemptions from restriction on administration

Registered midwives may also administer parenterally (not through the oral route), in the course of their professional practice, POMs that contain any of the substances in Box 5.2. It is important to remember that midwives may not administer any other substance specified in column 1 of Schedule 1 of the Medicines for Human Use Order 2011.

Midwife's supply order

As already explained, a registered midwife may administer in her own right, so far as is necessary for the practice of her profession, POMs for parenteral administration containing any of the substances in Box 5.2. However, the supply of controlled drugs may only be made to the midwife on the authority of a midwife's supply order signed by the appropriate medical officer who is a doctor authorised in writing by the Local Supervising Authority (LSA), or more commonly a Supervisor of Midwives (SOM). The order must specify the name and occupation of the midwife obtaining the drug, the purpose for which it is required and the total quantity needed. The pharmacist must retain the midwife's supply order for 2 years. A midwife is required to keep a record of supplies of diamorphine, morphine and pethidine received and administered in a book used solely for that purpose. The midwife must not destroy surplus stock but should surrender it to the supplying pharmacy. This is not to be confused with discarding any drug remaining in an ampoule after use. Diamorphine, morphine and pethidine are Schedule 2 Controlled Drugs; therefore, an appropriate entry is required in the Controlled Drug Register. Temazepam is a Schedule 3 Controlled Drug and therefore no entry is required in the Controlled Drug Register.

A midwife's records relating to the administration of medicines should be regularly audited by her named SOM and any concerns should be reported to the Accountable Officer for Controlled Drugs and the LSA Midwifery Officer.

Student midwives and exemptions

Student midwives are allowed to administer medicines on the midwives' exemptions list, except for controlled drugs, under the direct supervision of a sign off midwife. Direct supervision means direct visual contact by the midwife during the act of administration of the medicine by the student midwife. Student midwives may participate in the checking and preparation of controlled drugs on the midwives' exemption list for administration under the direct supervision of a registered midwife.

6 Women's choice and care options

Figure 6.1 Women's human rights and childbearing.

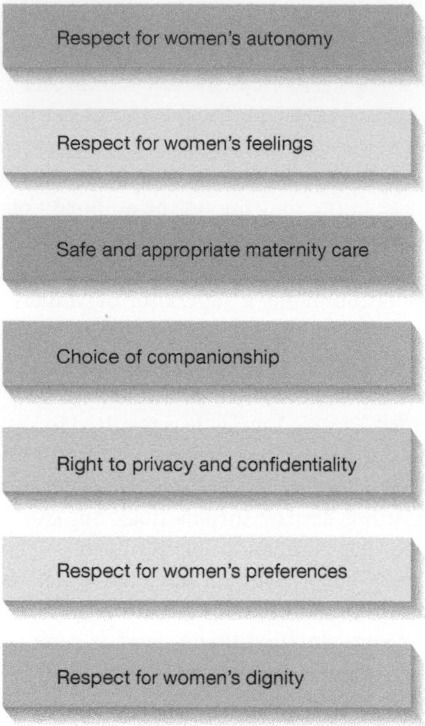

Figure 6.2 Dilemmas faced by women's lack of choice in birth.

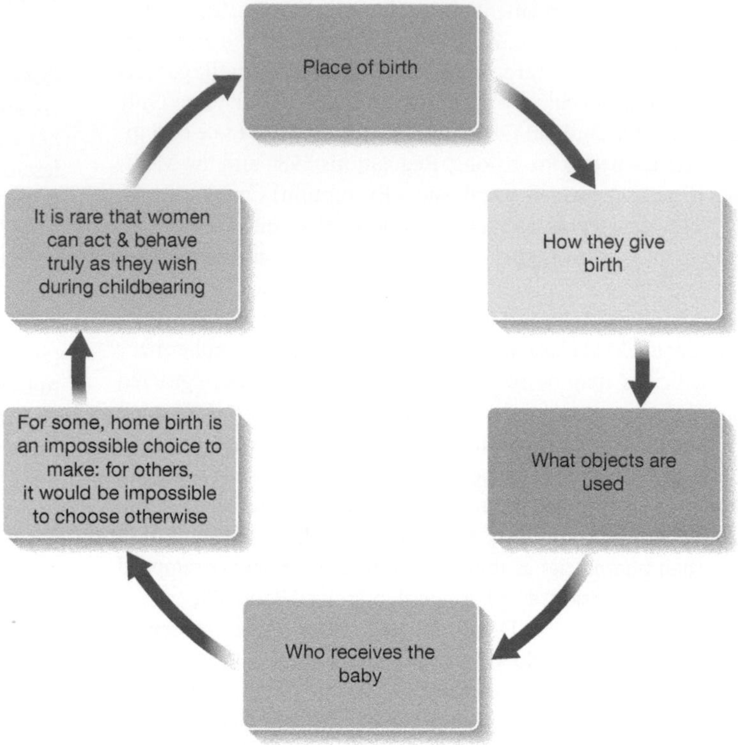

Figure 6.3 Women's choice of care options.

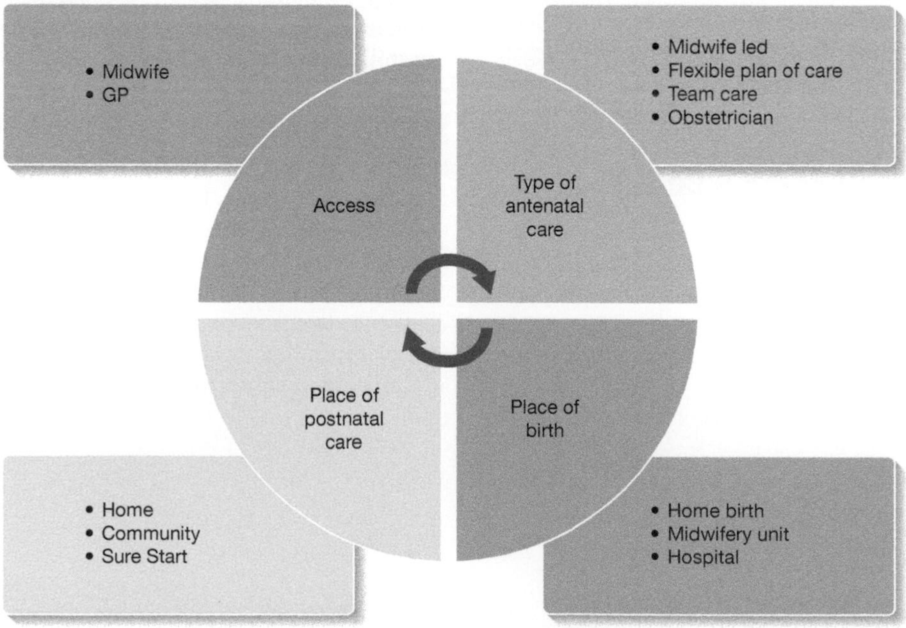

Midwifery at a Glance, First Edition. Edited by Eleanor Forrest © 2019 John Wiley & Sons, Ltd. Published 2019 by John Wiley & Sons, Ltd.
Companion website: www.wiley.com/go/forrest/midwifery

Contemporary healthcare policy within the Western world has become focused on embracing women's right to choice within the provision of maternity services. However, childbirth in the UK still mainly occurs within a medical paradigm. The relationship a woman has with maternity care providers and the maternity care system during the childbearing period is essential as a woman's experience of her care may impact on her confidence and self-esteem. This can influence how empowered she might feel and affect her potential to uptake essential services.

People are entitled to fundamental human rights as recognised by societies and governments nationally and internationally (Chapter 3). Although no specific charter exists that outlines how human rights are applied to childbearing, it is widely accepted that in respecting women's basic human rights, they should have choices (Figure 6.1).

It has been opined that obstetrics and childbirth have historically been medically defined within a culture of risk and safety which precludes a woman's ability to having full choices. Beliefs driven by a culture of risk become norms within society and influence issues such as women's place of birth and how they give birth (Figure 6.2).

Although women want to have choices within maternity services, the reasons for the choices they make are often multifactorial and influenced by many issues. For example, although the obstetrician may respect the woman's wishes, ultimately these will only be carried out within the medical perception of risk to the woman and the fetus and as such upholds the role of expert who takes ultimate responsibility over the woman. In this context, childbirth is viewed as a medical event rather than a social one.

Having choices implies that the onus to make a decision is on women opting for one particular choice. Women's decision making in relation to maternity care can be more informed if evidence-based information is provided and the support and care planning from midwives and other maternity healthcare professionals is woman centred and flexible. This includes respect for individual requirements and offering guidance on best and current options. Available services may vary in different areas, such as screening (Chapter 16), and giving women a choice of birthing place implies that home birth should be an option for all women.

Despite general awareness that women have choice, evidence suggests that many women still follow the belief that for safety reasons hospital is the best place in which to give birth, demonstrating a degree of fear and apprehension and that childbirth is perceived as unsafe. Women often do not exercise their right to informed choice due to constraints such as the opinions of doctors and midwives and the institution or environment within which maternity care takes place, such as the NHS in the UK. A re-evaluation of maternity care to focus on normality in childbearing may change the emphasis from risk to a more social and woman-led model of care.

Access

Although most women access services which are hospital based, there are choices available regarding how and where to access maternity care. Traditionally, once a woman initially suspects or confirms that she is pregnant, she will visit her GP. Women and their partners can choose to go straight to a midwife. By direct self-referral to their local midwifery service, their access to maternity services will be quicker; care planning and involvement in essential services can be initiated early (Figure 6.3).

Type of antenatal care

Women are being offered the option of attending a midwife as their first professional contact; however women should also be informed that they have the choice of seeing their GP at any point during pregnancy. Choice exists for women and their partners between midwifery care or care provided by a team of maternity health professionals, such as midwives and obstetricians. However, in most areas, this will be dependent upon their circumstances such as health and wellbeing factors. Following the initial history taking/booking visit, a flexible plan of care is usually made by the midwife in conjunction with the woman. Although women may choose midwife-led care, obstetric or team care may be deemed the safest option. As the pregnancy advances, this plan may alter, depending on individual circumstances. An example of this might be a woman who had been deemed initially suitable for midwife-led care, but who developed hypertension later in pregnancy and required transfer to joint obstetrician- and midwife-led care, or vice versa. Women with more complex needs should have joint care with other agencies such as social services or special needs in pregnancy teams (Figure 6.3).

Place of birth and postnatal care

Choice of place of birth is available to women and their partners. Midwives, obstetricians and other maternity care professionals should recognise that women have the right to choose their place of birth, in order to support them in their choice. This choice will again depend on a woman's particular circumstances. Options for place of birth are:

- A home birth whereby the midwife supports a woman at home for the birth
- A local midwifery unit, including a designated birth centre, with care led by a midwife, promoting normality
- A hospital supported by a local maternity care team: midwives, obstetricians and anaesthetists (Figure 6.3).

Postnatal care can be provided at home or in the community and may include options such as Sure Start. At home, women will have a choice of how and where to access postnatal care. Most midwives visit at home initially and can provide advice about local community supports such as breastfeeding groups in the community (Figure 6.3).

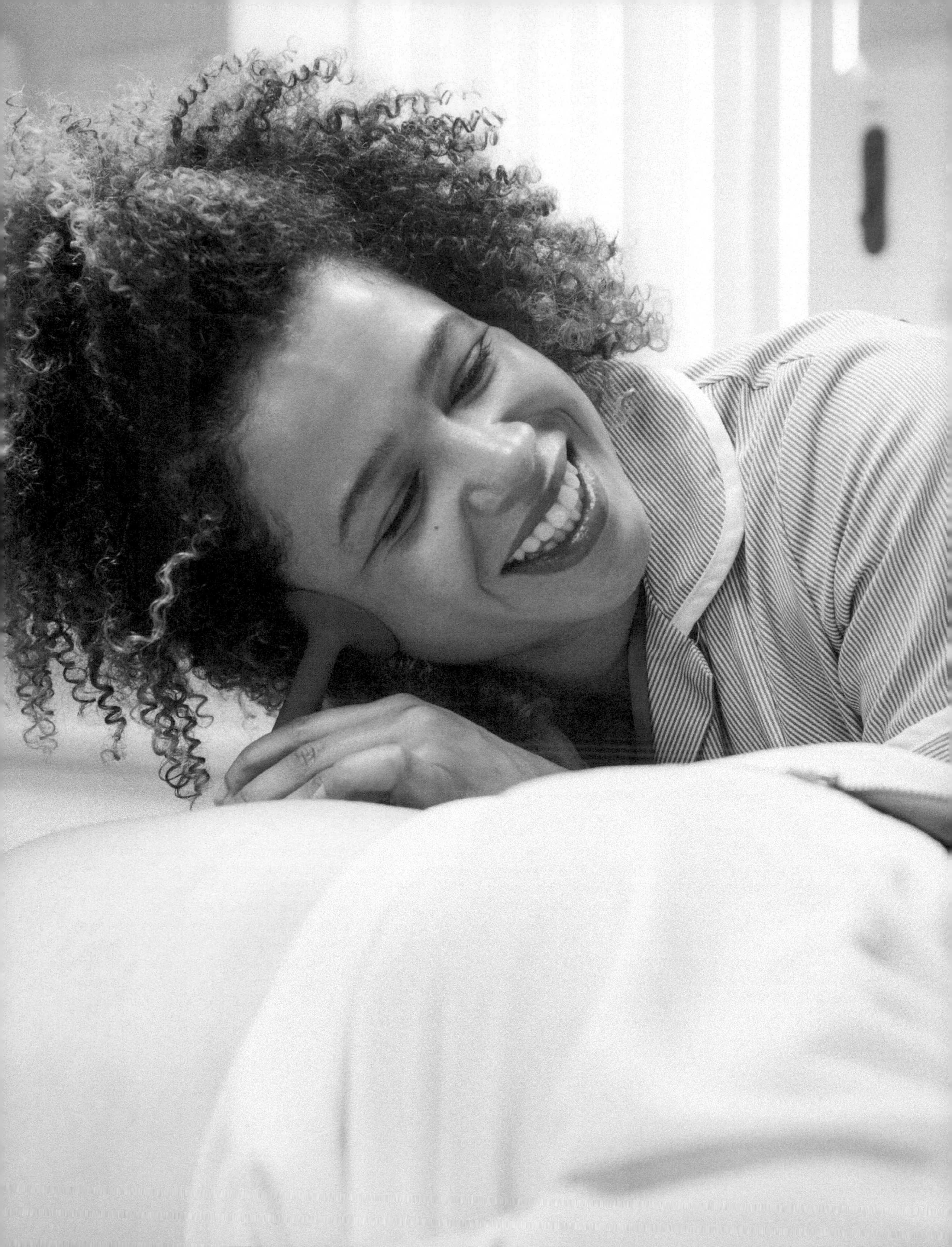

Anatomy and physiology

Chapters

7 Breast

Figure 7.1 Original anatomy of the breast.

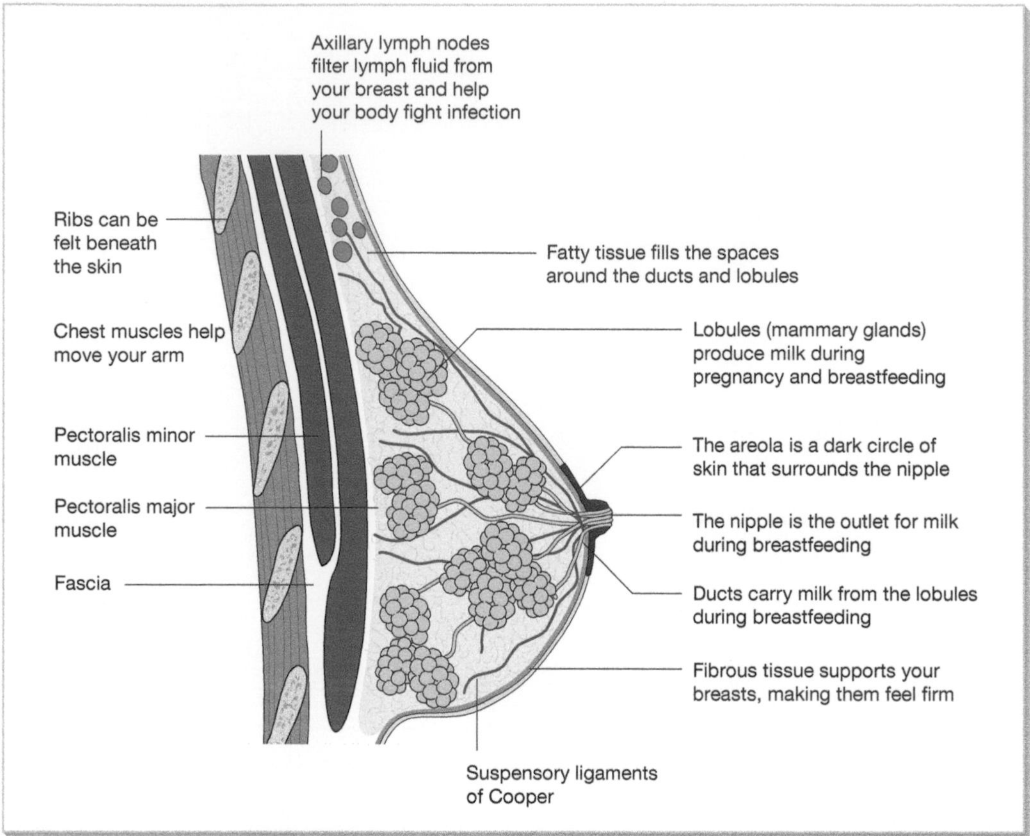

Figure 7.2 Feedback inhibitor of lactation (FIL) increased milk production.

Breast milk is removed
Level of FIL reduced
Pituatry stimulates prolactin
Milk production stimulated

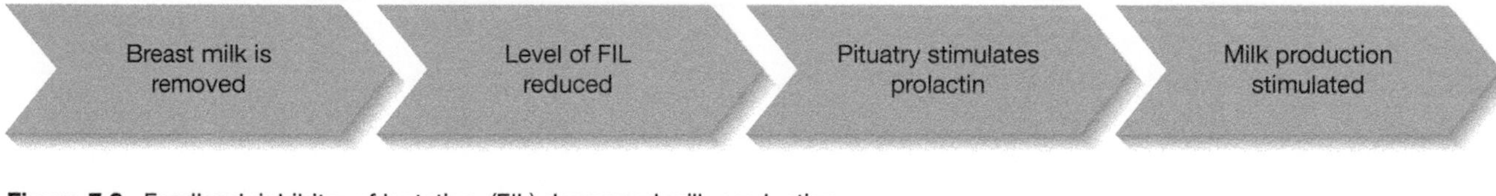

Figure 7.3 Feedback inhibitor of lactation (FIL) decreased milk production.

Milk stasis → Level of FIL increases → Pituitary decreases prolactin levels → Milk production decreases

Box 7.1 Contemporary accepted changes to anatomy of the breast.

- Ducts branch closer to the nipple
- The conventionally described lactiferous sinuses do not exist
- Glandular tissue is found closer to the nipple
- Subcutaneous fat is minimal at the base of the nipple
- The ratio of glandular to fat tissue is 2:1
- 65% of the glandular tissue is located in a 30 mm radius from the base of the nipple
- The range of milk ducts exiting the nipple is 4–18
- Complex ductal network, not always arranged in a radial or symmetrical pattern

Breast development

Female breast development begins between 8 and 13 years of age under the influence of the female hormone oestrogen (Chapter 9) and continues through puberty (Figure 7.1). Further maturation of the breasts takes place during pregnancy when glandular tissue proliferates. The primary function of the breasts, as mammary glands, is the feeding and nourishing with breast milk during the maternal lactation period.

Breast development starts with the flat area around the nipple (areola) becoming enlarged and some breast tissue forms under the nipple (Figure 7.1). When breast development is complete, each breast is distinct and the areola no longer appears swollen. In a healthy adult female, the breasts lie either side of the sternum between the second and sixth ribs. The breasts are anchored to the pectoralis major muscle by the suspensory ligaments. These ligaments relax with age and time, eventually resulting in the breasts drooping, or ptosis. The lower pole of the breast is fuller than the upper pole and the tail of Spence extends obliquely up into the medial wall of the axilla.

Until recently, the commonly accepted anatomy of the breast was as described by Sir Astley Parson Cooper in 1840 (Figure 7.1). More recent anatomical research involving imaging of the lactating breast using ultrasound has challenged a number of commonly accepted conclusions derived by Cooper (2005). These findings of breast anatomy have important implications for the way the breast is cared for, especially during surgery, and how breastfeeding is effectively supported. The major differences between the two models are (Box 7.1):

- Milk ducts branch closer to the nipple
- Lactiferous sinuses do not, in fact, exist
- Glandular tissue is found closer to the nipple
- Subcutaneous fat is minimal at the base of the nipple
- The external shape or size of the breast is not predictive of its internal anatomy or of its lactation potential
- The ratio of glandular to fat tissue rises to 2:1 in the lactating breast, compared to a 1:1 ratio in non-lactating women
- 65% of the glandular tissue is located within 30 mm from the base of the nipple
- Between four and 18 milk ducts exit the nipple
- The network of milk ducts is complex, not homogeneous. It is not always arranged symmetrically, or in a radial pattern
- The milk ducts near the nipple do not act as reservoirs for milk.

Physiology of lactation: how the breasts lactate and produce milk

Lactation is under the control of two hormones, oxytocin and prolactin. *Oxytocin* is responsible for the ejection of milk from the breast and *prolactin* is responsible for the production of breast milk:

Oxytocin …

- Is secreted by the posterior lobe of the pituitary gland in response to the baby suckling at the breast
- Causes the myoepithelial cells within the alveoli to contract and force milk into the lactiferous ducts, which is then ejected from the breast via the nipple. Some mothers feel this 'let down' of milk as tingling within the breast and it may be experienced as pain or discomfort
- Acts similarly on the uterus causing contraction, facilitating uterine involution and reducing uterine blood loss post-delivery. These uterine contractions are commonly referred to as 'after pains'. These are characterised by 'cramping' pains usually experienced in the first few days after delivery and are more noticeable following second and subsequent births.

Prolactin …

- Is secreted by the anterior lobe of the pituitary gland as maternal oestrogen and progesterone levels fall following the expulsion of the placenta
- Is produced in response to effective removal of milk from the breast
- Returns to prepregnancy levels around 7 days post-birth if the mother does not breastfeed, or milk is ineffectively removed from the breast
- Suppresses ovulation
- Is secreted more at night
- Levels peak at the end of each breastfeed to secure milk for the next feed.

In addition to hormones, the feedback inhibitor of lactation (FIL) is involved in milk synthesis (Figures 7.2 and 7.3).

sFIL …

- Is a whey protein within breast milk
- Is removed with effective breastfeeding resulting in increased milk supply
- Is increased in ineffective milk removal from the breast, resulting in a decrease in milk supply. The solution is decreasing the frequency of feeds, supplementing/substituting breastfeeds with formula milk or water or using a dummy to increase the time between breastfeeds
- Allows the breasts to function independently of each other
- Prevents the breasts from becoming over full.

8 Female reproductive system

Figure 8.1 Uterus and uterine tubes.

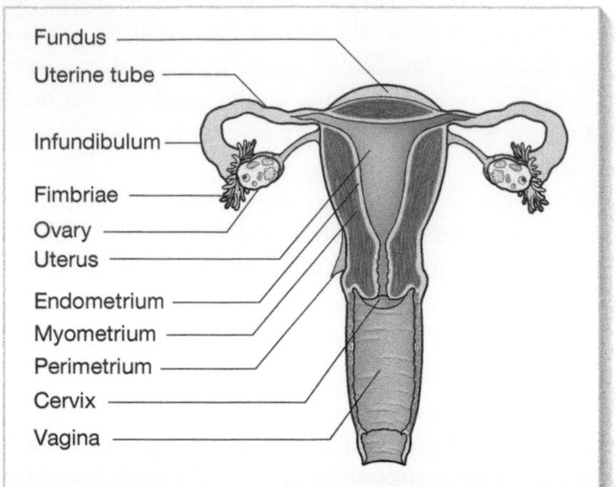

Figure 8.2 The uterus.

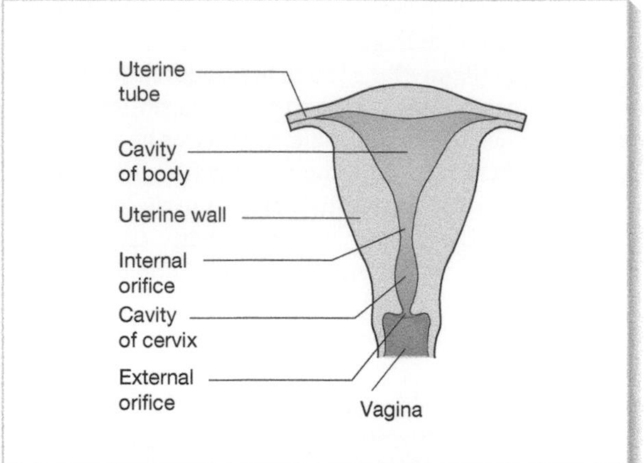

Figure 8.3 The uterus in relation to the bladder (in front) and rectum (behind).

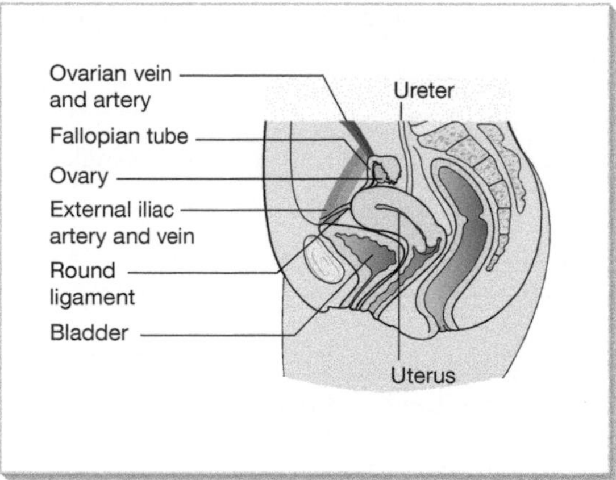

Figure 8.4 The ligaments.

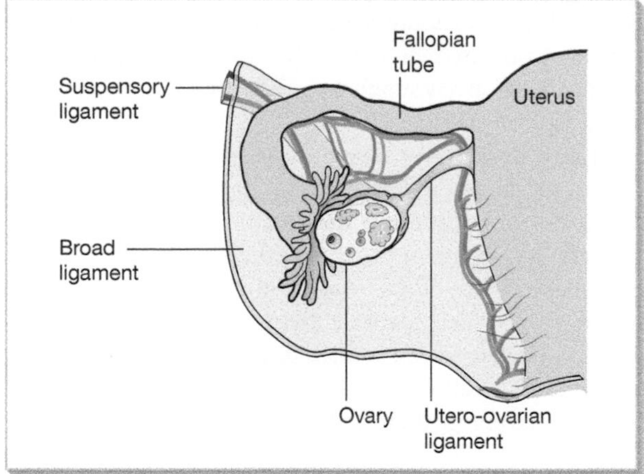

Figure 8.5 The broad ligament.

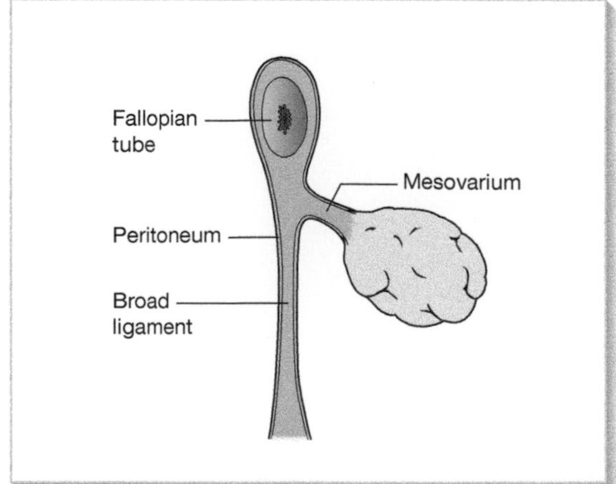

Figure 8.6 The vulva.

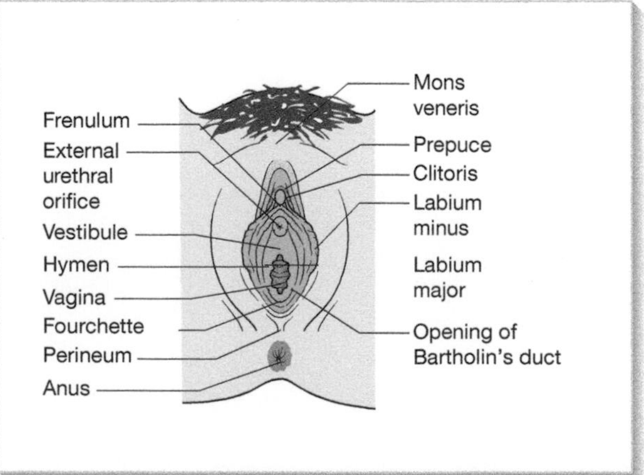

The female organs of reproduction may be classified as internal (uterus, uterine tubes and ovaries and vagina) or external (vulva) organs.

Internal organs of reproduction

The uterus is a hollow muscular organ (Figures 8.1 and 8.2) located within the true pelvis between the bladder, in front, and the rectum, behind (Figure 8.3). The uterus is described as leaning forward, anteverted, and also bending forward upon itself, anteflexed. In some women, the uterus leans backwards, a position described as retroverted. The position of the uterus within the pelvis is maintained by ligaments (Figure 8.4). A fallopian (uterine) tube is located on either side of the upper portion of the uterus at the cornua. The uterine tubes facilitate the passage of sperm from the uterus below and ova from the ovaries.

The uterus measures 7.5 cm long × 5 cm wide × 2.5 cm thick and is divided into the following areas:

- Body: upper two-thirds of the organ
- Cervix: lower one-third of the organ
- Fundus: curved upper margin of the body between the insertions of the uterine tubes
- Cornua: area at either side of the fundus where the uterine tubes join the body. The round ligament which helps to maintain the uterus in a position of anteversion and the ovarian ligament which anchors the ovaries near the uterus are also attached to the uterus at the cornuae
- Isthmus: narrow area between the body and the cervix.

A potential triangular space exists within the body of the uterus called the cavity. The vagina is situated below the uterus, but the lower half of the cervix protrudes into the vagina. A canal exists within the cervix that allows communication between the vagina below and the uterine cavity above. Narrow openings are located at either end of the cervical canal; the internal os, which is the opening between the cervical canal and the uterine cavity, and the external os, which is the opening between the cervical canal and the vagina. The vagina is a muscular tube that extends from the cervix to the external genitalia. This arrangement creates a continuous duct between the external genitalia and the ovaries, with the uterus situated in the middle. The uterus is therefore designed to prepare for the possible reception of a fertilised ovum on a cyclical basis, to provide a nurturing environment for the developing fetus, and to expel both fetus and placenta at the end of pregnancy. The walls of the uterus are composed of three layers:

1 **Endometrium** – an inner layer of ciliated epithelium that lines the uterine cavity. The thickness of this layer alters throughout the menstrual cycle in response to the ovarian hormones.

2 **Myometrium** – a muscular middle layer composed of multidirectional muscle fibres. The thickness of the myometrium varies in different areas of the uterus and is thickest in the upper portion of the body and thinner in the area of the isthmus.

3 **Perimetrium** – a fold of peritoneum that covers the anterior uterine wall, the fundus and the posterior uterine wall. The perimetrium extends laterally to form a double fold over the uterine tubes, known as the broad ligament (Figure 8.5).

The blood supply to the uterus is mainly from the uterine artery with corresponding venous drainage. The nerve supply is derived from the inferior hypogastric plexus. The uterus is supported from below by the pelvic floor and three pairs of ligaments located at the level of the cervix.

The ovaries are situated one either side of the uterus below the uterine tubes. They are attached to the uterus by the ovarian ligaments which extend from the cornuae on either side. Each ovary has a central medulla of fibrous tissue and an outer cortex from which ovarian follicles develop. The fringed end of the uterine tube is attached to the ovary by the ovarian fimbria. This facilitates entry of the ovum to the uterine tube. Fertilisation of the ovum usually occurs within the widest portion of the uterine tube (ampulla). Transportation of the ovum within the muscular uterine tube to the uterine cavity is by a combination of peristalsis and the action of the ciliated epithelial lining.

Vulva

The structures that compose the external reproductive organs are illustrated in Figure 8.6. The mons veneris (pubis) is a pad of fat that overlies the symphysis pubis and is covered in pubic hair. Below the mons pubis, the two labia majora extend backwards. The labia majora are composed largely of fatty tissue and on the outer surface are covered by skin and pubic hair, their inner surface is smooth. Two smaller folds of subcutaneous tissue known as the labia minora lie within the labia majora. These join anteriorly to form a double fold, within which is located the clitoris. The clitoris is a small, sensitive structure composed of erectile tissue. The fold of the labia minora that overhangs the clitoris is the prepuce, and the fold that joins underneath the clitoris is known as the frenulum. Between the folds of the labia minora that extend backwards is an area known as the vestibule in which the urethral orifice and vaginal introitus are located. Bartholin's glands are situated within connective tissue on either side of the vagina. Ducts from these glands are located on either side of the vagina. Posteriorly, the labia minora unite to form the fourchette. Anterior to the fourchette may lie the hymen, a membrane that partly occludes the vaginal introitus and which is usually ruptured at the time of first intercourse.

9 Menstrual cycle

Table 9.1 Calculation of the EDD.

This is an estimate only! The majority of babies will be born 10 days either side of the EDD. The expected date of delivery is calculated by adding 7 days and 9 months to the date of the last menstrual period. This is based on the average duration of pregnancy being 265 days from time of conception. In most menstrual cycles ovulation occurs on the 14th day and fertilisation around the 15th day. The expected date will be 280 days from the first day of the cycle. In asking the date of the LMP it should be ascertained that the bleeding was normal in amount and duration. Some women experience slight bleeding around the time of implantation that may be mistaken for a period and will, if this date is used, give an inaccurate LMP. Adjustments also have to be made for women whose menstrual cycle is routinely shorter or longer than 28 days. If the cycle is short, the number of days difference between the short cycle and 28 is subtracted from the calculation. If the cycle is longer than 28 days then the difference in days is added to the calculation.
For example: LMP 7th June 2010. Cycle normally 25 days. EDD 11th March 2011

LMP	Usual cycle length	EDD
2nd August 2010	28 days	9th May 2011
28th June 2010	28 days	5th April 2010
11th August 2010	21 days	11th May 2011
23rd August 2010	33 days	4th June 2011
23rd August 2011	33 days	3rd June 2012 (This pregnancy occurs over a leap year period so a day is deducted to allow for the extra day in February)

Figure 9.1 Control of the menstrual cycle.

Hypothalmus
FSH-RH & LH-RH
Anterior lobe of pituitary gland
1. Produces FSH & some LH
2. Produces LH & some FSH
Development of Graafian follicle
Ovulation
Rising levels inhibit FSH & triggers surge in LH
Produces oestrogen & some progesterone
Corpus luteum formed
Proliferation of endometrium
Produces progesterone & some oestrogen
Rising progesterone & oestrogen levels inhibit pituitary hormones
Secretory changes in endometrium OR PREGNANCY
Corpus luteum degenerates progesterone & oestrogen
Corpus luteum maintained by HCG
MENSTRUATION
Oestrogen & progesterone continue to be produced and endometrium not shed

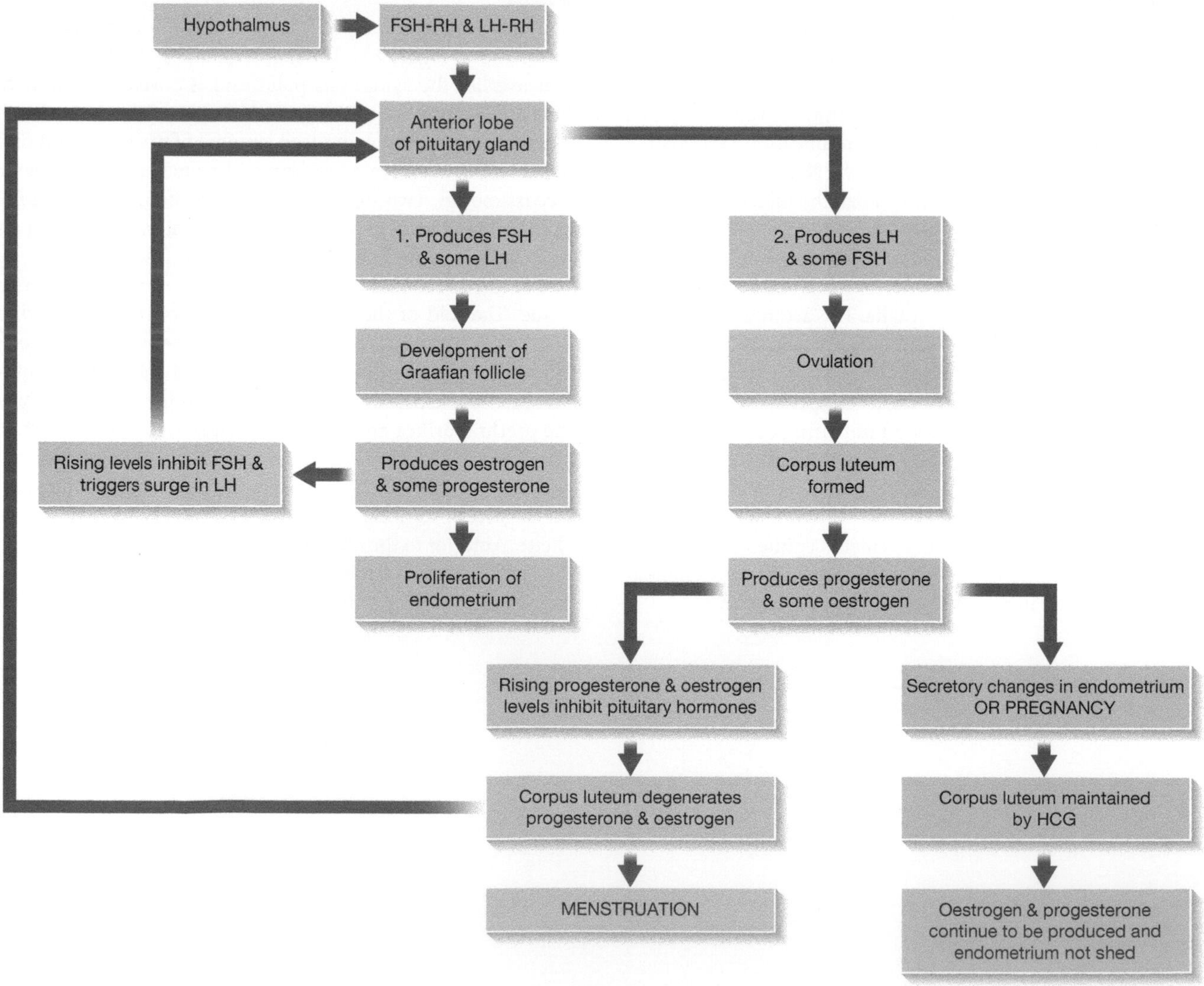

Figure 9.2 Endometrial change. Source: Chris 73, https://commons.wikimedia.org/wiki/File:MenstrualCycle.png. Licensed under Creative Commons CC BY SA 3.0

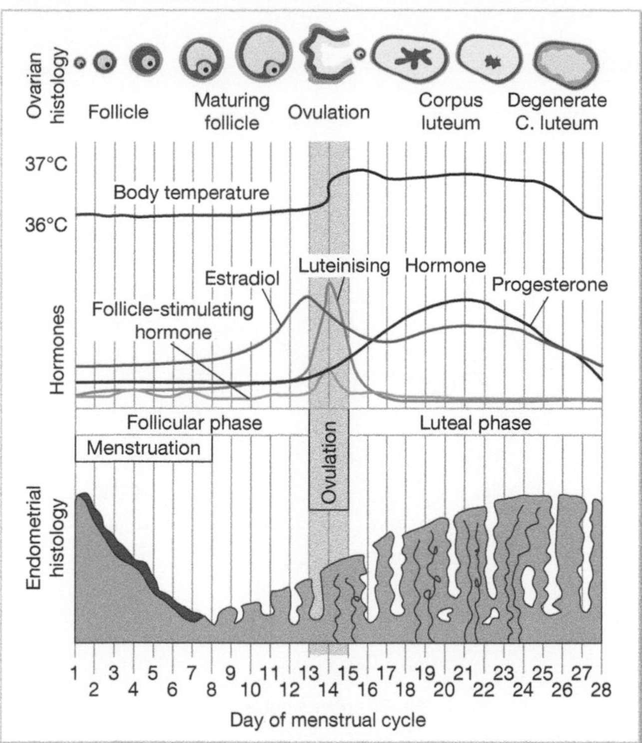

An understanding of the menstrual cycle is useful in midwifery practice as it relates closely to issues around fertility, conception and contraception. The date of the last menstrual period (LMP) prior to conception can be used to calculate the expected date of delivery (EDD) (Table 9.1).

Control of the menstrual cycle

The ovarian activity responsible for the changes in the endometrium that occur throughout the menstrual cycle is controlled by hormones from the anterior lobe of the pituitary gland (Figure 9.1). The functioning of the anterior lobe of the pituitary gland is influenced by gonadotrophic-releasing hormones (GnRH) from a nearby area of brain, the hypothalamus. The production of GnRH can be affected by a range of factors such as stress, emotional factors, disease and nutritional status and it is this mechanism that allows the menstrual cycle to be disturbed by external influences such as significant changes in lifestyle. There are two GnRHs produced by the hypothalamus:

- Follicle-stimulating hormone-releasing hormone (FSH-RH)
- Luteinising hormone-releasing hormone (LH-RH).

FSH-RH and LH-RH act upon the anterior pituitary lobe to produce follicle-stimulating hormone (FSH) and luteinising hormone (LH), respectively. Both these hormones are produced throughout the cycle, but the amounts vary at different points. At the start of a cycle larger amounts of FSH are produced than LH. These hormones are then carried via the bloodstream to the ovary, where FSH stimulates a few Graafian follicles to start enlarging. The ovum within each follicle is surrounded by a clump of cells known as the granulosa cells. Under the influence of FSH these cells start to produce the ovarian hormones known as oestrogens. To a lesser extent LH stimulates small amounts of another ovarian hormone, progesterone. The levels of oestrogens rise in the first half of the cycle. One Graafian follicle tends to be more active than others and produces larger amounts of oestrogen. In response to the rising levels of oestrogen, the amount of FSH produced by the anterior pituitary lobe is reduced and this probably inhibits the growth of the less active follicles. The more active follicle now produces rapidly increasing amounts of the oestrogenic hormone oestradiol, which triggers a rapid increase in the production of LH and to a lesser extent FSH. The sudden surge in LH results in changes to the follicular wall that allow the ovum to be released and ovulation occurs. The release of the ovum into the peritoneal cavity, usually mid-cycle, may be accompanied by a sharp pain known as mittelschmerz.

Following ovulation the remaining granulosa cells undergo change, resulting in the formation of a solid yellow area on the surface of the ovary, the corpus luteum or yellow body. The cells of the corpus luteum then start to produce increasing levels of progesterone and small amounts of oestrogen, reaching a peak of production about 9–10 days after ovulation. The high level of progesterone now circulating has a negative effect upon the hypothalamus and FSH and LH levels now decline. The pituitary hormones are required to maintain the corpus luteum. Unless the ovum becomes fertilised and pregnancy becomes established, the corpus luteum will degenerate and production of oestrogen and progesterone will fall. As these hormones are required to maintain the uterine endometrium, this results in disintegration of the endometrium and menstruation occurs. The fall in oestrogen and progesterone levels also initiates hypothalamic activity again and another cycle starts.

Endometrial change

The endometrium is composed of three layers:

1 A basal layer that remains unchanged throughout the cycle.
2 A superficial layer that alters constantly throughout the cycle.
3 A single cell of layer of epithelium.

The menstrual cycle can be divided into three phases according to changes that take place within the endometrium (Figure 9.2). Day 1 of the menstrual cycle occurs with the first day of menstrual bleeding and the three phases are categorised as follows:

Menstruation

Days 1–5. The superficial layer of the endometrium and the epithelial layers degenerate in response to the alteration in the balance of ovarian hormones. Oestrogen tends to dominate at this point in the cycle, causing the myometrium to become more contractile which aids the separation and expulsion of the endometrium. On average women will lose about 35 ml of blood during the process of menstruation.

Proliferative/follicular phase

Days 6–14. Under the increasing influence of FSH, the developing follicles produce increasing amounts of oestrogens. This leads to rapid growth and proliferation of a new superficial layer of endometrium from the basal layer. By mid-cycle the thickness of the superficial endometrium will have increased to 6 mm, whilst the epithelial covering will remain only one cell thick.

Secretory/luteal phase

Days 15–28. Following ovulation increasing amounts of progesterone, and to a lesser extent oestrogen, are produced from the corpus luteum. As a result the endometrium becomes increasingly vascular in order to provide a suitable environment for implantation of the ovum, should fertilisation occur. Without fertilisation occurring the corpus luteum will start to degenerate and the levels of progesterone and oestrogen will rapidly fall, resulting in disintegration of the endometrium and another episode of menstrual bleeding.

10 Maternal pelvis

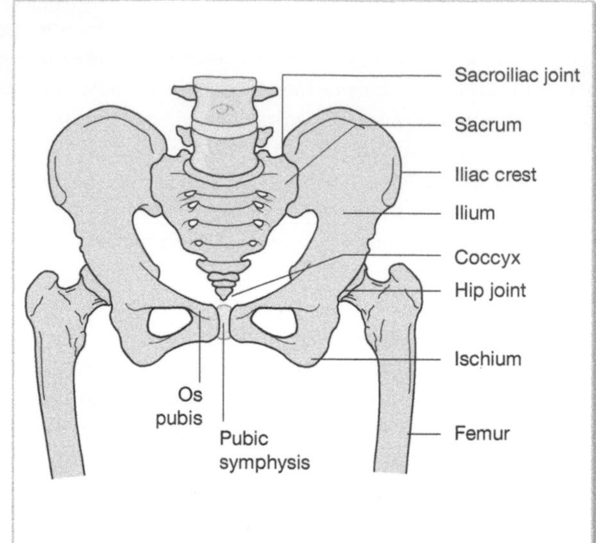

Figure 10.1 Female pelvis.

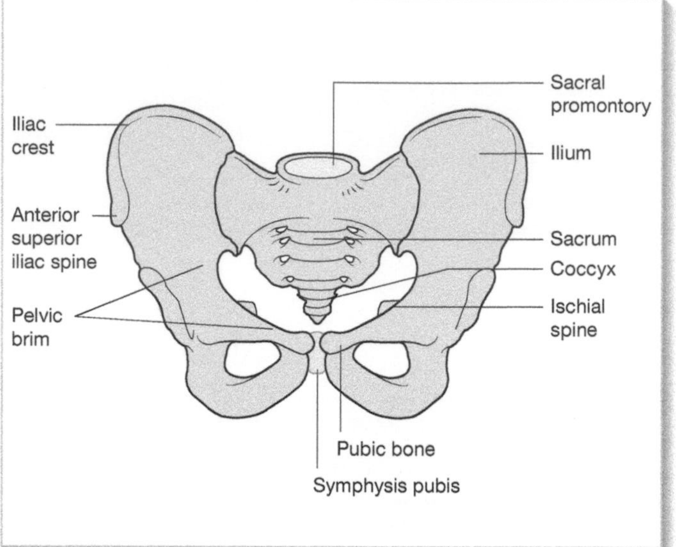

Figure 10.2 Landmarks of the pelvic brim.

Table 10.1 The pelvic joints.

Pelvic joints	Location	Comment
Sacroiliac × 2	Between sacrum and ilium	May be a site of backache
Symphysis–pubis × 1	Between the two pubic bones	A pad of cartilage exists between the articulating surfaces of the two pubic bones. Some separation of the joint may occur in late pregnancy causing pain
Sacrococcygeal × 1	Between sacrum and coccyx	Hinge joint that allows for backward movement of the coccyx during birth; increasing the anterior–posterior diameter of the outlet

Table 10.2 Pelvic types.

Type	Features	Brim shape	Comments
Gynaecoid: typical female pelvis	Round brim with accommodating anterior Straight side walls Blunt ischial spines Subpubic angle 90°		Found in 50% of female population Most conducive to childbearing
Android: male type pelvis	Heart-shaped brim with narrow anterior Side walls may converge Prominent ischial spines Subpubic angle <90°		Found in 20% of female population Associated with occipitoposterior positions of the vertex Converging side walls may inhibit descent & rotation of vertex Prominent ischial spines may prevent rotation Narrow subpubic arch prevents head fitting snugly under arch & may increase chances of perineal trauma
Anthropoid	Oval brim with extended anterior posterior diameter Narrow anterior Long sacrum & deep cavity Blunt ischial spines Subpubic angle >90°		Found in 25% of female population More common in non-white populations Associated with tall women Position of vertex usually direct occiput anterior or posterior & will not change during labour
Platypelloid	Kidney bean-shaped brim Reduced anteroposterior diameter & increased transverse diameter at brim Flat sacrum & shallow cavity Blunt ischial spines Subpubic angle >90°		Fetal head can only engage as an occipitolateral position Asynclitism of fetal head may occur to allow head to enter brim of pelvis

Companion website: www.wiley.com/go/forrest/midwifery

The relationship between the fetus and pelvis may be determined within the prenatal period by abdominal examination (Chapter 76). This may have implications for care, whilst the shape of the pelvis can have a significant impact on the progress of labour. The changing relationship of the fetus to the pelvis in labour provides an indication as to how labour is progressing. This may be determined through abdominal examination and examination per vaginam.

The pelvis is constructed from four bones (Figures 10.1 and 10.2):

- Two innominate bones which form the lateral and anterior aspects of the pelvis
- The sacrum and coccyx which form the posterior aspect of the pelvis.

The innominate bones are formed by the fusion of three smaller bones: the ilium, ischium and os pubis.

The ilium is a flat, flared, wing-shaped bone with a smooth concave anterior surface called the iliac fossa. The upper border of the iliac fossa is a curved ridge called the iliac crest which provides an attachment for muscles of the abdominal wall. The lower border of the iliac fossa is bounded by a ridge, the iliopectineal line. The anterior aspect of this line ends in a prominence called the iliopectineal protruberance. This is an important landmark on the pelvis as it is used to determine anterior positions of the vertex and is also an endpoint of the oblique diameters of the pelvic brim. The iliopectineal line is also important as it form the boundary between the false pelvis above, which is of lesser relevance to midwifery practice, and the true pelvis below, which is of great relevance to midwifery practice. Below the level of the iliopectineal line, the ilium forms the side wall of the pelvis.

The ischium is a strong, triangular bone that lies below the ilium. The lower border is a thickened prominence known as the ischial tuberosity, and is the part of the pelvis on which we sit. A small triangular inward projection is located above the posterior aspect of the tuberosity, the ischial spine. This is an important landmark as it can be felt during vaginal examination and provides a baseline to which the level of the fetal head can be compared in labour. The ischial spine is also significant because it narrows the birth canal and provides a landmark for locating the pudendal nerve. From the ischial tuberosity a shaft of bone passes upwards to join the pubic bone, forming the pubic arch and the large hole found at the front of the innominate bone; the foramen ovale.

Each innominate bone has an os pubis that articulates with the os pubis of the opposite innominate bone, forming the front of the pelvis. A pad of cartilage lies between the articulating pubic bones (symphysis pubis). Two shafts of bone project from the os pubis. The superior shaft (ramus) projects laterally to join the ilium at the iliopectineal prominence and forms the upper boundary of the foramen ovale. The lower ramus passes downwards to join the shaft of bone projecting from the ischium, thus forming the upper part of the pubic arch.

The sacrum is composed of five fused sacral vertebrae and forms the posterior aspect of the pelvis. It articulates with the iliac bones, forming the sacroiliac joints. The outer aspect of the sacrum is rough and provides attachment for muscles and ligaments. The inner aspect is smooth and concave and is called the hollow of the sacrum. The centre of the first sacral vertebra overhangs the hollow of the sacrum slightly. This is the sacral promontory and is an important pelvic landmark. The lower border of the sacrum articulates with four smaller fused vertebrae, the coccyx, at the sacrococcygeal joint.

The joints that exist between the different bones of the pelvis are summarised in Table 10.1. Ligaments support the pelvic joints. In addition there are two important ligaments that run between the sacrum and the ilium: the sacrotuberous ligament and the sacrospinous ligament. Although soft tissue, these ligaments form part of the posterior wall of the pelvic outlet.

Due to the curvature of the sacrum, the true pelvis is a curved tube consisting of three parts: the brim, which forms the boundary with the false pelvis, the cavity and the outlet. The brim of a normal female pelvis is round; the landmarks of the brim are summarised in Figure 10.2. Knowledge of the landmarks of the brim is important in determining the position of the fetal head.

The cavity is bounded anteriorly by the pubic bone and posteriorly by the sacrum and coccyx. Consequently, it is curved and deeper at the back than the front as the depth of the pubic bone is 4 cm compared with the length of the sacrum and coccyx, which is 12 cm. During the birth of a baby, its body will still be following the curve within the cavity once the head is born. Due to the undulating nature of the structures forming the pelvic outlet there is a difference between what is known as the anatomical outlet and the obstetric outlet. In practice the obstetric outlet is the true space that exists to allow for the passage of the fetus.

Space within the pelvis is limited and, combined with the shape of the brim, cavity and outlet (Table 10.2), means that the fetus has to adapt to the alterations in pelvic shape that occur as it descends through the pelvis. The normal female pelvis is known as the gynaecoid pelvis. Whilst this is the type of pelvis seen most commonly in women, some women have differently shaped pelves that may result in the shape and diameters of the brim, cavity and outlet being altered. This in turn may have an impact on the progress of labour. Table 10.2 summarises the different types of pelves.

11 Maternal pelvis and fetal skull

Figure 11.1 Relationship of the occiput to the pelvis.

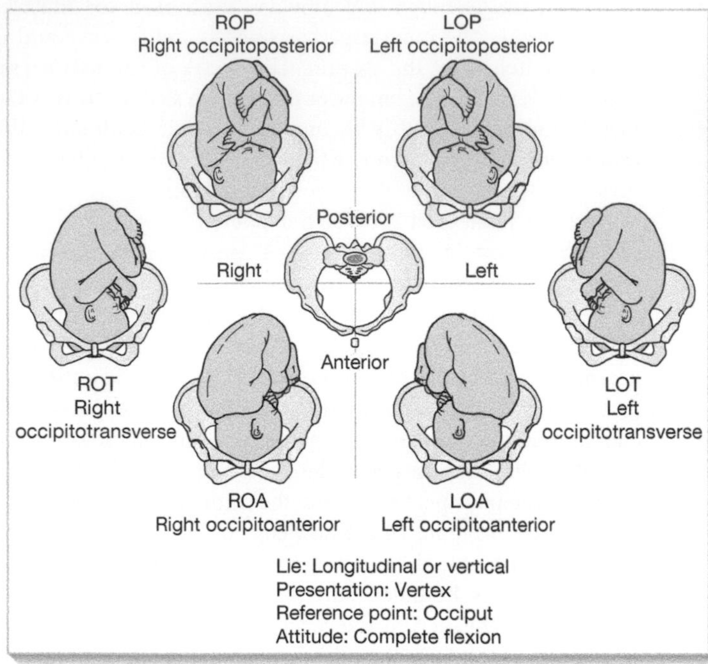

Figure 11.3 Vertex positions related to findings on examination per vaginam.

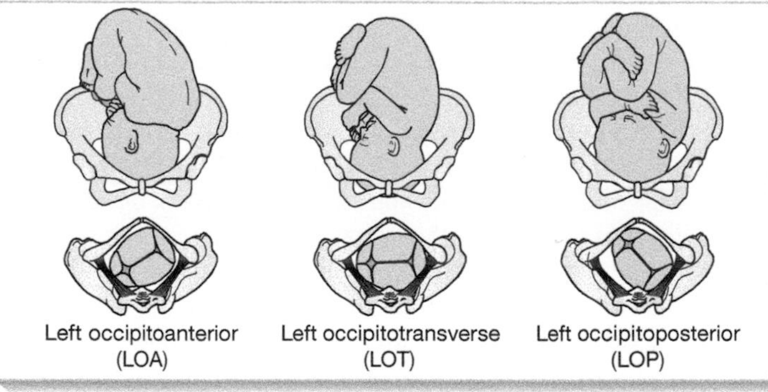

Figure 11.5 Moulding of fetal head occipitoanterior position.

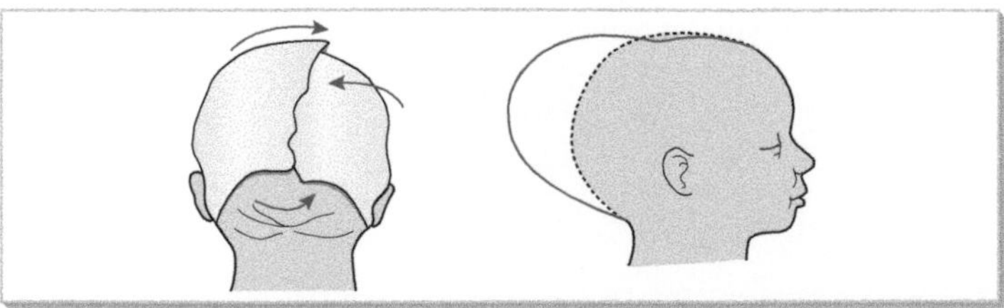

Box 11.1 Structures affected by moulding.

- The fold of dura mater that lies between the two cerebral hemispheres
- The falx cerebri
- The fold of dura mater that lies between the cerebrum
- The cerebellum
- The tentorium cerebelli

Figure 11.2 Rotation of occipito-anterior position from LOA to direct OA on examination per vaginam.

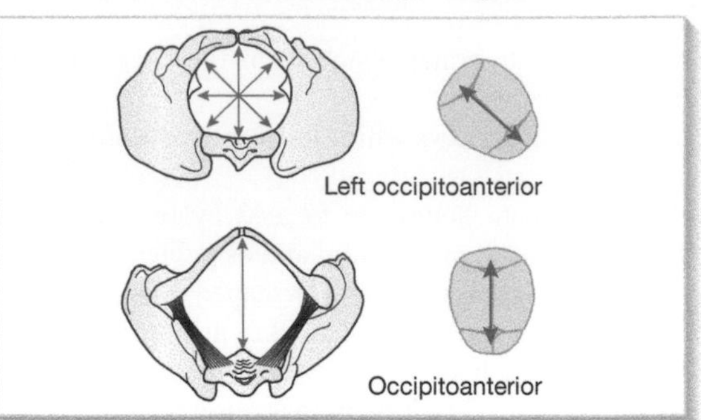

Figure 11.4 Level of fetal head in relation to ischial spines.

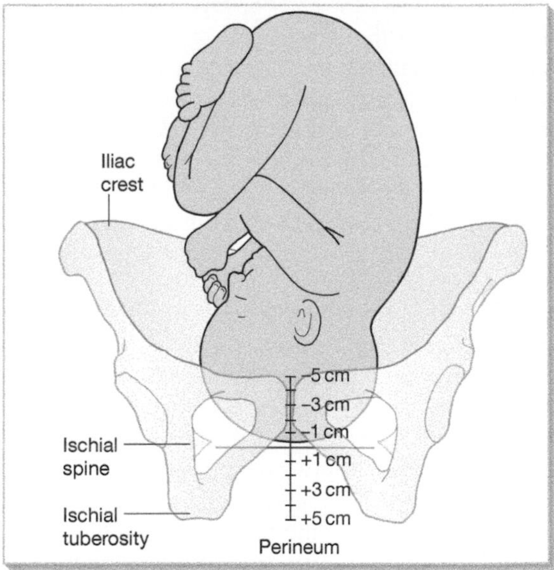

Figure 11.6 Caput succedaneum and cephalhaematoma.

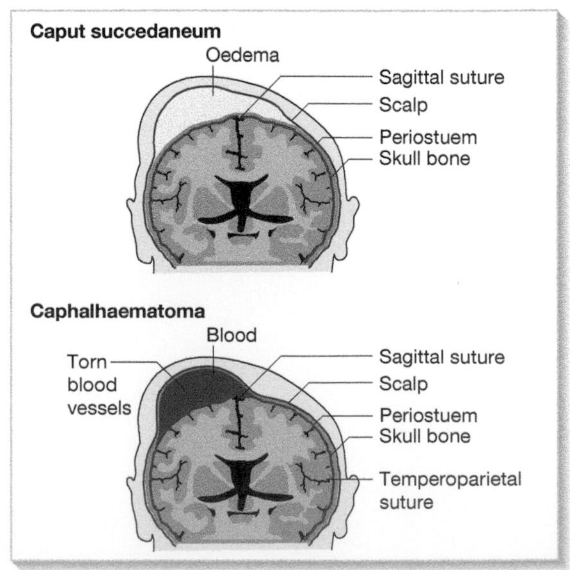

Understanding of the interplay between the fetal skull and maternal pelvis is important to midwifery practice. In this chapter this will be considered in relation to positioning of the vertex, examination per vaginam in labour, moulding and swellings on the head.

Position of the vertex

In a cephalic presentation the most likely presenting part is the vertex. The vertex is defined as the part of the fetal skull bounded by the anterior and posterior fontanelles and the parietal eminences, and generally this will be the part of the baby that will be born first. The position of the fetus is defined by the relationship of the denominator of presentation to the brim of the maternal pelvis. The denominator in a vertex presentation is the occiput. The brim of the pelvis is divided into six areas (Figure 11.1). Note right and left are *maternal* right and left:

1 Left anterior
2 Left lateral
3 Left posterior
4 Right anterior
5 Right lateral
6 Right posterior.

Position is therefore determined by the relationship of the occiput to the six areas of the pelvic brim. The possibilities are: left occipitoanterior (LOA), right occipitoanterior (ROA), left occipitolateral (LOL), right occipitolateral (ROL), left occipitoposterior (LOP) and right occipitoposterior (ROP). Position of the vertex may be determined through abdominal examination (Chapter 76) or examination per vaginam.

Examination per vaginam

Findings on abdominal examination in relation to the position of the vertex, degree of flexion and level of the fetal head can be confirmed through examination per vaginam. Position is determined by locating the posterior fontanelle and relating this to the brim of the maternal pelvis. The fontanelles can be differentiated by their shape and the number of sutures that join to form the fontanelle.

The ideal position for the fetal head is occipitoanterior. In this position the fetal head is usually well flexed and the posterior fontanelle will be palpable in the anterior aspect of the pelvis (Figure 11.2). Rotation of the fetal skull will occur with descent so that the location of the posterior fontanelle will alter indicating rotation of the occiput and position of the vertex. Before birth, the fetal head will usually rotate so that the occiput lies directly under the symphysis pubis. This is known as a direct occipitoanterior position and is confirmed by feeling the posterior fontanelle directly below the symphysis pubis. In practice locating the fontanelles is often difficult due to the thickness of the cervix, insufficient dilatation of the cervical os and moulding. In posterior positions of the occiput, the fetal head tends to be poorly flexed and the posterior fontanelle may not be felt whilst the anterior fontanelle is likely to be palpable in the anterior aspect of the pelvis (Figure 11.3). If flexion increases and anterior rotation of the occiput occurs, the posterior fontanelle will be increasingly felt whilst the anterior fontanelle becomes less palpable. In addition, the level of the fetal head in relation to the ischial spines can be determined (Figure 11.4).

Moulding

In labour the sutures allow the bones of the fetal skull to override each other slightly. This can decrease the engaging diameter by 1.25 cm. It is important that the total volume of the fetal skull is not reduced as this would compress the brain. Consequently, the diameter at right angles to the engaging diameter will increase by an equivalent amount. This leads to a change in shape of the fetal skull that will vary depending on the position or presentation. Figure 11.5 outlines the typical moulding associated with an occipitoanterior position. Following birth the shape of the head will gradually return to normal. Whilst moulding is a normal adaptation that facilitates birth, extreme or rapid moulding may cause traction on structures within the fetal skull (Box 11.1). These structures, which are joined at right angles near the back of the brain, contain large venous sinuses. Extreme or rapid moulding can result in tearing of these structures, particularly the tentorium cerebelli, leading to interventricular haemorrhage. Extreme moulding is associated with malpresentations and malposition of the occiput.

Swellings on the head

Two forms of swelling may be observed on the head of a newborn baby as a result of the articulation that may occur between the fetal skull and maternal pelvis and other tissues during labour. These are caput succedaneum and cephalhaematoma (Figure 11.6).

Caput succedaneum

This is an oedematous swelling of the scalp tissue that has resulted from the dilating cervix causing pressure on the fetal head during labour. This interferes with the venous return from the scalp tissue and oedema develops in the scalp tissue overlying the dilating os. This swelling is apparent at birth and may be felt on internal examination, making palpation of the fontanelles and sutures difficult as it may cross a suture line. This swelling will pit when pressure is applied and will gradually become smaller, usually disappearing within 36 hours of birth.

Cephalhaematoma

Friction between the pelvis and fetal skull during labour may lead to separation of the periosteum from a skull bone and consequent bleeding between the skull and periosteum. As the periosteum is adherent to the borders of the bone, the swelling will be limited to a specific bone, usually a parietal bone, and consequently does not cross a suture line. A cephalhaematoma is not obvious at birth and gradually develops over the first 12–72 hours. This swelling persists for several weeks, becoming progressively harder and does not pit on pressure. Occasionally it may be bilateral, usually affecting both parietal bones and may contribute to the baby developing jaundice or anaemia.

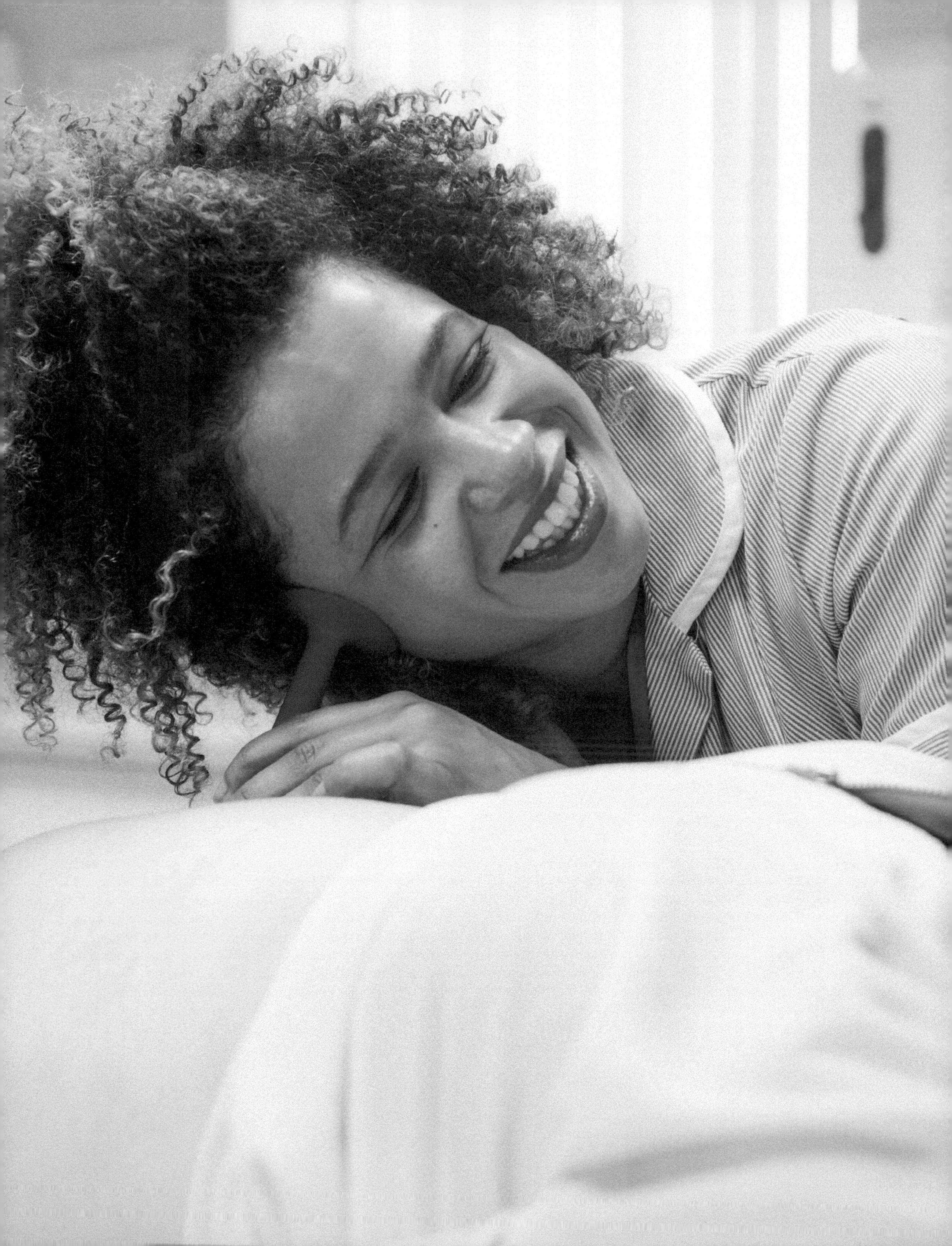

Preconception

Chapters

12 Preconception care

Figure 12.1 Conditions that require prepregnancy counselling.

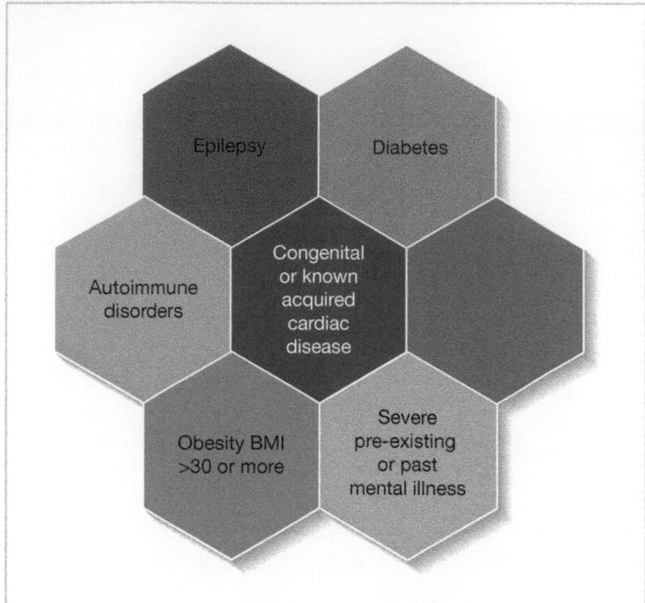

Figure 12.2 Issues for mental health review.

Relapse of illness

- Risks: to fetus & those related to stopping/changing medication

Women of childbearing potential who have an existing mental disorder and/or who are taking psychotropic medication

- Discussion: impact of the disorder & effect of treatment on health (own & fetus/baby)
- Contraception use & pregnancy plans
- How pregnancy/childbirth can affect a mental health problem; risk of relapse; how a mental health problem & its treatment might affect the woman and fetus/baby

Figure 12.3 Multidisciplinary approach to mental health care in prepregnancy counselling.

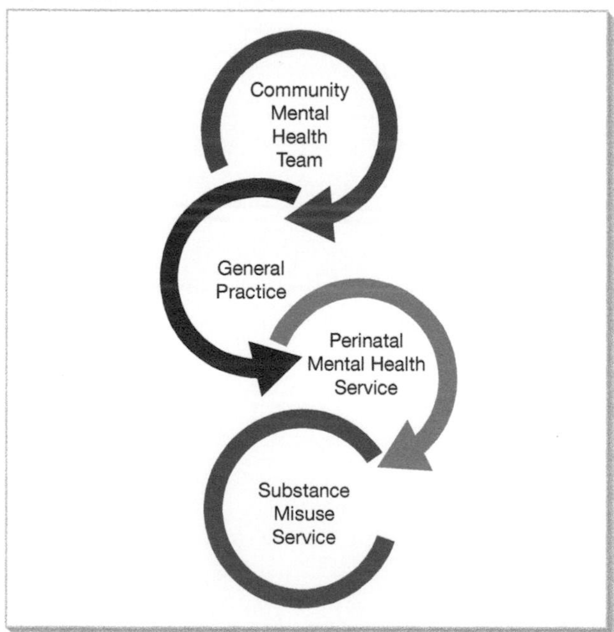

Midwifery at a Glance, First Edition. Edited by Eleanor Forrest © 2019 John Wiley & Sons Ltd. Published 2019 by John Wiley & Sons, Ltd.
Companion website: www.wiley.com/go/forrest/midwifery

Preconception care is known to affect maternal and child health outcomes in a positive way. Providing care before conception occurs can provide necessary interventions for women and partners and help in planning for pregnancy. The ultimate aim of preconception care is, both short and long term, to improve maternal and child care. This is also relevant to men as the pregnancy outcome can be affected by their lifestyle and health. However, many people do not present for preconception advice as not all pregnancies are planned and the opportunity to receive important prepregnancy information is lost.

Preconception advice is about providing encouragement to women and their partners to be proactive and prepare for pregnancy, to be as healthy as possible to promote the optimal chance for a healthy pregnancy and baby and reduce perinatal and maternal mortality. Examples of this are:

- Promoting informed choice and decisions: helps women and partners to focus on conception, pregnancy, their readiness to be parents and health issues that could affect this, thus creating an environment most conducive for conception and organogenesis
- Provision of lifestyle advice: such as promoting healthy eating, smoking cessation and limiting alcohol intake and drug use
- Guidance on taking folic acid supplements
- Advising on when to discontinue contraception and enabling a planned conception
- Provision of best management and planning to optimise care for women with chronic health problems including mental health problems
- Offering genetic counselling: screening and identification of couples with an increased risk of having a baby with a genetic or chromosomal malformation and providing them with knowledge to enable them to make informed decisions.

Guidance for preconception care

Parents who have lost a pregnancy but hope to have another baby often have many concerns, such as the risks involved in another pregnancy and the chance of a healthy baby, or even when it would be appropriate to plan another pregnancy. Therefore, it is important to understand that such parents may still be experiencing grief and are worried about the pain of another loss (Chapter 66). A couple may have differing views about when it is right to have another pregnancy and this can affect sexual relationships as there can be concerns about conceiving or their inability to conceive if they try.

For women with a pre-existing history of medical health problems (Part 7), previous pregnancy loss or mental health issues, their prepregnancy planning is likely to be initially provided by their GP or mental health team. To reduce maternal mortality the most common conditions that require prepregnancy counselling and advice are medical and psychiatric conditions (Figure 12.1).

When a woman attends for preconception care, an assessment will be required to establish her needs; it will be based on the following in order to offer appropriate advice:

- Timing of planned pregnancy
- Smear history
- Taking folic acid
- Lifestyle history: smoking, alcohol intake, illicit drug use, and whether overweight or obese
- Health history: miscarriage, risk or concern regarding chromosomal abnormalities or inherited genetic disorders, health problems, risk of hepatitis B, rubella immune status, history of chickenpox or shingles, risks of exposure to radiation or hazardous substances
- Medication: prescribed, over-the-counter or herbal.

Consideration needs to be given to the mental health of women as part of preconception care and pregnancy planning. The provision of preconception care in order to reduce the risk of maternal deaths from all causes, including from suicide, has been advocated. Many women are particularly vulnerable to mental health problems during childbearing, for example those having assisted reproduction or other fertility treatments. Also, mental health conditions may be aggravated by pregnancy and guidelines recommend that counselling and support, whether planned or opportunistic, should be provided for all women capable of childbearing.

Ideally, women should discuss pregnancy plans with their doctor. Referral can be made to specialist perinatal mental health services for those with a mental health problem newly diagnosed, pre-existing or with a family history of a mental health problem. Issues such as contraception and pregnancy risks will be discussed (Figure 12.2).

Multidisciplinary preconception care

Childbearing women often have differing healthcare needs and this requires a multi-disciplinary approach to their care. For example, women with previous medical or obstetric problems require follow-up appointments to help provide information to explain what has happened, from those professionals relevant to their care: physicians, obstetricians, midwives, geneticists and the voluntary sector. However, clear answers may not always be possible and the distress and disappointment of parents must be acknowledged.

For those women with a pre-existing or previous mental health problem, or a family history of mental ill health such as bipolar disorder or schizophrenia, a multidisciplinary approach to care is of particular relevance. This is to ensure that appropriate care planning is implemented prior to pregnancy (Figure 12.3).

Liaison between professional groups and services requires good communication, which is crucial to ensure that women with mental health problems and the individual health needs of couples planning a pregnancy are met when planning a pregnancy. As this requires a multiprofessional approach, a wide range of health and voluntary sectors and stakeholders are required to ensure appropriate access to preconception care.

13 Follow-up after pregnancy loss

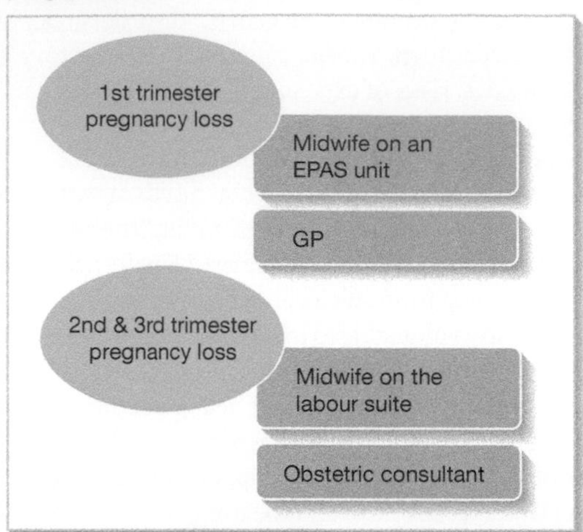

Figure 13.1 Main referral routes following pregnancy loss.

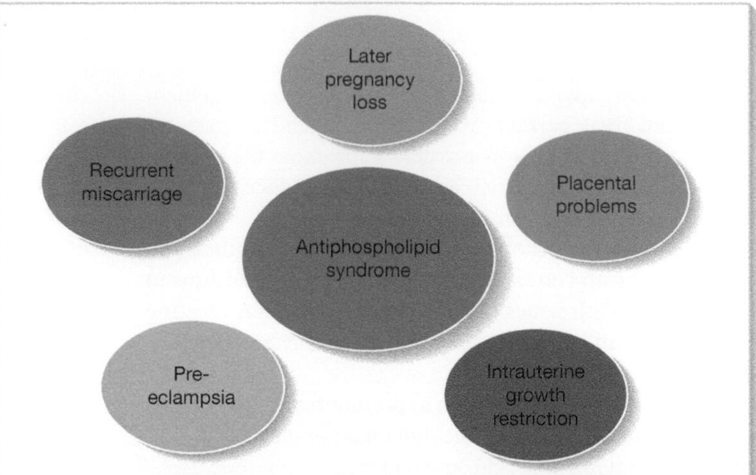

Figure 13.2 Antiphospholipid syndrome.

Figure 13.3 Treatment for antiphospholipid syndrome.

Low dose aspirin taken when a woman has a positive pregnancy test → Scan to confirm intrauterine pregnancy → Low molecular weight heparin from approximately 6 weeks' gestation onwards → Other general wellbeing investigations to optimise wellbeing: full blood count, ferritin, folate, vitamin B12, thyroid function tests, HbA1C

Box 13.1 Example of support by charity groups.

- Free telephone support group facility
- Website
- Downloadable information leaflets:
  - trying again
  - men and miscarriage
  - antiphospholipid syndrome
  - pregnancy loss
  - talking to the children

Box 13.2 Eight-week post loss appointment.

Before appointment
- Encourage the couple to write down questions and bring them along to the appointment.
- Perhaps meet the couple whilst in the labour suite to make personal contact, though this is not always possible
- Telephone after 3–4 weeks rather than send an appointment letter. This timing will allow for the funeral (if one is taking place) to have occurred

Appointment
Explain:
- why this happened
- postmortem results
- placenta pathology, and other investigations
- future management plan

Box 13.3 Examples of support groups.

SANDS (Stillbirth and Neonatal Death Society)
Child Bereavement UK
These organisations can offer further support and information to individuals with the use of telephone helplines, 'one to one' or group meetings, websites and forums

Box 13.4 Meeting the couple.

- Ask how they both are and acknowledge how difficult it must be to come back to the hospital/unit
- The couple's response will often be a guide to what issue needs to be addressed initially
- There can then be a natural flow to the discussion covering all aspects of their antenatal care, the diagnosis of maternal and/or fetal problems, previous obstetric and medical history & the subsequent events of the delivery of their baby & the care received
- Allow questions as they wish & give them the time they need
- Check that the couple understand any answers although there is not always an answer to why it happened to them and their baby
- It can be worthwhile for the midwife to offer the choice of a further appointment at the hospital with her or direct telephone contact to discuss results & to reinforce herself as a point of contact if any other concerns or questions arise or in the event of a new pregnancy

Box 13.5 Discussion of results.

- Approximately 50% of couples will consent to a postmortem examination which can lead to a clear diagnosis in some cases or an incidental finding with a dual pathology in others
- Sometimes nothing is revealed and this can lead to further feelings of frustration but in these cases this can be positive as it has excluded other problems and therefore reduce recurrence
- Placental pathology reports are becoming more informative and can be very important when trying to gather as much information about possible causes. This can inform plans of treatment in a future pregnancy, for example including the use of low dose aspirin (75 mg) to improve placental implantation and function

Midwifery at a Glance, First Edition. Edited by Eleanor Forrest © 2019 John Wiley & Sons, Ltd. Published 2019 by John Wiley & Sons, Ltd.
Companion website: www.wiley.com/go/forrest/midwifery

It is of upmost importance that women suffering recurrent first trimester miscarriage or pregnancy loss in the second or third trimester know there will be a definite plan for follow-up and investigation in the following weeks. This should involve a midwife who has specialist skills and experience in pregnancy loss and counselling. Women and their partners need to have appropriate support tailored to their individual circumstances and reassurance that everything will be done to find out why this has happened to them and their baby. They need to know that there is help and hope for a future pregnancy, albeit that it is likely to be a very anxious and fearful event. Research has demonstrated that acknowledging pregnancy loss and providing a genuine caring approach with follow-up, at the right time can significantly reduce and enhance recovery of the woman's long-term emotional state. Relationships with partners, other children, family members and friends can be affected, along with work and lifestyle activities. Follow-up will depend on the maternity unit's organisational processes and resources. The following is a suggested process for follow-up care. The key is to be sensitive, flexible and mindful that not all individuals and couples will respond to pregnancy loss in the same way and within the same timeframe.

Referral process

Early Pregnancy Assessment Services (EPAS), the labour suite, GPs, community midwives and health visitors should refer the woman and her partner to a pregnancy loss follow-up service (Figure 13.1). Normally, labour suite/EPAS units ensure that communication systems and processes are in place at the time of the loss.

First trimester miscarriage

One in four pregnancies end within the first 12 weeks of pregnancy. The most likely cause is a sporadic chromosome or genetic problem with the pregnancy which will naturally miscarry rather than anything the woman has been doing. The incidence of first trimester miscarriage rises with increasing maternal age from 1:2 to 1:3. Women can alter their lifestyle to promote a positive effect on pregnancy outcomes by, for example: smoking, drug and alcohol cessation; improving BMI, diet and exercise; and optimising any predisposing medical disorders (Chapter 12).

It is very common for women to have one or two miscarriages, less common to have three miscarriages – particularly three miscarriages in a row. Recurrent miscarriage is defined as three consecutive miscarriages and it is often not until this point that women are referred for investigations. Historically, it is thought that 1:100 women will suffer three miscarriages; however, anecdotally it is more common than this. Some midwife-led clinics may offer to see women after two miscarriages for reassurance, investigation and a prepregnancy discussion regarding health, lifestyle and the significance of increasing maternal age. It has also been suggested, that women who have had one miscarriage which reached a 10-week size in growth (not gestational age) should also have investigations performed.

Investigations

Fifteen percent of women who have three or more miscarriages will have a condition called antiphospholipid syndrome ('sticky blood syndrome') which can lead to many complications (Figure 13.2). Investigations can often produce false positive results and it is therefore important to check this blood test at least 8 weeks after pregnancy. A positive result will require a second test to confirm the condition and, if confirmed, subsequent pregnancies should be appropriately treated (Figure 13.3).

Providing support is important; this can be by follow-up through a hospital clinic or from the primary care service. There are also well-recognised miscarriage support charities available for extra support and information (Box 13.1). Often when miscarriage is diagnosed women are offered a scan in their next pregnancy for reassurance via the EPAS. This can sometimes be organised by self-referral or by the GP. Most EPASs allow for self-referral in cases of abdominal pain or vaginal bleeding in a pregnancy, which can allow women to feel more in control and empowered.

Late miscarriage and stillbirth

Ideally, follow-up 8 weeks' post loss is provided by a specialist midwife; she will then become the woman's point of contact to deliver information, support and above all hope for the future. This can be a particularly emotional and sometimes physically traumatic time for women and their partners and they require clear information (Box 13.2). Partners have often returned to work and women sometimes find themselves at home alone for periods of time. A telephone call allows the midwife to introduce herself and acknowledge the loss of the baby, explain the process of investigation and follow-up and to reassure the woman that she will be supported as much as possible through the coming months. It is also an opportunity to find out how much support she has from family, friends and support groups (Box 13.3). to the midwife can also assess whether the grief and bereavement reactions are within an expectant pattern for this early stage or if the grief appears more complicated and requires earlier review from the GP or referral to the clinical psychology services for further support (Chapter 66).

The appointment

A clear arrangement of when and where the midwife will meet the women and her partner should be made in advance. A sensitive, warm and welcoming greeting should aim to relax the couple. Meeting at the entrance of the maternity unit is helpful as it can be very difficult entering the unit for the first time since previously leaving the hospital after losing their baby (Box 13.4). Ideally, the named consultant will also be present to greet the couple, having reviewed the case notes, maternity hand-held notes, placental pathology report and postmortem examination, if performed (Box 13.5). In the process of gathering information, a thrombophilia screen will be offered at this appointment.

Expect expressions of anger, frustration and feelings of blame. They may blame others for not looking after them well enough or even themselves for something they did or did not do, and often there is an overwhelming sadness.

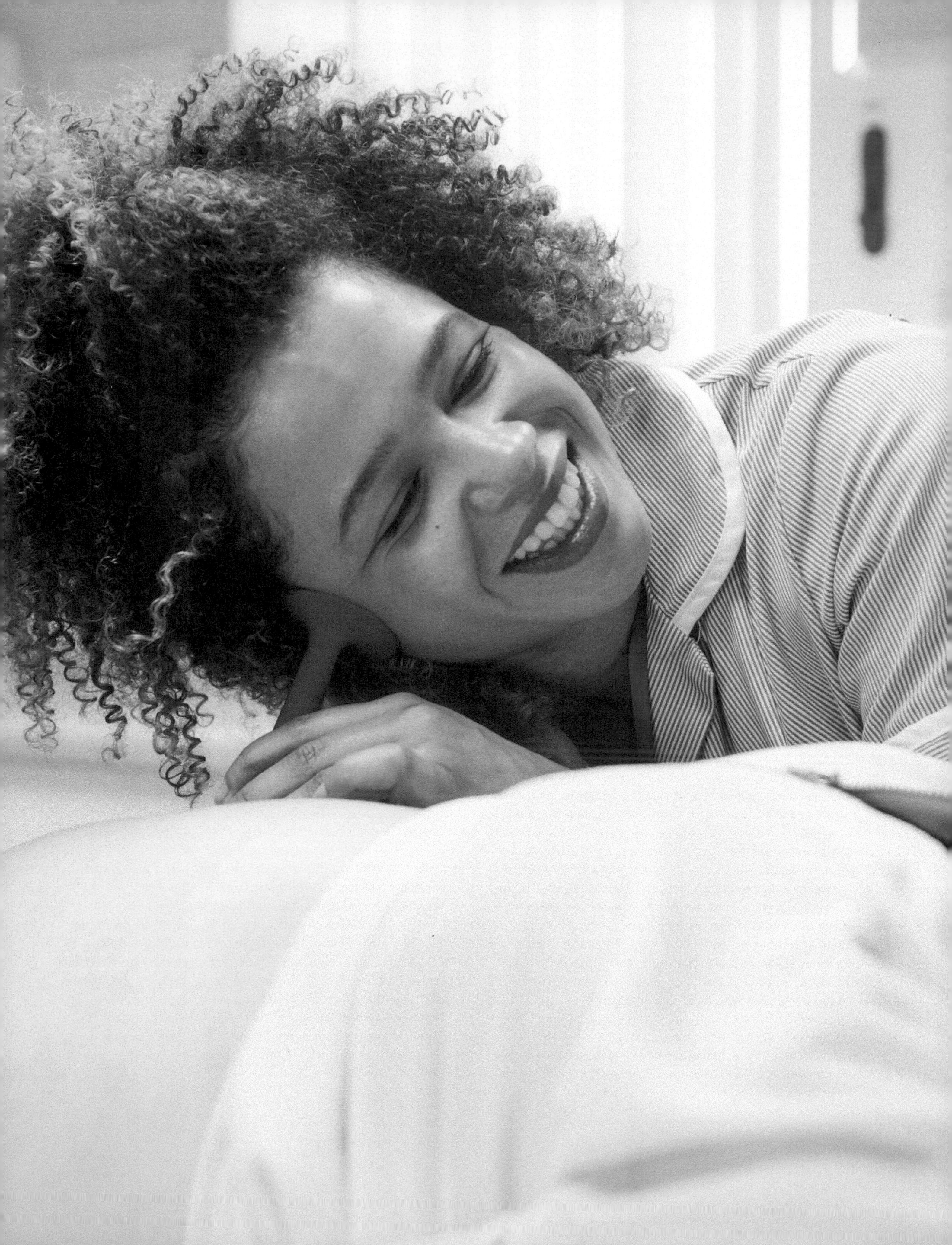

Antenatal

Chapters

14 Maternal physiological adaptation to pregnancy

Box 14.1 Hormonal influences (oestrogen and progesterone).

Muscle layer of the uterus
- Reduces muscular activity of the uterus

Blood vessels
- Reduces muscular activity of the muscular layer of the blood vessels
- Due to increased amounts of circulating blood volume, contributes to the development of varicose veins

Respiratory
- Increased breathlessness caused by progesterone, making the respiratory centre more sensitive to carbon dioxide levels in the blood

Urinary system
- Dilatation of the renal pelves and ureters
- Relaxes the detrusor muscle in the bladder resulting in urgency to pass urine
- Increased relaxation of the internal urethral sphincter combined with pressure from the uterus leads to stress incontinence

Gastrointestinal system
- Generalised reduction of muscle tone combined with the pressure from an enlarged uterus contribute to the common problems of heartburn, constipation and haemorrhoids

Body fat
- Increase in body fat during pregnancy

Ligaments
- Backache due to relaxed ligaments that normally stabilise the joints of the pelvis – this is beneficial at the time of delivery but a source of discomfort to the pregnant woman

Box 14.2 Changes due to increased blood volume.

- The plasma volume increases by about 50%. This increase starts gradually during the first trimester but continues at a more rapid pace during the second trimester
- The red blood cell volume increases by 20% between the 2nd & 3rd trimesters. Although the number of red blood cells is increasing, the disproportionately greater & earlier increase in the plasma volume leads to a state of haemodilution in which the haemoglobin, haematocrit & red blood cell volume appear to be reduced
- Increasing levels of plasma protein & white blood cells also appear to become reduced
- The increase in blood volume leads to a 40% increase in cardiac output by the 30th week of pregnancy
- The heart rate also increases by 11–17%, peaking at around the 30th week

Figure 14.1 Respiratory anatomical and functional changes.

Anatomical changes
- Flaring of the lower ribs
- Increase in the transverse diameter of the chest by 2 cm
- Increased activity of the diaphragm which rises by 4 cm

Functional changes
- Tidal volume gradually increases from 500 to 700 ml
- Expired volume increases by 100–200 ml
- Reduction in residual volume which results in a lower $P\text{co}_2$ & increased $P\text{o}_2$
- 18% increase in oxygen-carrying potential of the blood

Box 14.3 Changes to offset blood pressure rising.

- The relaxant effect of progesterone on blood vessel walls
- Cutaneous vasodilation
- Increased blood flow to the kidneys
- Increased blood flow to the uterus and placental bed. This is estimated to increase from 50 ml/min in the 10th week of pregnancy to 700 ml/min by term

Box 14.4 Uterine changes.

- Perimetrium acts to protect the uterus
- Myometrium allows dilatation of the cervix, shortens upper uterine segment (1st stage of labour), helps with expulsion of baby (2nd stage) & controls bleeding (3rd stage), shortens & pulls up the cervix, which in turn helps to expel the fetus during labour
- The uterus becomes vertical in pregnancy. As it rises in the abdomen it leans towards the right. It has a prepregnancy size of 7.5 × 5 × 2.5 cm, whilst at term it grows to around 30 × 23 × 20 cm. As the uterus grows, it leaves the pelvic cavity at around 12 weeks & eventually fills the abdominal cavity by 40 weeks. It reaches the umbilicus by the 24th week & by the 36th week reaches the anterior abdominal wall at the level of the xiphisternum. It now weighs about 1100 g, which is a 20-fold growth. The uterus capacity changes from 6 to 5000 ml

Pregnancy is the period from conception to birth when a woman carries a developing fetus in her uterus. The duration is 280 days or 40 weeks: 9 calendar months + 1 week taken from the first day of the last menstrual period. During this time physiological adaptation to pregnancy involves changes to every system within the woman's body. These changes are all designed to nurture the fetus and prepare the body for labour and lactation. Genetic factors and hormonal effects are influential in underpinning most of the physiological changes in pregnancy (Box 14.1).

Cardiovascular system

By the 20th week of pregnancy the circulating blood volume will have increased by 40–50%. The increases in blood components vary and occur at different rates (Box 14.2). The red blood cell volume increases by 20% between the second and third trimesters, however the disproportionately greater and earlier increase in the plasma volume makes it appear that the haemoglobin, haematocrit and red blood cell volume appear to be reduced (haemodilution). A 21% increase is also noted in the stroke volume, which peaks between the 16th and 22nd weeks of gestation. The increase in blood pressure that would result from such a large expansion in circulating blood volume is offset by several factors (Box 14.3). As a consequence the blood pressure should remain normal throughout the pregnancy, with a slight drop often noted mid-trimester. The heart increases slightly in size, and slight upward and lateral displacement occurs as a result of pressure from the growing uterus. Plasma protein increases with reduced concentration (haemodilution). A reduction in albumin reduces osmotic pressure leading to physiological oedema. Clotting factors increase in fibrinogen, factor 7, factor10 and platelets leading to a change in coagulation time from 12 to 8 minutes. This increases the risk of thrombosis, embolism and disseminated intravascular coagulation (DIC) (Part 8); this is particularly important for the third stage of labour.

Respiratory system

During pregnancy, both anatomical and functional changes occur within the respiratory system (Figure 14.1). Overall there is a 40–50% increase in ventilation and an 18% increase in the oxygen-carrying potential of the blood, which together support the increase in oxygen consumption required. Some women find that nose bleeds are more common in pregnancy as a result of increased vascularity.

Renal system

The glomerular filtration rate increases in early pregnancy. As a result of the increased circulating blood volume the kidneys enlarge and dilatation of the renal calyces, pelves and ureters, particularly on the right side, is noted in the first trimester. Pressure on the bladder, from the enlarging gravid uterus, leads to frequency of micturition in early pregnancy. This situation resolves as the gravid uterus rises out of the pelvis in the second trimester. However, in later pregnancy frequency of micturition often becomes a problem again when lightening occurs.

Gastrointestinal system

Increasing progesterone levels lead to relaxation of the intestinal musculature. As a consequence gut motility is reduced and constipation can become a problem. Relaxation of the cardiac sphincter leads to heartburn and this situation is exacerbated further by the upward displacement of the stomach by the gravid uterus as pregnancy progresses. The combination of hormonal changes and pressure from the growing uterus also contribute to delayed stomach emptying and the development of haemorrhoids.

Musculoskeletal system

Increasing progesterone and relaxin levels lead to increased mobility and flexibility of joints. This can cause softening of the symphysis pubis and the sacroiliac joint. The effects of progesterone in later pregnancy may lead to a degree of destabilisation of the pelvic joints. The centre of gravity alters in pregnancy and many women develop a lordosis of the lumbar spine in later pregnancy which contributes to the development of backache.

Breast changes

The breasts enlarge and veins appear more obvious as vascularity increases. The nipples also enlarge with the surrounding sebaceous glands, Montgomery's tubercules, becoming more obvious with alterations to pigmentation. Colostrum is produced by 16th week. See Chapters 7, 34 and 62 for more information on the breasts and infant feeding.

Skin changes

Various skin changes can occur in pregnancy, mostly as a consequence of hormonal activity. Hair and skin become greasier and spots can be a problem. Hair can feel thicker in pregnancy as natural hair loss is delayed. Increasing levels of the melanocyte-stimulating hormone lead to areas of increased pigmentation. Striae gravidarum may appear, particularly on the lower abdomen and breasts.

Uterus, cervix and vagina changes

The uterus forms a protective and highly nutritive environment which supports the growth and development of the fetus (Box 14.4). It prepares a bed and nourishes the fertilised ovum for the gestational period and expels the products of conception at full term; involuting after childbirth. The cervix length remains almost unchanged but the blood supply increases and it becomes softer and bluish in colour. More mucous is secreted to form the operculum, blocking the cervical canal of the uterus in pregnancy to prevent ascending genital tract infection. The pH becomes more acidic and acts as a barrier.

Weight gain

Maternal weight usually increases by 0.5 kg/month for the first 20 weeks of pregnancy and then by 0.5 kg/week for the second 20 weeks of pregnancy. Metabolism alters in pregnancy so that there is little need to increase the calorie intake. Inadequate weight gain in pregnancy may contribute to low birth weight, whilst excessive weight gain may contribute to the amount the woman has to lose postnatally. It has also been attributed as a risk factor for shoulder dystocia. Long-term obesity may lead to cardiovascular disease and diabetes (Part 7).

15 Taking a history

Figure 15.1 The why, who, where, when, how and what of a booking visit.

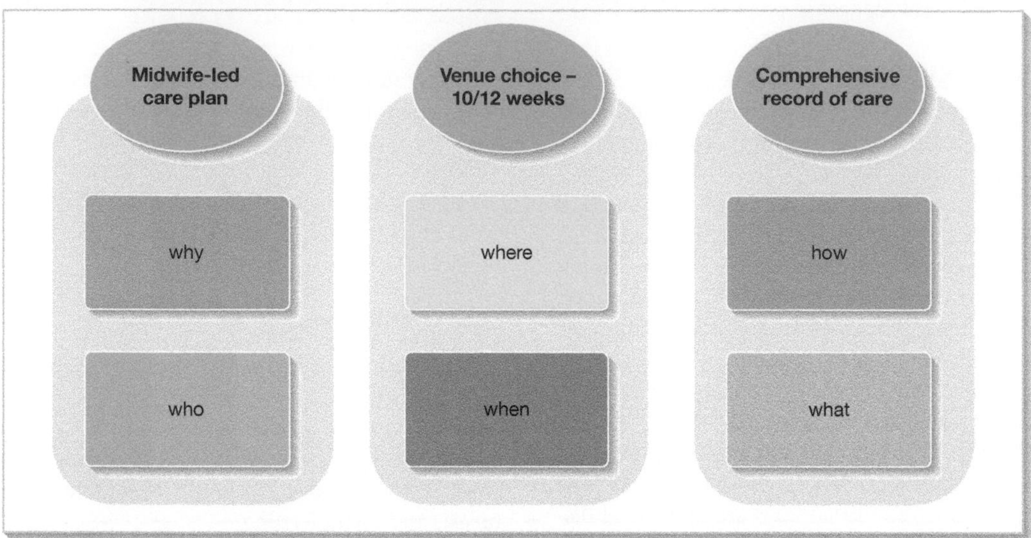

Figure 15.2 Key components of booking history.

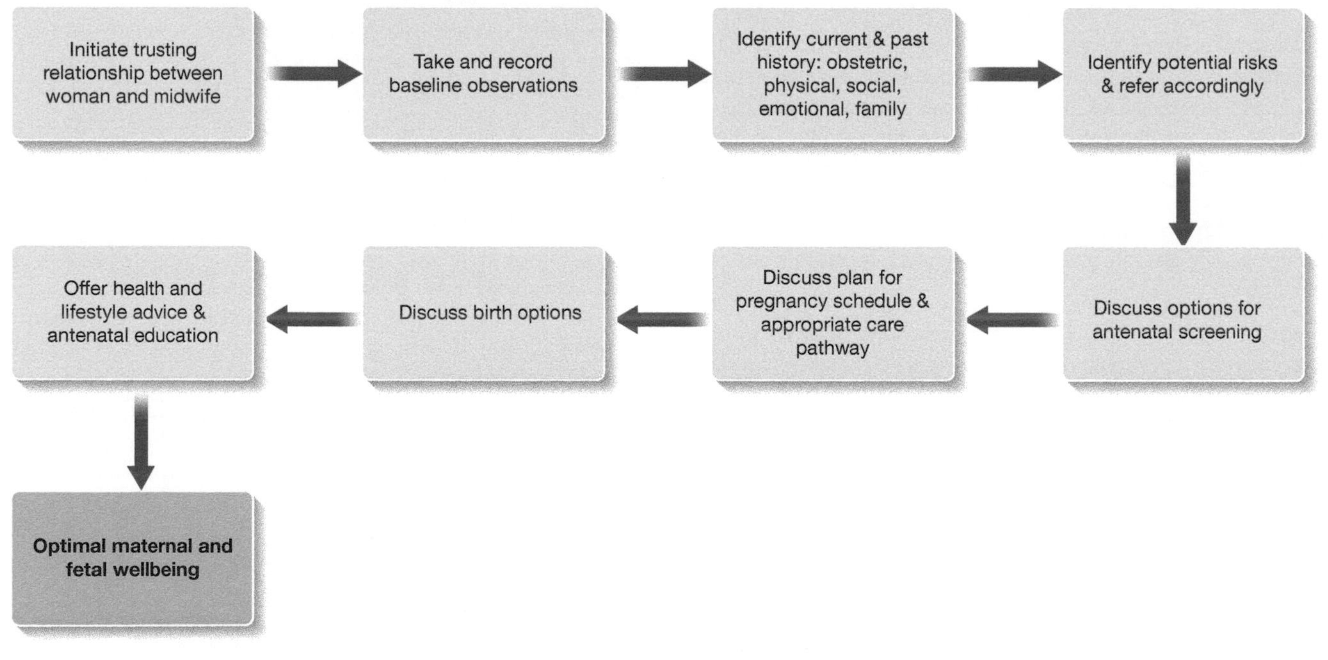

This chapter will focus on the initial booking history; however, the same principles of communication and relationship building, risk assessment and care planning will apply when having to elicit a history at any time in the childbearing continuum (Figure 15.1).

Why

The booking visit is important for many reasons, but is most likely to be the crucial visit to building initial relationships and establishing a plan of care for the woman. It forms the basis for all antenatal care and sets guidelines and timescales for follow-up visits. Antenatal care ensures the health and wellbeing of the mother and fetus by monitoring physical and emotional parameters and the provision of information about pregnancy, birth and the postnatal period.

Who

The midwife should be the main professional taking the history in a normal pregnancy due to the important nature of taking a history and the skill required. Midwives have the communication skills to build a rapport with women in order to obtain the relevant information. Midwives can individualise care, taking into account women's physical social, emotional and educational needs and those of their families. Liaison with appropriate health professionals may be necessary to ensure all needs are met.

Where

Women should be offered a choice of venue for taking their booking history – either a hospital, local community-based healthcare clinic or the woman's home. It is important that the venue is convenient for the woman and that she is able to feel comfortable. Some hospital or clinic venues may be difficult places for women to attend, perhaps due to the association of previous experiences, or their location. In the woman's own home, the balance of power shifts from the professional to the woman and becomes more equal, encouraging communication. The home booking history may take longer, but affords the midwife the opportunity to get to know the woman in her home environment and to acknowledge any social issues. The development of mutual respect can best be forged in the home environment; however, the woman must feel that she has a choice of venue. The venue for taking a history should be private and, ideally, free from interruptions.

When

It is recommended that all women be seen before 10 weeks' gestation and the booking history taken by 12 weeks' gestation. This allows for the identification of any problems or potential risks, whilst giving health advice and information such as available screening tests. Recording a history early allows information to be recorded from the outset. Care planning can be initiated and the appropriate care pathway commenced, with immediate consultant referral if deemed necessary. Women with more complex needs can be cared for by the appropriate multidisciplinary team. Booking later than 12 weeks' gestation can lead to increased morbidity. If women contact maternity services later in pregnancy, a full history should be taken within 2 weeks.

How

Throughout the UK many areas now use an electronic system which provides a platform to collect, record and store live data throughout the perinatal period for both mother and the neonate. Some regions provide an App for women to download, allowing them access to their maternity notes electronically. Other areas of the UK will have their own national documentation but the principles of accurately recording a detailed booking history still apply.

A holistic approach to taking a history is recommended to ensure that all aspects of a woman's needs are addressed. Women are encouraged to make informed decisions about their care (Chapter 6) so the booking history must be comprehensive. Information provided to women should be accessible and time given to clarify understanding. Consideration should be given to the need for interpreter services in some instances.

Although some private time should be offered to all women when taking a history to discuss sensitive issues, (e.g. gender-based violence or child abuse), the midwife should involve partners and family members as they can impact positively on a woman's pregnancy. Whilst respecting confidentiality, a sensitive, non-bias approach in which assumptions are avoided, must be adopted by the midwife taking the history.

What

Comprehensive information about the woman's current and past physical, obstetric, psychiatric and social history should be noted, in addition to any family history. Appropriate referral can then be made, for example when there is increased BMI or mental health problems. With the woman's consent, an ultrasound scan should be offered at this appointment to ensure gestational age. An appropriate plan of care is initiated. The booking history provides an opportunity for the midwife to discuss public health issues such as the effects of smoking, drinking alcohol and substance use in order to promote healthy living. Health promotion advice such as diet, exercise, benefits of vitamins and local antenatal education and exercise classes should be offered (Figure 15.2). When taking a history with vulnerable women, their particular needs should be addressed: teenagers, unsupported women, homeless or asylum-seeking women and those with disabilities or mental health problems (Part 10).

16 Antenatal investigations and screening

Table 16.1 Antenatal screening tests.

Blood	Ultrasound scan
FBC	Diagnose pregnancy
ABO & Rh group	Assess growth & liquor volume
Infections	Placental position
Haemoglobinopathies	Fetal anomalies
Fetal anomalies	

Table 16.2 Countries with prevalent haemoglobinopathies.

South Asia	East & SE Asia	Others
India	China	Middle East
Pakistan	Hong Kong	Mediterranean
	Malaysia	Poland

Table 16.3 Antenatal diagnostic tests.

Chorionic villus sampling	Amniocentesis
From 11 weeks' gestation	From 15 weeks' gestation
Usually transabdominal	Transabdominal
Chorionic villi obtained; chromosomes analysed	Amniotic fluid obtained
Small risk of pregnancy loss	Fetal cells cultured; chromosomes counted
Diagnose fetal chromosome variations	Small risk of pregnancy loss
	Diagnose fetal chromosome variations

Women are offered information about the many routine screening and diagnostic tests available in pregnancy – generally discussed at the first visit. National guidelines and local policy should be followed in order that midwives provide the best possible information to women. Midwives also require skills to be effective communicators, especially when discussing screening for issues such as fetal anomalies. Referral may have to be made to the fetal medicine team for on-going testing, discussion of results and women's options regarding continuation or termination of pregnancy for fetal anomaly.

Screening tests

These assess the likelihood or risk of a condition, health problems or disabilities of the mother and baby (Table 16.1). It is always the woman's choice to accept the tests and they should be conducted with the woman's consent. The results from some screening tests may result in more invasive diagnostic tests being offered and women need to be informed of this possibility in order that informed decisions can be made (Chapters 6 and 16).

Blood tests

Blood is taken to assess maternal and fetal wellbeing.

Full blood count (FBC)

Initially taken at booking and at intervals during pregnancy; detects a fall in haemoglobin (Hb). Serum ferritin may also be assessed. Platelet levels may fall in pregnancy and need to be tested. White cell count normally rises in pregnancy, but an abnormal rise may be indicative of an infection.

ABO and rhesus (Rh) blood group

Taken at booking to determine which main blood group a woman belongs to and whether any antibodies exist. Rhesus factor will also be determined with this test. Rhesus negative results may require the woman to have anti-D immunoglobulin if the fetus is rhesus positive. Guidelines advise all non-sensitised rhesus negative women should receive routine anti-D prophylaxis.

Infectious diseases

Screening for infectious disease is important because treatments are relatively simple and can reduce risks to the mother and baby. Most women are now protected against rubella, so it is not routinely tested for unless the woman is unsure if she has been immunised. The hepatitis B virus (HBV) status of all pregnant women should be ascertained at the booking visit as HBV affects the liver and can be carried to the fetus and by body fluids to others. Although not common in the UK, women are still routinely screened for syphilis as the untreated condition can damage maternal and fetal health. Routine testing for human immunodeficiency virus (HIV) is recommended as HIV can be passed to the fetus, damaging the immune system, which can lead to acquired immunodeficiency syndrome (AIDS). All tests require informed consent and a tactful approach to this topic is necessary. Some maternity units may have a resource person identified to meet the more complex needs of some women.

Haemoglobinopathies

Sickle cell and thalassaemia disorders are amongst a range of inherited single gene, recessive disorders that affect haemoglobin. As these conditions arise predominantly in people with family backgrounds from particular countries (Table 16.2), women are asked to complete a family origin questionnaire to guide the midwife in deciding who requires to be screened. Women with assisted pregnancies may require screening, especially if sperm or egg donation has occurred. If the woman is a carrier of sickle cell or thalassaemia, her partner also requires testing. The preferred time for testing is prior to 10 weeks' gestation.

Down's syndrome

This blood test is available to all pregnant women, regardless of age. It is a personal decision whether the test should be taken and may require in-depth discussion with the midwife. Testing can be screening and diagnostic. Screening is by a blood test and nuchal translucency (NT) ultrasound scan (less than 14 weeks' pregnant) or blood test alone (14–20 weeks' pregnant). Screening results can be altered if the mother smokes or has an assisted pregnancy. Diagnostic testing is mentioned below.

Ultrasound scans

Early pregnancy scans are performed to diagnose pregnancy, assess the growth and development of the fetus and estimate the stage of pregnancy. Fetal anomalies may also be noted and the woman should be made aware of this, as she may not wish to know. The NT scan can also be performed between 11 and 14 weeks of pregnancy. Mid-pregnancy scans are performed between 18 and 21 weeks of pregnancy. A scan at this gestation can detect placental position and many fetal anomalies (e.g. neural tube defect), but not all anomalies can be assessed and these may require later scanning. Third trimester scans are conducted to assess fetal growth and amniotic fluid volume. Most routine scans performed on the NHS are 2D black and white images, but 3D colour image scans are available.

Diagnostic tests

Chorionic villus sampling (CVS)

CVS is a first trimester test, usually carried out from 11 weeks' gestation within a specialist centre. A fine needle is guided transabdominally (or via the cervix, but this is rarer), under ultrasound visualisation of the placent, and chorionic villi are obtained. These are examined for fetal chromosomal abnormalities. This test carries a small risk of pregnancy loss which varies within units. Rhesus negative women will require anti-D immunoglobulin following this procedure.

Amniocentesis

This test is carried out after 15 weeks' gestation, usually within a specialist centre. About 20 ml of amniotic fluid is extracted via a fine needle inserted through the abdominal wall into the uterus. The fetal cells are cultured and diagnosis of chromosomal abnormalities, fetal infections and genetic diseases can be made. The pregnancy loss risk is low (approx. 0.5–1%), but women must be informed of this (Table 16.3).

17 Preparation for childbirth

Figure 17.1 Grantly Dick-Read.

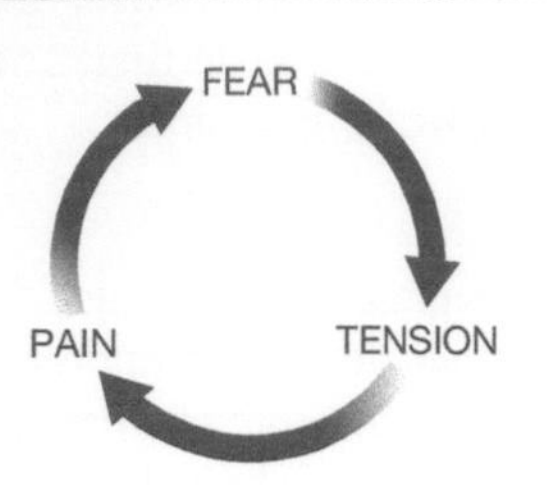

If women eliminate fear they would diminish the pain experienced during childbirth. The focus should be on peace, calm and relaxation to promote coping styles regardless of birth outcome

Figure 17.2 Positions for labour and birth.

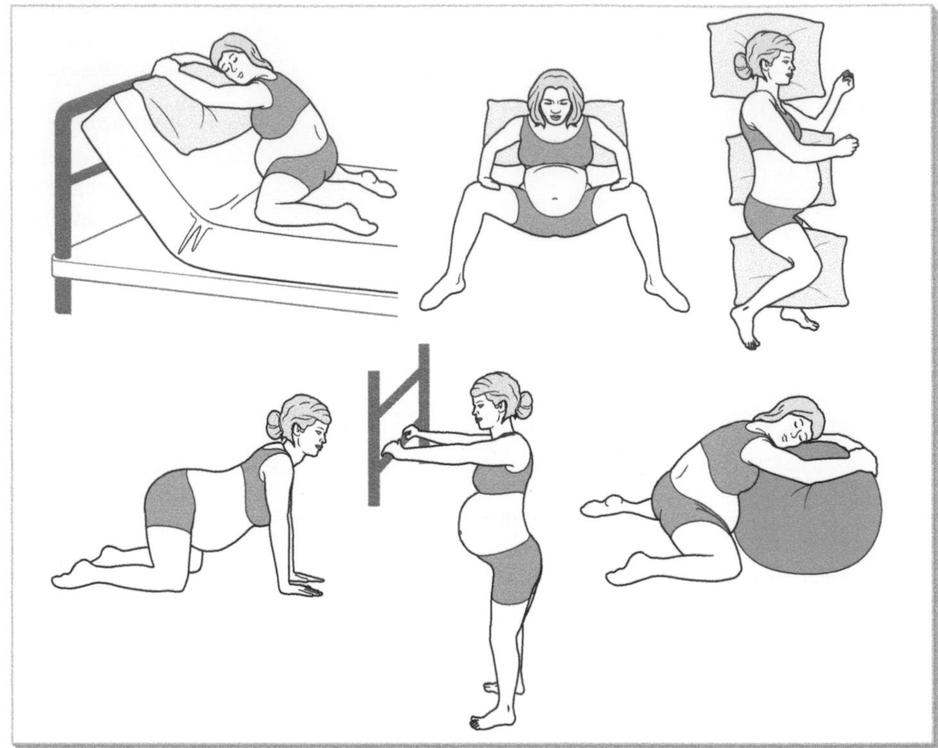

Figure 17.3 Maslow's hierarchy of needs.

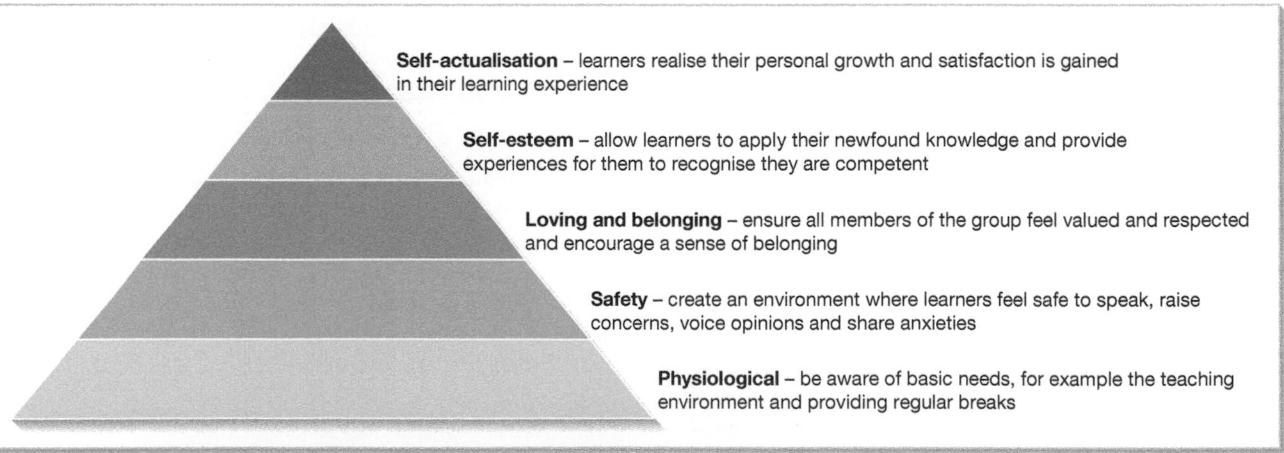

Box 17.1 Keeping active for birth. Source: YogaBellies, Reproduced with permission.

Exercise and yoga during pregnancy has many benefits:

- Increased circulation of blood and oxygen throughout the body
- Strengthened core muscles and birthing muscles resulting in reduced back pain and easier birth
- Improved digestion and sleep
- More energy
- Yoga in particular brings the focus to breathing. Concentrating on breathing correctly enables relaxation even in frightening or high stress situations
- New friendships

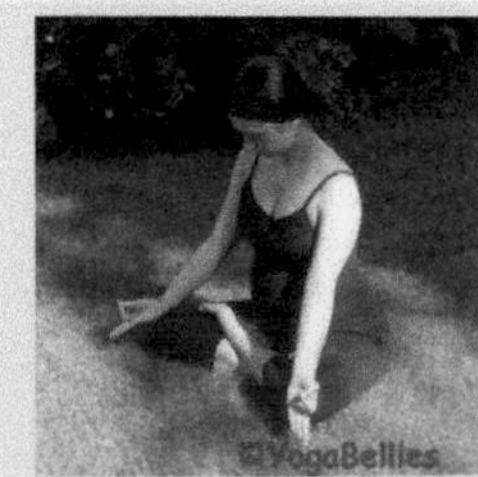

Midwifery at a Glance, First Edition. Edited by Eleanor Forrest © 2019 John Wiley & Sons, Ltd. Published 2019 by John Wiley & Sons, Ltd.
Companion website: www.wiley.com/go/forrest/midwifery

Childbirth is a momentous life changing event for any woman as she welcomes her baby to the world; it is a journey of self-discovery, hard work and achievement. Preparing for childbirth should be regarded as beneficial and essential. Women should feel supported by their midwife and their needs or fears recognised and understood. It is important that midwives understand that women will have different views with preconceived ideas of what her birth will be like; she may be influenced by her cultural, social, religious and previous birth/s.

Throughout history pregnant women have gained knowledge from their mothers, sisters and other women in the community about labour and parenting. The trend of moving birth from home to the hospital setting has allowed this insight to be diluted. The now medicalised event of childbirth has forced instinctive, cultural and family birth rituals to be second place. Education and informed choice are fundamental aspects of modern maternity healthcare policy; it is therefore essential that midwives and childbirth educators support women with their birth choices.

There are three areas to consider when providing a birth preparation session: understanding the psychological impact of birth, being active in birth and adult learning.

Psychological birth preparation

Grantly Dick-Read in 1944 first highlighted the need for antenatal education after he recognised that fear and anxiety had a direct impact on a woman's birthing ability and her birth outcomes. He concluded through his observations that should women have a fear of childbirth it lends to tension which often results in pain (Figure 17.1). Fear is an essential response to any emotional or physical danger, if fear was not experienced humans would be unable to protect themselves from actual threats. However, humans often fear situations that are far from life-or-death; birthing a child is an example of this. One of the main causes of fear in childbirth is women associating pain with childbirth. Fear of childbirth is often generated in today's society via the media as television shows almost exclusively promote birth in a medicalised model involving intervention and doctors. These programmes depict birth as a dramatic, edge-of-seat story unfolding and women observing these shows are at risk of becoming anxious about their upcoming birth.

If a woman approaches labour with fear then her body is already adopting a defensive stance, this then alerts the body to release the 'stress hormone' catecholamine (adrenaline and noradrenaline). The stress hormone prepares the body for a flight, fight or freeze mode. As labour does not require fight or flight it will often choose the third option of freeze mode and labour consequently slows down and in some cases stops altogether. This sympathetic response to pain will increase the heart rate and respirations as well as reducing uterine blood flow, which may lead to a reduction in uterine activity and oxytocin production. Oxytocin is required for normal labour to progress.

As a midwife it is essential that women are informed that labour is a sensation that may indeed cause discomfort. However, provided with the right supportive and positive input women can be encouraged to embrace their birth, not fear it.

Active birth preparation

Traditionally it is midwives who are considered to be the guardians of active natural birth; they have the skills to ensure the correct physical environment for a physiological birth. It is important that women are encouraged to consider the benefits of remaining active and upright during labour. Being able to change position and moving around freely helps cervical dilatation and aids the position of the baby to come through the pelvis (Figure 17.2 and Box 17.1). The concept of women lying on their backs can be in part attributed to the invention of forceps 300 years ago; if women were lying on their backs it gave the doctor more control over the birth. It is important that the 'control' is given back to women and that they are encouraged to trust in their body and to adopt whichever position they like during the early stages of labour and during the birth of their baby.

A review of existing studies in 2012 concluded there was greater efficiency when giving birth in an upright position, with evidence showing that there is a reduced risk of assisted delivery and episiotomy. However, a lower rate of episiotomy comes with a higher risk of second degree tear but research has shown that tears are less traumatic to tissues and heal more easily than episiotomies. Women should be encouraged to birth in whatever position they feel comfortable in and not the position the midwife would prefer. Midwives should be able to adapt the principles of care during labour to work with the woman and her partner to ensure a positive birth experience.

Adult learners

Being pregnant is a great motivator for women and their birth partners to seek out information and attend courses to prepare them for the birth of their baby. As a course facilitator it is essential that midwives meet the basic needs of the learners and Maslow's hierarchy of needs illustrates this concept (Figure 17.3).

When designing a childbirth preparation course careful consideration should be given to the provision of relevant teaching materials; clear aims and an agenda should be set and feedback obtained. Adult learners have different learning styles and also bring their own life experiences and as a facilitator it is the midwives place to be mindful of these factors and build upon them.

18 Post-term pregnancy

Box 18.1 Naegel's rule.

Using Naegel's rule, gestation is calculated by:

- Taking 1 week after the last menstrual period and counting 9 months' gestation from then

Box 18.2 Fetal and maternal complications.

- Restricted fetal growth
- Fetal malformations
- Decline of placental function, reducing oxygen and nutritional supply to the fetus
- Meconium aspiration
- Neonatal hypoglycaemia
- Increased risk of cerebral palsy
- Fetal macrosomia
- Birth injury
- Increased risk of caesarean section

Figure 18.1 Key points to consider in post-term pregnancy.

Key point
- Membrane sweep should be offered after 40 completed weeks of pregnancy

Key point
- To ensure induction of labour is offered at the appropriate gestation, accurate dating of pregnancy is required

Key point
- Midwives should remain up to date with recent guidelines for post-term pregnancy and induction of labour. Therefore, familiarise yourself with your department's policy for post-term pregnancy and induction of labour

Midwifery at a Glance, First Edition. Edited by Eleanor Forrest © 2019 John Wiley & Sons, Ltd. Published 2019 by John Wiley & Sons, Ltd.
Companion website: www.wiley.com/go/forrest/midwifery

The incidence of post-term pregnancy is 5–10%, but a previous prolonged pregnancy increases the likelihood. There is also a familial tendency. All pregnant women should be given adequate information so that they can make informed decisions about their care and any recommended treatment. As post-term pregnancies can be associated with complications, informed decision making in conjunction with a healthcare professional is of particular relevance. Approximately 70% of women will have given birth by 40 weeks' gestation and more than 80% will have given birth by 42 weeks' gestation.

Definition

Post-term pregnancy is when pregnancy continues beyond a gestation of 41 weeks plus 3 days or 10 days or more beyond the estimated date of delivery (EDD).

Accurate dating

The expected due date of the baby is of significant social and emotional importance to a woman and her family. The significance of the EDD for key professionals such as midwives, obstetricians and neonatologists is to enable them to evaluate fetal development and general wellbeing.

Last menstrual period (LMP) dating using Naegel's rule (Box 18.1) has long been used by women and professionals when making decisions such as when a pregnancy has become post-term. However, a more accurate method of dating is recommended as it can be difficult to remember exact LMP dates so they are therefore not always reliable. As around 70% of pregnancy inductions are due to the pregnancy being considered post-term, dating by ultrasound scan in developed countries is most often used to ensure a more accurate prediction of birth date. However, unless performed early in pregnancy, within the first trimester, accuracy cannot be guaranteed. Crown–rump length, or head circumference measurement if the crown–rump measurement is > 84 mm, should be used.

Factors increasing the risks of post-term pregnancy

- Primigravid pregnancy
- Previous post-term pregnancy
- Maternal raised prepregnancy weight and increased weight gain during pregnancy
- Raised maternal BMI
- Increased maternal age
- Fetal and maternal complications (Box 18.2).

Features

Fetal macrosomia occurs as the fetus continues to grow in utero, and by 42 weeks' gestation babies are more likely to weigh more than 4000 g. A large baby increases the likelihood of prolonged or dysfunctional labour with subsequent injury to the mother and baby.

Post-maturity features are often evident in babies born post term. These can be a combination of decreased subcutaneous fat, loose skin which is dry and flaky, an absence of lanugo and vernix, longer nails, which, with the umbilical cord, are often stained with meconium. Although these babies appear mature, they are often malnourished.

As there is a general reduction in fetoplacental circulation from 35 weeks onwards, the post-term baby can be subjected to varying degrees of growth restriction. The post-term baby has been shown to have changes to its circulation in Doppler studies. In addition, the placenta often has calcifications beyond term.

Oligohydramnios can occur in the post-term pregnancy, which reduces the supportive environment of the uterus for the baby. The reduced liquor volume can cause the cord to become compressed, leading to changes in fetal heart rate. Subsequent meconium staining can then result in meconium aspiration.

Management and midwifery care

There is a slightly greater risk of perinatal morbidity and mortality when the pregnancy is post term and although the overall risk remains low, greater care must be taken to avoid complications. Midwives should be involved in making sure that communication and information is adequate to ensure women make informed decisions regarding their post-term care. This should include induction and the implications of this, but also any associated risks with continuing the pregnancy, whilst expecting labour to commence spontaneously. Consideration should be also be given to the emotional and social implications of induction of labour to ensure an individual plan of care can be implemented for women. Care should include the following:

- Symphysis–fundal height should be measured and recorded
- Blood pressure should be measured and urine tested for proteinuria
- Give verbal and written information
- Provide an opportunity for women and their families to discuss issues and ask questions
- Membrane sweep should be offered
- Vaginal examination offered to determine Bishop's score
- Discuss options and choices for induction of labour
- Offer induction of labour as a safer management option for obese women to avoid potential caesarean section
- Cardiotocography (CTG) performed and recorded to ensure fetal wellbeing
- Advise women to call their midwife or maternity hospital if they have any concerns regarding their baby or birth.

Key points

The key points that midwives must consider in relation to post-term pregnancy and the care of women are outlined in Figure 18.1.

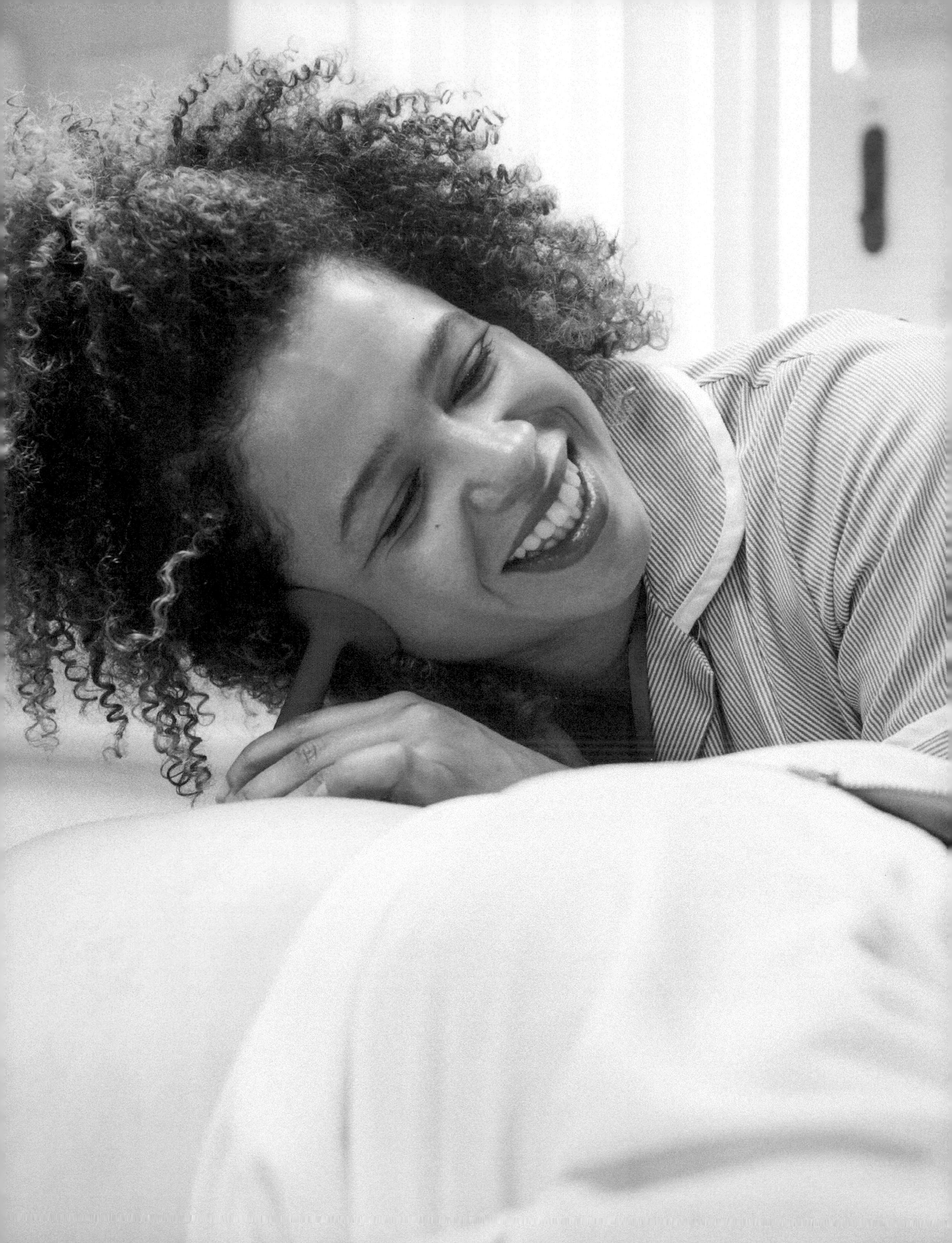

Intrapartum

Chapters

19 Physiology of labour

Figure 19.1 Progesterone/oestrogen ratio.

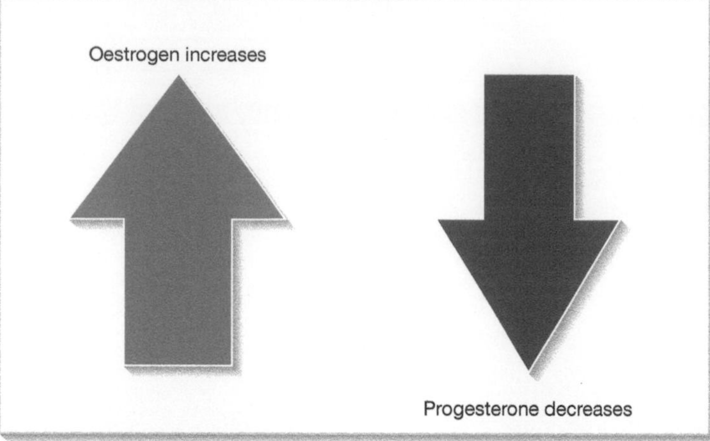

Figure 19.2 Gap junctions.

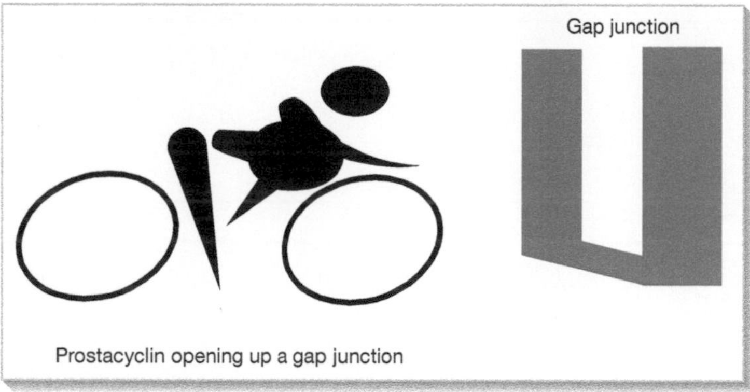

Figure 19.3 Oxytocin receptors.

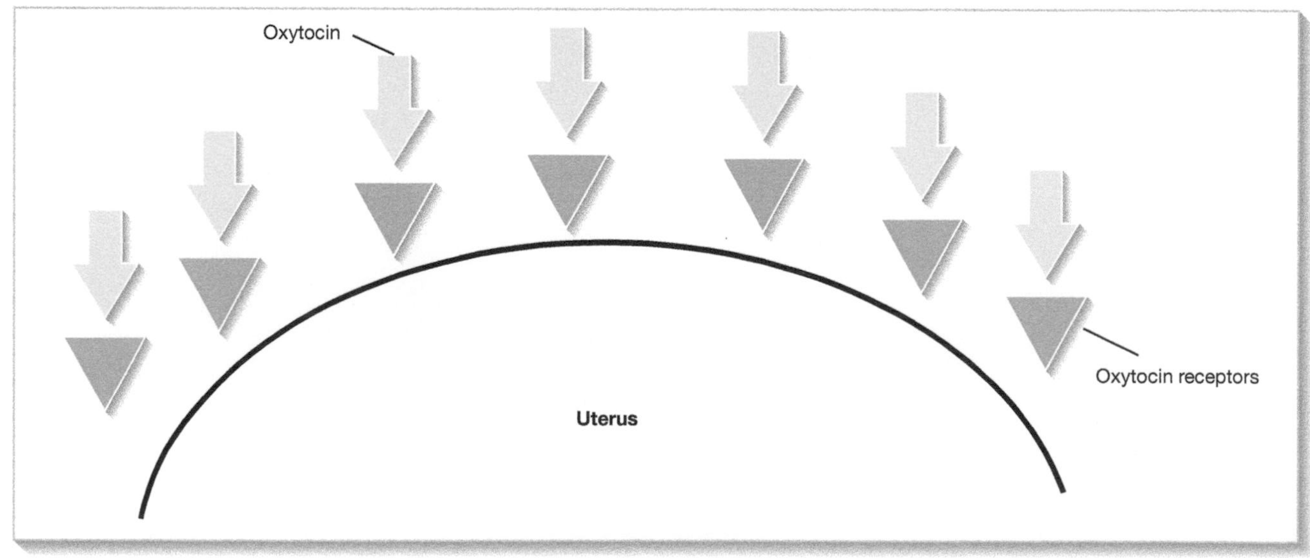

The physiology of labour is a complex interplay of maternal hormones, proteins and enzymes. The commencement of labour is affected by factors of fetal and placental origin.

The uterus is a unique muscle in the body which, in pregnancy, increases by up to 20 times its usual size. It develops in pregnancy to accommodate the fetus through hyperplasia and hypertrophy. It maintains relative quiescence until birth when, due to co-ordinated suppression and expression of hormones, it contracts to dilate the cervix and expel the fetus. The uterus, unlike other muscles, has the ability to contract and retract to open and hold the dilatation of the cervix, facilitating the birth of a baby. It consists of three distinct layers – the peritoneum, myometrium and endometrium. In pregnancy the endometrium is called the decidua. The myometrium comprises three muscle layers – longitudinal, circular and oblique. Myocytes in the myometrial cells work in a co-ordinated rhythm creating uterine contractions. The initiation of labour is not completely understood but there is a decrease in the inhibitory hormone progesterone, an increase in oestrogen and the procontractile hormone oxytocin, together with increased prostaglandin levels. The impact of these four important hormones and others on the onset of labour, are discussed here. Stretch receptors in the uterus activate the uterus in late pregnancy and stimulate contractions and increase oxytocin receptors. The onset of labour is influenced by the fetus and the woman. An important endocrine pathway, the fetal hypothalamic–pituitary–adrenal (HPA) axis, is activated at the onset of labour.

Fetal initiation

Cortisol from the fetal adrenals enables progesterone to convert to oestrogen, decreasing the inhibitory function of progesterone (progestation). As the progesterone/oestrogen ratio increases in favour of oestrogen, the uterus becomes sensitive to oxytocin, a contractile hormone. Fetal dehydroepiandrosterone (DHEAS) enhances the production of oestrogen too. Oestrogen has an important role in 'priming' the myometrium to increase sensitivity to oxytocin; it increases the formation of gap junctions and enhances the production of prostaglandins, which 'ripen' the cervix. The ratio of oestrogen to progesterone changes in late pregnancy, with oestrogen becoming the dominant hormone (Figure 19.1). Progesterone is also produced in the placenta, and together with human chorionic gonadotrophin (HCG) and relaxin, inhibits the release of oxytocin and the formation of gap junctions, necessary for the myocytes to message each other to promote uterine contractions. In addition, relaxin has a quiescence impact on myoctyes and inhibits oxytocics, as do melatonin, nitric oxide and corticotrophin-releasing hormone (CRH).

Prostaglandin

Prostaglandin is significant in promoting 'softening' and dilatation of the cervix, in membrane rupture and in contraction of the myometrium. Prostaglandin can be stimulated via an inflammatory response to tissue trauma such as coitus or membrane sweeping post 40 weeks. The level increases from 36 weeks and prostacyclin enables the opening of gap junctions that increase contractibility of the myocytes (Figure 19.2). Prostaglandin is produced in the membranes, decidua, myometrium and cervix. Oxytocin stimulates the synthesis of prostaglandins, which aids relaxation of the lower segment of the uterus during labour to facilitate passage of the fetus.

Corticotrophin-releasing hormone

CRH is an important hormone that potentiates the hormones prostaglandin and oxytocin and is found in the placenta and pituitary gland. In pregnancy its levels are low due to CRH-binding protein but the levels rise towards the end of pregnancy and during labour when CRH-binding protein falls. CRH levels are high in premature labour, which indicates its role in stimulating labour, and it has been described as a placental 'clock' which may impact on pregnancy duration. It aids in the opening of calcium channels in myocytes to facilitate action potentials across the cell membranes to stimulate contractions.

Oxytocin

The most significant hormone, oxytocin, has its origins in the fetal and maternal posterior pituitary gland. The uterine receptors for oxytocin increase greatly in the late stages of pregnancy and the second stage of labour as the pelvic floor is stretched and displaced by the descending baby. Oxytocin surges occur at night from 32 weeks onwards, which increases gap junctions and oxytocin receptors in readiness for labour. As the fetus grows, stretch receptors in the uterus are activated in late pregnancy and stimulate contractions, increasing the number of oxytocin receptors (Figure 19.3). With aligned hormonal influences, the uterus is ready for the onset of labour. The calcium balance in myocytes is altered enabling contraction and retraction of the myometrium. During a contraction, calcium ions within the intercellular space rise, adenosine triphosphate (ATP) breaks down and myocytes are shortened due to the cross-bridges of actin and myosin reducing the length of the cell (causing the myometrium to contract). This creates synchronous contraction and retraction of the uterine muscle which acts upon the cervix enabling dilatation.

The cervix is influenced by hormonal and enzyme activity and needs to 'soften' and efface to increase its ability to dilate. The cervix comprises a matrix of connective tissue, collagen and muscle fibres, held together tightly by dermatan and decorin. Towards the end of pregnancy the cervix changes; the matrix is broken down due to hormonal and enzyme activity which destabilises the connective tissue. The cervix becomes favourable to the uptake of water molecules which 'soften' it before the onset of labour. Prostaglandin levels rise due to an increase in hyaluronic acid and 'prime' the cervix for labour. This change in the rigid cervix to a softened state together with increasing uterine contractions, enable effacement dilatation. The contracting uterus enables the softened cervix to efface and dilate. This intricate system initiates labour and enables birth.

20 Mechanism of normal labour

Box 20.1 Mechanism of normal labour – the dynamic factors.

- Lie – how the fetus lies within the maternal abdomen: long, transverse or oblique
- Presentation – what is at or within the brim of the pelvis; this could be cephalic (vertex) or breech (buttocks)
- Denominator – the area of the presenting part that is best applied to the cervix; this could be the occiput, frontal (brow) or face of the fetal skull, fetal sacrum or lower limbs (breech)
- Position – where the denominator relates to the position of the pelvis: left/right; anterior/posterior, e.g LOA (left occipitoanterior)
- Attitude – flexed or deflexed
- Engagement – how much of the fetal skull has descended into the brim of the pelvis; some may occur before onset of labour

Box 20.2 Ferguson's reflex.

- Spontaneous urge to push during labour that occurs when the presenting part of the fetus reaches the pelvic floor
- May occur without full cervical effacement (shortening and thinning of the cervix)
- Woman is discouraged from pushing until the cervix has dilated completely to prevent damage to the cervix

Box 20.3 And so the normal birth story goes...

- With a long lie and
- Cephalic presentation in a
- LOA position, well flexed and engaged
- With onset of strong regular contractions
- Descent of the fetus takes place through the pelvis
- With further descent after transition and full dilatation of the cervix
- The head rotates on the pelvic floor
- As the occiput pivots and becomes deflexed under the pubic arch, the face sweeps the perineum and the head is born
- Internal rotation of the shoulders occurs, described as restitution
- At the next contraction the anterior shoulder can also pivot under the pubic arch with the posterior shoulder spontaneously birthing
- The body follows by lateral flexion following the curve of carus within the pelvis

Figure 20.1 Asynclitism (a, c) can resolve and allow delivery (b).

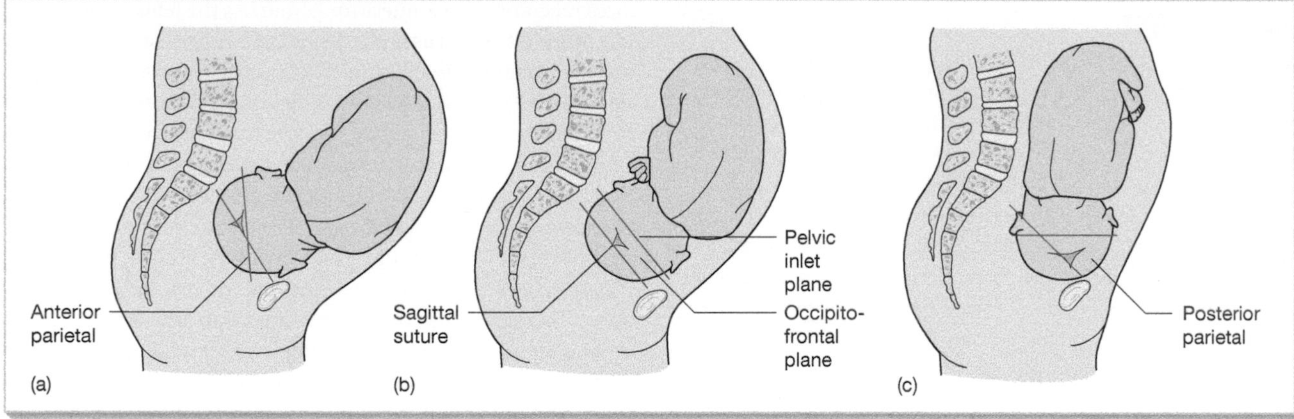

Fetal journey in labour and birth

During the process of labour (Chapters 19 and 21), the fetus descends through the maternal soft tissues and bony structures. There are a number of aspects that form a description of that journey – the *mechanism of labour.* This is the interplay between the fetal skull and the maternal pelvis (Chapter 11) and is demonstrated in how the fetal skull descends and rotates through the pelvis and birth canal, before emerging through the vaginal opening to be born.

Passenger, power and passage

Three elements are involved in the success of this journey: the passenger (fetus), the power of the expulsive forces and the shape and adequacy of the passage to get through. The fetus is not a passive passenger, it is active, aware and reactive to its situation and able to move and wriggle. The power of the co-ordinated rhythmical contractions (Chapters 19 and 21) is sensitive to influences in the environment and delivery of care which can hinder that power.

The progress of passing through the pelvis and soft tissues which are formed into a birth canal is monitored by professionals; the length of time this takes can impact on the wellbeing of both the mother and the baby. The fetus may fail to fit through a pelvis, resulting in an arrest of progress or complete obstruction within the passage. Therefore, determining fetal descent within the mechanism of labour is essential. A mobile woman following active birth principles with reduced anxiety provides the best opportunity for this mechanism to occur spontaneously (Chapter 21).

Fetal positioning and descent

Assessment of the fetal position and the descent through the pelvis and birth canal in labour is made by undertaking abdominal palpation and vaginal examination (VE). When palpating the pregnant abdomen (Chapter 76) in labour, a midwife needs to specifically recognise and determine these dynamic factors; lie, presentation, denominator, position, attitude and engagement (Box 20.1).

Occasionally on VE with a longitudinal lie, an umbilical cord presentation is discovered; although this does not alter the mechanism of labour, the birth should be expedited. The pressure on the cervix and vaginal soft tissue from the denominator is fundamentally influential in the progress of labour (Box 20.2).

A left occipitoanterior (LOA) position of the fetal skull is regarded as the most likely to result in a normal birth. In this position the fetal skull is well flexed due to its relationship to the pelvic curves below the brim. Engagement is said to have occurred when the fetus has begun to descend. In a cephalic presentation this is when the biparietal diameter of the fetal skull enters the brim of the pelvis. On palpation this can be felt and documented as how many fifths of the head remain palpable above the brim or how many fifths are engaged; the midwife needs to be clear which measurement is being used.

It is very important to closely follow engagement in the pelvic brim as this means descent in the parturient woman and the overall progress of the labour and birth can be carefully monitored.

Progress through the mechanism

Abdominal palpation and VE enable a midwife to assess progress. With the onset of strong, regular contractions of labour (Chapter 21), further descent of the fetus through the pelvis takes place. When the cervix is fully dilated and the soft tissues in the birth canal become distended, further descent occurs during the transitional phase. Internal rotation of the fetal head occurs on the pelvic floor from a transverse position commonly to an occipitoanterior (OA) position. An occipitoposterior (face to pubes) position is also possible, although seen less frequently. A brow presentation is believed to have a diameter that is too great to pass through the diameters of the pelvis and be deliverable.

In the OA position as the head pivots under the pubic arch, the head becomes deflexed and the occiput emerges. By further extension of the fetal head, the face sweeps the perineum and the head is born beyond the maternal perineum. Internal rotation of the shoulders then occurs from a transverse to an anteroposterior position, demonstrated by and described as restitution.

Birth

In spontaneous unassisted birth, such as in water, at the next contraction the anterior shoulder can also be seen to pivot on the pubic arch, with the posterior shoulder spontaneously birthing. The body follows by continued lateral flexion, following the curve of carus within the pelvis, directing the baby naturally towards the arms and breasts of its mother (Box 20.3). Assistance of the birth of the shoulders is commonly seen where traction is applied to release the anterior shoulder from beneath the pubic arch of the pelvis.

Detecting deviations

Descent should be determined by palpation not just during a VE. This is paramount as moulding and caput may give the appearance at the introitus that the vertex is low in the birth canal; however the widest diameter of the presenting part may be obstructed within the bony structure. A common description of the internal presentation of descent is where the head relates to the pelvic ischial spines. Although these are generally undetectable, a skilled birth attendant gains experiential knowledge of whether the fetal head is above (high), at or below (low) the spines. A fetal head may adopt a synclitic position (asynclitism); this can only be detected on VE although it can resolve and allow delivery (Figure 20.1).

This underpinning knowledge and ability to recognise these determinants on palpation is a fundamental midwifery skill and core to monitoring progress in childbirth. It is important that midwives do not rely solely on cervical dilatation measurements. Any delay in the fetal journey should be quickly assessed, with timely medical intervention when appropriate; this may be a matter of life and death if medical assistance is far away.

21 Promoting normal labour

Figure 21.1 Requirements for normal childbirth.

Normal childbirth

Abnormal childbirth

Clinical intervention

Medical pathology

Grounded physiologically, psychologically & spiritually

Controlled physiological, psychological & spiritual needs

Figure 21.2 Midwives' role.

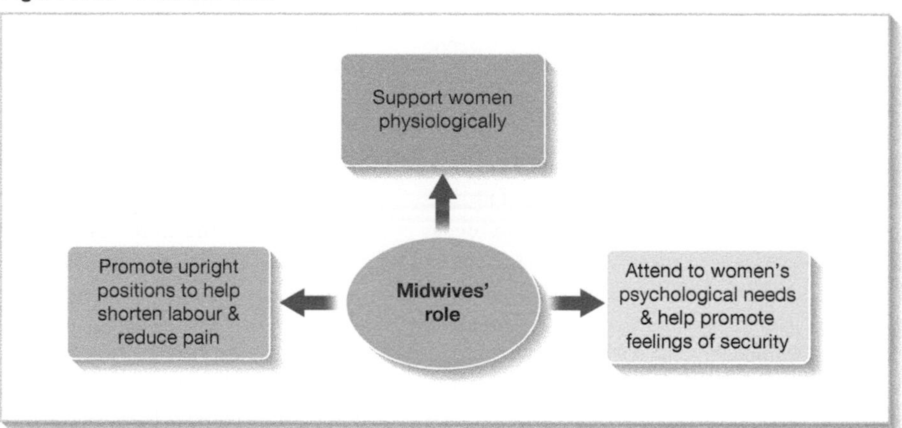

Figure 21.3 Surge of oxytocin and contractile forces.

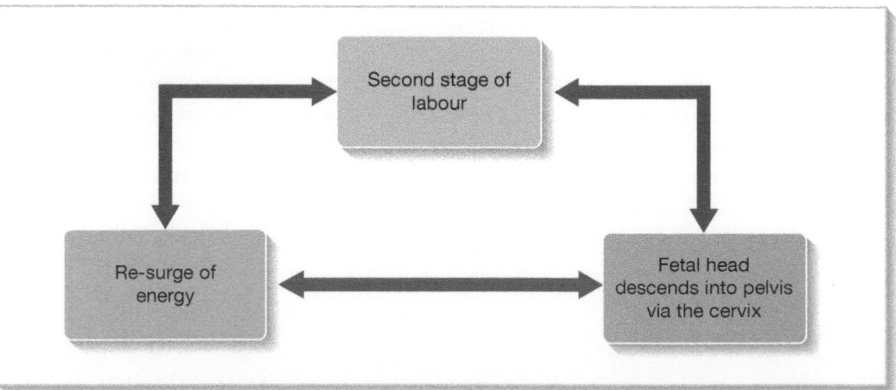

The onset of pregnancy is a normal physiological function of female reproduction and the majority of women will progress to have a normal labour and birth. It is generally agreed that normal childbirth is spontaneous in onset with the vertex presenting and occurring at term without any medical, pharmaceutical or surgical interventions.

The birth of a child is a profound event for a woman and her partner. Normal childbirth occurs when a woman gives birth with the labour physiologically, psychologically and spiritually grounded – as opposed to the labour being controlled by a prevailing medical pathology or by clinical intervention (Figure 21.1).

Physiology

In terms of the physiology of normal birth, the woman and fetus should be in optimum health, the fetus presenting in a vertex, favourable position and able to negotiate the maternal pelvis. The woman should have optimal hormonal responses at the onset of labour and her body responds and is suffused with oxytocin, enabling a contracting uterus and a dilating cervix (Chapter 19).

The Midwife's role

The midwife has a pivotal role in facilitating normality in childbirth – supporting women physiologically to maintain advantageous upright positions during labour to decrease the length of labour and to help women cope with painful contractions. Upright positions can increase the pelvic diameter during the birth of the baby and ease the passage through the birth canal. A supporting, caring midwife attends to the psychological needs of women, enabling them to feel safe in their environment and prepared for the demands of labour (Figure 21.2).

Stages

Traditionally, childbirth has been divided into three stages. The *first stage* comprises release of the operculum (show) and the onset of regular contractions. This facilitates a dilating cervix with membrane rupture as the fetal head descends into the pelvis. The cervix effaces, dilates and becomes continuous with the uterus and vagina. This physiological process results in the formation of a birth canal, a passage for the emerging baby. At this point the fetal head is able to move through the birth canal in preparation for the second stage of labour.

It is normal for women at this *transition stage* to feel overwhelmed by the huge waves of contractions and the pressure of the fetal head on the pelvic floor. This is characterised by women wanting to stop the process of birth and becoming fearful and floundering. Midwives are mindful of this transitional stage and encourage the woman by acknowledging her powerful feelings and informing her of the closeness to the birth of her baby – the onset of the second stage of labour.

The *second stage* of labour creates a surge of oxytocin (Figure 21.3) as the fetal head descends into the pelvis and through the cervix and a new energy emerges. The woman's diaphragm fixes and the increased uterine contractions generate an urge to push the baby through the birth canal – the fetal ejection reflex (Ferguson's reflex; Box 20.2). Birth occurs when the fetal head and shoulders traverse the pubic arch and the newborn emerges.

Oxytocin continues to increase as the baby is placed onto the mother's body and is stimulated by skin to skin contact. The distended uterus continues to contract, this time to expel the placenta and membranes. These strong uterine contractions create living ligatures as the muscle layers of the uterus close and tighten around the blood vessels at the placental site. The umbilical cord remains attached and is left to pulsate for up to 3 minutes before it is cut to ensure transfusion of blood to the baby together with important stem cells. The uterus continues to contract and decrease in size to ensure minimal loss of blood from the placental site. This normal process is unhurried and the placenta is expelled with maternal effort and gravity and without the use of any oxytocic drugs. The expulsion of the placenta, membranes and delayed cord cutting is called the physiological *third stage* of labour.

It should be noted that birth is a continuous process and dividing it into stages can create expectations of what should be 'normal' timeframes for each stage. The development of stages of labour is a construct to define the events of labour and should be, as mentioned, viewed with a critical eye to ensure that the natural, normal rhythms of labour and birth are undisturbed.

There has been recent recognition of a *fourth stage* of labour; this is the period when the woman and her newborn infant begin their exclusive bonding. It is a time when the woman's senses are enhanced as she smells her newborn infant, becomes aware of the softness of the baby's skin against her, gazes in wonder at her creation and commences breastfeeding. Oxytocin is at its peak and this facilitates initiation of a breastfeeding dyad and maternal–infant bonding. Extraneous noises or procedures can impact negatively on oxytocin production, therefore the midwife needs to be extremely sensitive to this period, remaining quiet and calm to enable breastfeeding and bonding.

The birth of a baby has a powerful physiological and psychological impact on a woman and her life will change irrevocably. Becoming a mother brings responsibility for the physical and psychological development of another human being. Pregnancy and labour are the beginning of a woman's journey to motherhood and a connectedness with eons of women's experiences. The woman's experience of childbirth will have an impact for life and the midwife needs to ensure that women are supported through the psychological transition of birth as well as the physiological action of birth with an emphasis on normality.

22 Pain relief

Table 22.1 Non-pharmacological methods of pain relief in labour.

Method	Advantages	Disadvantages
Acupuncture, acupressure, homeopathy, reflexology	• Accelerates physiological functions of the body (such as labour) • Reduces pain • Reduces anxiety • Stimulates endorphins and oxytocin • High maternal satisfaction	• Almost exclusively seen only in out-of-hospital settings • Requires an independent/private practitioner to instruct on the usage and/or be available to provide treatment in labour
Aromatherapy	• Promotes relaxation • Reduces pain • Reduces anxiety • May lower blood pressure • Regulation of contractions/accelerate labour • Reduce nausea and vomiting • Stimulates endorphins and oxytocin • Low cost and easy to train midwives in usage • High maternal satisfaction	• Use with caution in women with asthma/other allergies or sensitivities • Not recommended for use with some obstetric conditions • Contraindicated in preterm labours • Some aromatherapy oils may not be used in conjunction with other complementary therapies • Requires a midwife or private practitioner to be available to prescribe and provide treatment
Deep relaxation techniques/ hypnosis	• Promotes relaxation • Reduces fear and anxiety • Reduces pain • Stimulates endorphins and oxytocin • Low cost and easy to train midwives to teach as part of antenatal education • High maternal satisfaction	• Requires techniques to be learnt and practised by the woman and her birthing partner if to be successful • Requires a level of knowledge and understanding of the professionals caring for the woman in labour to maximise success

Table 22.2 Pharmacological methods of pain relief in labour.

Method	Advantages	Disadvantages
Entonox® (inhaled nitrous oxide and oxygen)	• As it is patient controlled, it may be used at any time in labour and the woman retains control • Safe and quick acting, does not pass through the placenta • Can easily be transported to any area of maternity including home births (via a cylinder) • Does not affect the length or progress of labour • Requires very little instruction on how it is to be used • May be used in conjunction with other non-pharmacological and pharmacological methods of pain relief	• Associated side effects should be discussed with the woman prior to administration, which may include: • Nausea and vomiting • Dizziness • Drowsiness • Ineffective if used incorrectly (timing with contractions is important as the relief is short lasting)
Opioid injection (pethidine/ diamorphine)	• May reduce anxiety • May induce sleep/very relaxed state • It may be prescribed in early labour or during labour and more than one dose may be given (typically 2–4 hours apart) • In normal circumstances a midwife may prescribe opioid injections for labour, making it easily accessible and available to all women • No additional resources or monitoring is required • May be used in conjunction with other pharmacological methods of pain relief	• Pain relief may be limited with opioid injections • Low maternal satisfaction • A woman would need to be admitted into a birthing unit or hospital in order to have it administered • Associated side effects should be discussed with the woman prior to administration, which may include: • Nausea and vomiting • Drowsiness • Effects of opioids on the fetus as it passes through the placenta (drowsy, sleepy, respiratory depression at birth, poor feeding) • Caution with women with allergies/sensitivities

The prevention and control of pain in labour is a major concern for women and professionals alike. This may be deemed as the physical elimination of labour pain or the prevention of suffering, increased satisfaction and empowerment with a primary goal of a positive experience, even when there is pain. The pain a woman experiences during labour may vary enormously; there are many physiological, psychological and psychosocial dimensions to what a woman feels and how she interprets it. The labour experience has many complex behavioural and cultural components, providing a highly personal and unique experience for the individual woman. Certain forms of pain relief may have different effects on one woman to another and her choices are personal based on beliefs, culture, religion, education and experience.

Non-pharmacological methods

Non-pharmacological approaches to pain in labour include a wide variety of techniques designed to target physical sensations of pain and psychoemotional and spiritual components of care through prevention of suffering. Pain is viewed as a normal part of the process, rather than as a sign of abnormality, injury or distress. The focus is on supporting the woman, building self-confidence and enhancing personal coping strategies. This midwifery model of care promotes satisfaction and overall wellbeing; the woman is actively involved in her pain management.

Changing position and remaining active may increase women's feelings of comfort and control as well as assisting the physiological process of labour. Upright, kneeling and squatting positions with the woman leaning forwards increase the transverse and anterior–posterior diameter of the pelvic outlet, creating more space and movement for the fetus to descend. By adopting a wide range of positions and remaining active and mobile in labour, a woman may prevent pain that is associated with prolonged labours and fetal malpositions.

Touch and massage may be used to promote relaxation and comfort in labour. Human touch by a birthing partner, professional supporter (doula) or midwife in labour can create a feeling of being cared for and reassurance that she is supported and loved. Expressions of anxiety (increase in blood pressure and heart rate) may reduce with touch and massage techniques and a woman may feel a decrease in pain in response to reduced anxiety. Additional non-pharmacological therapies are given in Table 22.1.

Hydrotherapy may be used during labour (water immersion) but must be deep enough to cover the woman's abdomen to reduce labour pain and promote labour progression. Water immersion may promote relaxation, aid mobility as the water increases buoyancy and enhance feelings of control and satisfaction. Optimum timing of pool entry may accelerate labour, whereas if used in early labour, contractions may decrease in strength and intensity causing labour to slow or stall. Consideration should be given to maintaining an optimum water temperature (36–37°C), availability to women in the local area and having robust procedures in place (training of all professionals involved in the safe evacuation of a woman in the pool in an emergency). There are very few absolute contraindications to the use of water immersion in labour; therefore this should be a viable option for most labouring women.

Transcutaneous electrical nerve stimulation (TENS) is the transmission of low-voltage electrical impulses from a handheld, battery-powered generator to the skin via surface electrodes. Specific TENS units, convenient for a labouring woman's use, are available to rent or buy and may provide a safe and effective method of reducing labour pain. Pain signals are interrupted by the electrical impulses sent out by the TENS machine before they reach the spinal cord and brain. The body's natural painkillers-endorphins may also be stimulated whilst using a TENS machine, which has traditionally been used for chronic back pain, neck pain, sports injuries and arthritis.

Non-pharmacological methods of pain relief in labour may be popular with women and especially useful in settings where resources are low. Cost is often minimal and although there is overall a lack of high-quality evidence regarding their use and effectiveness, interventions are viewed as being safe and maternal satisfaction high.

Pharmacological methods

Regional anaesthesia, such as epidurals, spinals or a combination of the two, has been shown to be the most effective form of pharmacological pain relief in labour. An epidural is when high concentrations of local anaesthetic drugs or a combination of low-dose anaesthetic and opioid drugs are inserted via a fine catheter into the epidural space around the spinal column. A spinal is analgesic drugs being inserted directly into the fluid surrounding the nerves in the spinal column. Traditionally, when higher doses of anaesthetic drugs have been used, side effects have been more severe, including; leg weakness and numbness, hypotension, fetal heart rate anomalies and poor mobility or inability to change positions with a subsequent impact on the woman giving birth (longer first and second stages of labour, increased instrumental deliveries, increased perineal trauma due to higher levels of intervention and subsequent pain, bruising and problems with incontinence). More recently, opioids are used in conjunction with lower levels of anaesthetic drugs but this has an impact on the fetus as opioids pass through the placenta.

Regional anaesthesia is complex and there are many other potential, rare but potentially life limiting or threatening, side effects. All regional anaesthesia must be administered by an anaesthetist; the availability of which must be explained to all women requesting this form of pain relief, and the woman given the opportunity to make an informed decision based on a consultation with the anaesthetic team. Regional anaesthesia does not always work and may need to be re-sited or it may not work very quickly or provide adequate pain relief. Continuous electronic fetal monitoring will also be advisable in order to monitor the fetal heart rate and record timings of contractions. Table 22.2 lists further pharmacological methods of pain relief in labour.

23 Water birth

Figure 23.1 Typical birth pool.

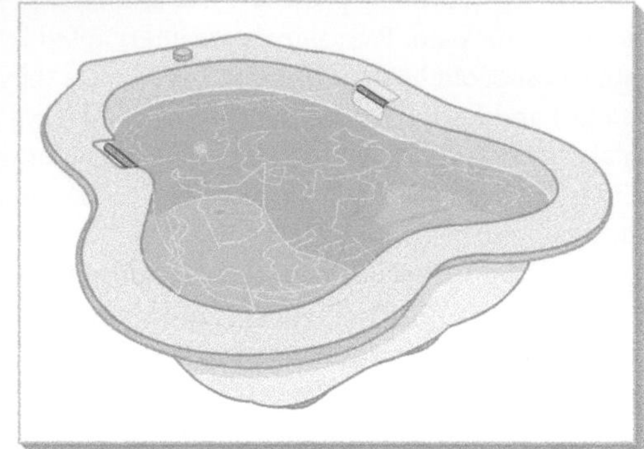

Figure 23.2 Care in labour.

1st stage

- Someone always with woman
- Hourly check of water temp (33–37°C)
- Hourly maternal temp check
- Standard labour care for women

- Vaginal examination can be carried out in the water
- Avoid dehydration – woman to drink 500–1000 ml fluid/hou (+ midwife)
- Urine voiding standing in a container or out to toilet

2nd stage

- Water temp 36–37°C; checks every 15 minutes
- Physiological pushing; bottom under water
- Presence of second midwife
- Hands 'off' approach

- Do not feel for the cord
- Baby born completely under the water
- Once head emerged, not to be submerged again
- Keep baby's body under water
- No clamping or cutting cord under water

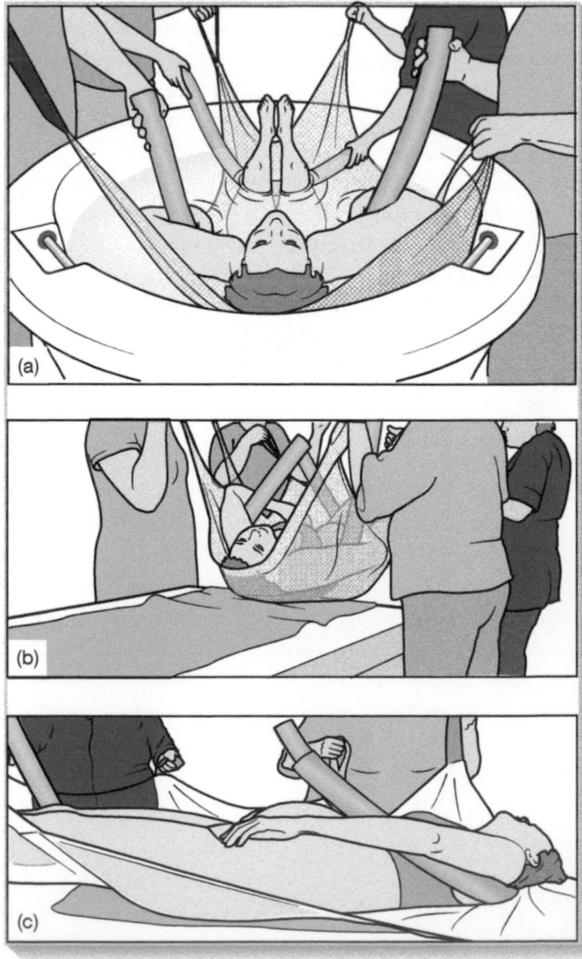

Figure 23.3 Evacuation procedures and equipment.

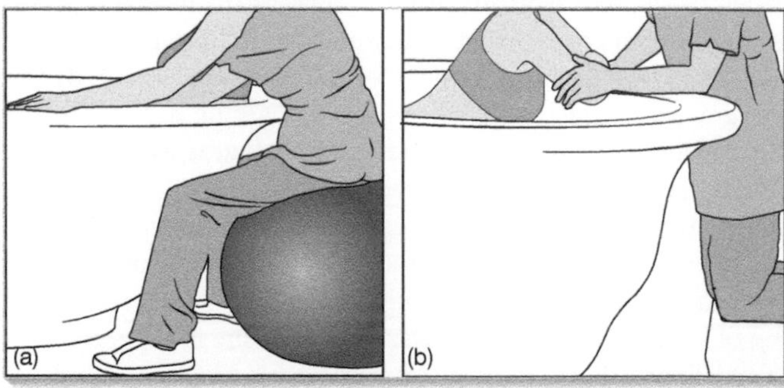

Figure 23.4 Support positions for mother & midwife/birth partner.

Box 23.1 Benefits of water for labour and birth.

- Promotes physiology of labour
- Lowers anxiety as contractions less painful
- Reduces the need for pharmacological analgesia
- Greater satisfaction for mother and midwife – one-to-one care, autonomy and supportive of physiological birth
- Shorter first stage of labour
- Reduced intervention contributes to more positive postnatal mental health
- Fewer instrumental deliveries and operative births, fewer third degree tears

Box 23.2 Equipment required.

- Bath and room thermometer
- Gauntlet gloves
- Portable underwater Doppler for fetal heart monitoring
- Disposable sieve
- Mirror
- Light source
- Evacuation equipment

Midwifery at a Glance, First Edition. Edited by Eleanor Forrest © 2019 John Wiley & Sons, Ltd. Published 2019 by John Wiley & Sons, Ltd.
Companion website: www.wiley.com/go/forrest/midwifery

Box 23.3 Exclusion criteria.

- Small for gestational age
- Fetal abnormalities
- <37 weeks or >42 weeks
- Multiple births
- Spontaneous rupture of membranes >24 hours
- Meconium-stained liquor
- Fetal distress
- Raised BP or temperature
- Earlier use of narcotic sedation (within 2 hours or if still drowsy)

Box 23.4 Situations requiring woman to leave the pool.

- Maternal request
- Concern regarding routine maternal or fetal observations
- Artificial rupture of membranes – can then return to pool
- Fresh thick meconium
- Failure to progress
- Water heavily soiled
- During 2nd stage if large baby suspected
- Mother experiencing excessive fear or loss of control
- Need for pharmacological pain relief (excluding Entonox®)

The use of water in labour and birth in home or hospital environments provides buoyancy and freedom of movement in labour that can support relaxation, pain relief and facilitates labour physiology and optimal positioning for birth within a midwifery model of care. Purpose-built pools can be used (Figure 23.1) or inflatable pools are suitable for home birth. As a result women may experience less need for pharmacological analgesia and be more likely to achieve a normal birth. All women in the antenatal period should be provided with information that enables an informed decision to be made on the use of water for labour and birth. This allows them to consider the benefits (Box 23.1) and possible disadvantages, although evidence on water birth lacks rigorous, transferable, good-quality data. Despite this, water births can empower women to feel in control of their birth experience and facilitate a 'better birth' with reduced use of epidural/spinal analgesia.

Immersion in water can be utilised in each phase of labour, if all observations remain within normal limits, with additional points of care (Figure 23.2) and with appropriate risk assessment and appropriate equipment available (Box 23.2). There is no evidence to suggest that women should only enter the pool once labour is established or that women should leave the pool at frequent intervals. However, women do require adequate hydration and regular observation to ensure they do not become pyrexial.

Water birth has typically been the domain of healthy women with uncomplicated pregnancies, with practice protocols frequently stating exclusion criteria (Box 23.3). However, given the benefits of buoyancy, vasodilatation and relaxation, labouring in water may be beneficial to women with a raised BMI, hypertension and previous lower segment caesarean section (LSCS). One-to-one care with a trusted midwife during water birth enables mothers to understand when pool evacuation may be required (Box 23.4).

The baby, birth and third stage

Neonatal wellbeing is not adversely affected by immersion in water, however care must be taken to ensure that the woman does not rise out of the water and then immerse herself again in the late second stage as this could initiate neonatal respiration. The baby should be born underwater and gradually brought to the surface. A nuchal cord can be slipped over the baby's head if required and care taken to avoid cord traction that could lead to rupture. Once the baby's head reaches the surface of the water it must remain above the water level and skin-to-skin care and early breastfeeding initiated as desired. Whilst some women may choose to leave the pool for the third stage due to blood loss into the water, a physiological third stage of labour can be offered to women. Estimation of blood loss may be more difficult as it is diluted in the water.

The midwife's role

Generally, women choosing to labour and birth in water require less intervention, giving midwives an opportunity to practice autonomously. Having confidence and belief in the physiology of labour and women's ability to give birth naturally will enhance the experience and help facilitate the process of birthing in water. Midwives can be further encouraged to facilitate women to labour and give birth in water through training, including pool evacuation techniques (Figure 23.3), the provision of practice-based protocols, appropriate equipment and clinical governance procedures. Midwives also need to be aware of local protocols for the separate uses of water for labour and birth, such as analgesia in the first stage of labour and birthing in water.

Additional observations are required to monitor the depth and temperature of the water which should be level with the woman's breasts when she is sitting and not exceed 37.5°C. Water and maternal temperature should be recorded hourly. Although there is often less intervention in water birth, attention to water cleanliness therefore becomes a key priority in maintaining asepsis. A sieve can remove most debris, but the woman may have to leave the pool temporarily to decontaminate it following a vomit, for example.

Adequate provision for a clean water supply and adherence to infection control procedures, including cleaning the pool after use, must be made. Chlorine-based solutions are often used but local policy should be adhered to; all cleaning solutions should be effective against hepatitis B and C and HIV infections.

Midwives and partners should be mindful of health and safety issues related to water and when supporting women in the pool to adopt positions compatible with moving and handling requirements (Figure 23.4). Assistance will be required in an emergency to help the woman out of the pool quickly. Management should be commenced immediately; therefore midwives should be proficient in dealing with such situations.

As women's experiences of water births are generally positive in terms of feeling relaxed, involved in decision making and being in control, midwives have a responsibility to be able to support women as required.

24 Augmentation of labour

Box 24.1 Oxytocin.

- Synthesised in hypothalamus
- Transported to posterior pituitary gland
- Released & acts on smooth muscle
- Increased oxytocin receptors in myometrium

Box 24.2 Considerations for labour progress.

- Parity
- Descent and rotation of the fetal head
- Changes in the strength, duration and frequency of uterine contractions
- Cervical dilatation and rate of change
- Station and position of presenting part
- The woman's emotional state
- Referral to the appropriate healthcare professional

Box 24.3 Note about the definition of delay.

It has been traditional practice to define delay largely by the rate of cervical progress without taking into account either maternal uterine activity or descent or rotation of the fetal head during labour

Figure 24.1 Phases of labour.

Latent phase
• Cervix dilates to 3 cm
• Cervix shortens & softens
• Cervix adopts a central position
Active phase
• Cervix dilates to 10 cm
• Rotation & descent of the fetal head

Figure 24.2 Midwives' role.

Encouragement
Support
Observation
Reassurance
Effective communication
Respect woman's decisions

Midwifery at a Glance, First Edition. Edited by Eleanor Forrest © 2019 John Wiley & Sons, Ltd. Published 2019 by John Wiley & Sons, Ltd.
Companion website: www.wiley.com/go/forrest/midwifery

Augmentation is an intervention to correct slow progress in labour. This process to enhance the progress of labour is facilitated by the administration of an intravenous infusion of oxytocin (Box 24.1). However, amniotomy or artificial rupture of membranes (ARM) may also be performed if the membranes are still intact.

As discussed Chapter 19, labour is considered in two phases; the latent phase and active phase (Figure 24.1). The latent phase can last 8–10 hours, and the cervix:

- Dilates to 3 cm
- Becomes shorter and softer (3 to < 0.5 cm)
- Adopts a central position.

The active phase is of shorter duration:

- The cervix dilates from 3–10 cm
- Rotation and descent of head occurs.

The active phase of labour is contentious because the expectation is that once labour has been diagnosed, progress is based mainly on a cervical dilatation of 1 cm per hour. However, there have been suggestions in the literature that 0.3–0.5 cm per hour might be more realistic and reflect the appropriate progress of normal labour.

Definition of delay

The definition of delay of labour differs depending on whether the woman is nulliparous or parous.

- In a nulliparous woman, delay can be defined when the cervix dilates < 2 cm in 4 hours
- In a parous woman, delay can be defined when the cervix dilates < 2 cm in 4 hours or there is a slowing in progress.

Although it is acknowledged that the duration of labour is dependent on parity, clinical practice and local guidelines regarding labour rarely make that distinction. A diagnosis of delay in the established first phase of labour must take into consideration all aspects of progress in labour (Boxes 24.2 and 24.3).

Suspected delay

Membranes intact

- Consider amniotomy
- Vaginal examination every 2 hours.

Membranes ruptured

- Vaginal examination every 2 hours
- If progress < 1 cm dilatation:
  - Diagnose delay
  - Support
  - Effective pain relief
  - Offer external fetal monitoring (EFM)
  - Vaginal examination every 2 hours.

Following membrane rupture

Once amniotomy has been performed, the midwife must consider the following.

Nulliparous

- Consider oxytocin
- Advise continuous EFM
- Vaginal examination 4 hours after oxytocin in established labour
- If progressing > 2 cm per hour, conduct vaginal examination 4 hourly.

Parous

- Abdominal palpation
- Consider oxytocin
- Advise continuous EFM
- Vaginal examination; if progressing < 2 cm per hour, consider caesarean section.

The midwife's role in prolonged labour

When labour has become prolonged or progress is slow, a woman can experience increased levels of stress, anxiety and fatigue. As such, the midwife has an important role in providing support, reassurance and encouragement to ensure that the woman's labour is a positive experience. To achieve this, the midwife must communicate effectively with the woman and her family whilst also observing her physical and emotional health and wellbeing to prevent complications.

The midwife needs to provide explanations and involve the woman in the decision-making process in order that she can fulfil her personal expectations. The midwife is required to provide care that is evidence based and woman centred to ensure that the woman's values and beliefs are considered. This will encourage flexibility when considering options for care, especially when labour has become prolonged. The midwife should respect a woman's opinion regarding her wish to decline interventions such as amniotomy or intravenous infusion of oxytocin to enhance her labour progress.

Prolonged labour increases the risk of infection, haemorrhage and the subsequent need for an emergency caesarean section to be performed. Midwives are therefore required to ensure accurate observation of maternal wellbeing and provide advice on suitable food and drink (Chapter 26), positions and any additional support (Figure 24.2).

25 Induction of labour

Figure 25.1 Possible consequences of induction of labour.

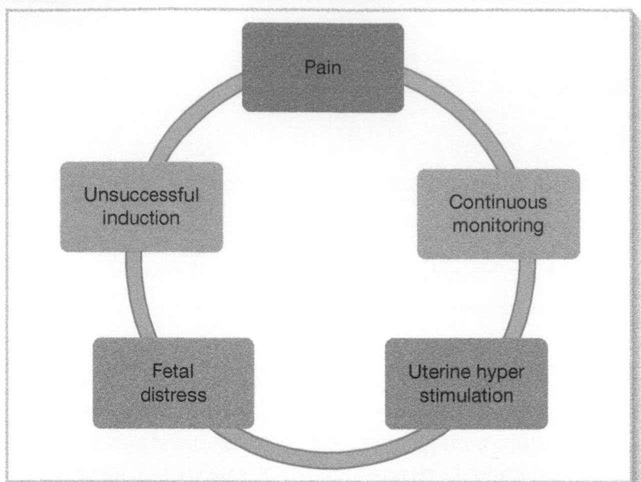

Figure 25.2 Membrane sweep.

Membrane sweep

40- & 41-week antenatal visits – nulliparous women should be offered a vaginal examination to sweep membranes

41-week antenatal visits – parous women should be offered a vaginal examination to sweep membranes

When a vaginal examination is carried out to assess the cervix – woman should be offered membranes sweep

Additional membrane sweep can be offered if no spontaneous onset of labour

Box 25.1 Contraindications to induction of labour.

- Parity
- Descent and rotation of the fetal head
- Changes in the strength, duration and frequency of uterine contractions
- Cervical dilatation and rate of change
- Station and position of presenting part
- The woman's emotional state
- Referral to the appropriate healthcare professional

Box 25.2 Non-pharmacological methods.

CAUTION

Women should be informed that the available evidence does not support the following methods for induction of labour:

- Herbal supplements
- Acupuncture
- Homeopathy
- Castor oil
- Hot baths
- Enemas
- Sexual intercourse
- Acupuncture

Box 25.3 Criteria for induction of labour.

- Lie – longitudinal
- Presentation – cephalic
- Placenta – normally situated
- Pelvis – Adequate
- Umbilical cord – not palpable on vaginal examination
- Bishop score ≥ 8
- Station – at least 0–3
- Cervix – favourable

Table 25.1 Bishop score.

	0	1	2	3
Dilatation	0	1–2	3–4	≥5
Length effacement	>2 0–30%	2–1 40–50%	1–0.5 60–70%	<0.5 >80%
Consistency	Firm	Medium	Soft	Soft/none
Position (cervix)	Posterior	Mid cavity	Anterior	Anterior/none
Station	−3	−2	−1/0	+1/+2
'Very ripe' or 'favourable' cervix: ≥ 8				

Induction of labour is an intervention to stimulate uterine contractions before the onset of spontaneous labour. It is a term used from 24 weeks of pregnancy.

Induction of the birth process must follow the woman's individual needs and preferences and include informed consent by the woman. Women who are being offered this procedure should have the opportunity to make informed decisions about their care and treatment, in partnership with their healthcare professionals. Midwives have an important role to ensure that women are fully informed of the reasons why induction is being offered. An explanation should be provided regarding how and where induction will take place, the provision of pain relief and the possible consequences and contraindications of this procedure (Figure 25.1 and Box 25.1). Before induction of labour is carried out, a Bishop score should be assessed and recorded and a normal fetal heart rate pattern should be confirmed using electronic fetal monitoring.

Reasons for induction of labour

Compromised maternal condition

- Prolonged pregnancy
- Pregnancy-induced hypertension and pre-eclampsia
- Medical conditions such as diabetes, cardiac disease and renal disease
- Maternal request.

Compromised fetal condition

- Pre-labour rupture of membranes at term (PROM)
- Preterm pre-labour rupture of membranes (PPROM)
- Twin or multiple pregnancy
- Fetal growth restriction/intrauterine growth restriction (IUGR)
- Fetal anomaly.

Methods of induction of labour

Membrane sweep

A membrane sweep is considered an adjunct to induction of labour and should be offered and conducted after 40 weeks of pregnancy. This involves a vaginal examination whereby the examining finger is passed through the cervix to rotate against the wall of the uterus in order that the chorionic membrane is separated from the decidua. If a finger cannot be inserted into the cervix, a similar effect can be elicited by massage of the vaginal fornices, around the cervix (Figure 25.2).

Pharmacological methods

Insertion of a vaginal prostaglandin E_2 (PGE_2) tablet, gel or a controlled-release pessary is commonly used for induction of labour. PGE_2 is a naturally occurring female hormone that helps to ripen the cervix. Recommendations are:

- One cycle of vaginal PGE_2 tablets or gel; one dose, followed by a second dose after 6 hours if labour is not established (up to a maximum of two doses)
- One cycle of vaginal PGE_2 controlled-release pessary; one dose over 24 hours.

Intravenous syntocinon is also commonly used to induce or augment labour; this is a synthetic version of the hormone oxytocin, which is naturally-occurring. The posterior pituitary gland releases oxytocin towards the end of pregnancy and causes the smooth muscle of the uterus to contract. Administer as per local guidelines and protocol. Contraindications for the use of syntocinon generally are:

- Pathological fetal heart rate (FHR) tracing
- Obstructed labour
- Hypertonic uterine contractions.

Non-pharmacological methods

Women should be informed that the available evidence does not support certain non-pharmacological methods for induction of labour (Box 25.2).

Surgical methods

It is not recommended that amniotomy be used as a primary method of induction of labour unless there are specific clinical reasons for not using vaginal PGE_2, in particular the risks of uterine hyperstimulation. Refer to Chapter 78 for more information.

Criteria for induction of labour

Criteria for the induction of labour are listed in Box 25.3, but consideration needs to be given to the Bishop score.

Bishop score

The Bishop score is the rating system used to assess suitability of the cervix for induction of labour and is made by doing a vaginal examination. The score is based on the dilatation, effacement (or length), consistency, position of the cervix and station. A score of 8 or more generally indicates that the cervix is ripe or 'favourable', indicating that there is a high chance of spontaneous labour or a positive response to induction interventions (Table 25.1). Reassess the Bishop score to monitor progress 6 hours after the insertion of a vaginal PGE_2 tablet or gel, or 24 hours after the insertion of a vaginal PGE_2 controlled-release pessary.

- **Dilatation** – occurs with effacement and is a measure of the diameter of the stretched cervix. This is an important indicator of progression through the first phase of labour
- **Effacement**– as the cervix becomes stretched it thins. Individual variation affects effacement
- **Consistency** – the cervix in primigravid and younger women is more resistant to stretching. Subsequent vaginal births soften the cervix and allows for easier dilatation at term
- **Position** – The position of the cervix varies between women. The anatomical location of the vagina faces downwards; anterior and posterior locations relatively describe the upper and lower borders of the vagina. As an anterior position is better aligned with the uterus, there is an increased opportunity of spontaneous birth
- **Station** – this is the position of the fetal head in relation to the distance from the ischial spines. Negative numbers indicate that the head is further inside, above the ischial spines.

26 Nutrition in labour

Figure 26.1 Energy metabolism.

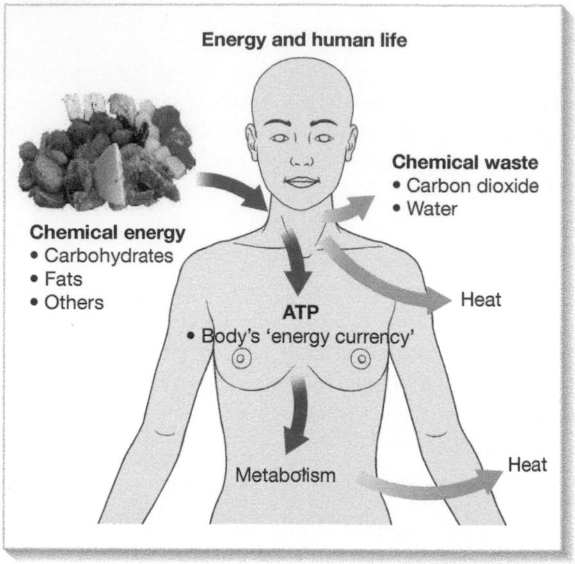

Energy and human life
Chemical waste
• Carbon dioxide
• Water
Chemical energy
• Carbohydrates
• Fats
• Others
ATP
• Body's 'energy currency'
Heat
Metabolism
Heat

Figure 26.3 Intravenous infusion risks.

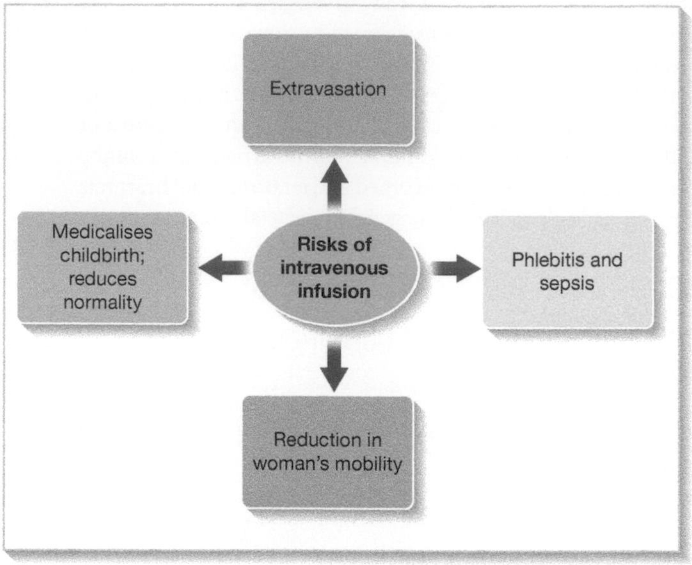

Extravasation
Medicalises childbirth; reduces normality
Risks of intravenous infusion
Phlebitis and sepsis
Reduction in woman's mobility

Figure 26.2 Maslow's hierarchy of needs.

morality, creativity, spontaneity, problem solving, lack of prejudice, acceptance of facts
Self-actualisation
self-esteem, confidence, achievement, respect of others, respect by others
Esteem
friendship, family, sexual intimacy
Love/belonging
security of body, of employment, of resources of morality, of the family, of health, of property
Safety
breathing, food, water, sex, sleep, homeostasis, excretion
Physiological

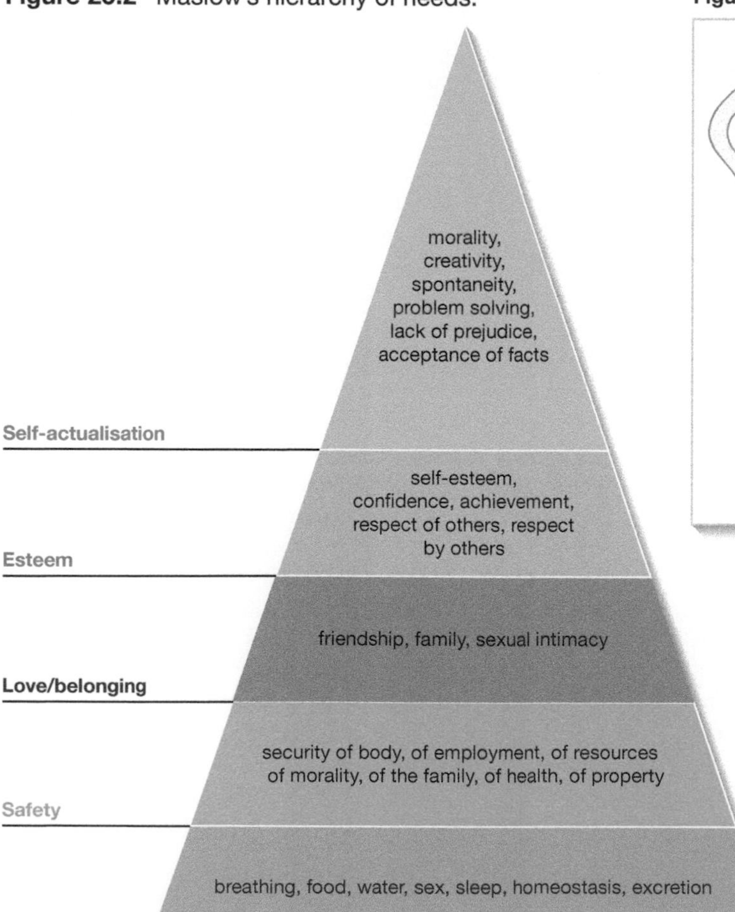

Figure 26.4 Appropriate foods in labour.

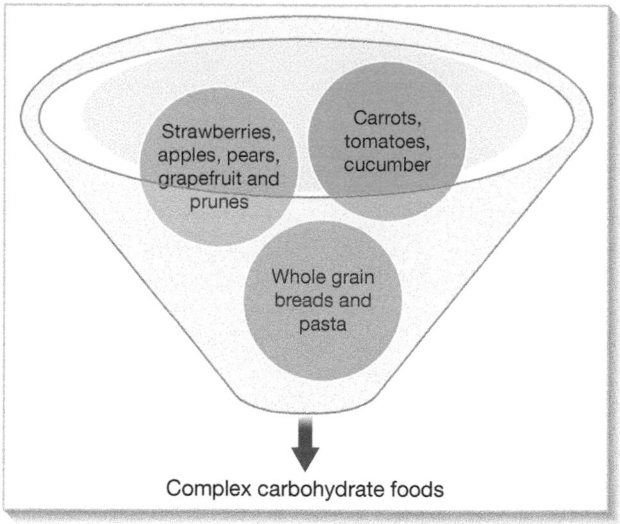

Strawberries, apples, pears, grapefruit and prunes
Carrots, tomatoes, cucumber
Whole grain breads and pasta
Complex carbohydrate foods

Midwifery at a Glance, First Edition. Edited by Eleanor Forrest © 2019 John Wiley & Sons Ltd. Published 2019 by John Wiley & Sons Ltd.
Companion website: www.wiley.com/go/forrest/midwifery

Nutrition is recognised as the food needed in response to dietary requirements; the more energy being utilised, the more kilocalories are needed. The kilocalories required in labour are vast, enabling the body to respond to the increased energy requirements due to uterine contractions and a corresponding increase in cardiac output due to maternal effort. Energy requirements in active labour are estimated to be 700 to 1100 kilocalories/hour.

Physiologically, gastric tone and motility decreases in pregnancy and labour leading to a mild delay in gastric emptying, especially following food being eaten. Other factors that influence gastric emptying are fear and pain, use of opioid medication and high fibre and high fat foods. When a woman has an opioid analgesia, consideration should be made regarding dietary intake as the opioid will reduce gastric absorption of nutrients from the diet.

Lack of nutrition

If insufficient glucose is available then body fat will be broken down in order to provide glucose (gluconeogenesis), with a subsequent development of ketosis and potentially ketoacidosis (Figure 26.1). Ketones are recognised as an indicator of metabolic imbalance; however the significance of this in labour has been undetermined. It has been suggested that the presence of ketonuria could lead to a longer labour and a possible ensuing intervention, although this has not yet been supported by research. However, it has been established that there is a negative psychological impact when there is a restriction of food and fluids. Food is a provider of nutrition, and oral intake is a form of comfort and control for women in labour. Maslow's hierarchy of needs recognised physiological factors, including air, food and drink, as basic needs and unless these are fulfilled then a person is unable to move up to the higher level growth needs (Figure 26.2).

Emesis

Restriction of eating in labour has been present in a variety of forms within UK maternity unit policies, based on the belief that eating and drinking in labour can increase the likelihood of regurgitation, leading to aspiration if a general anaesthesia is required. In 1946, Mendelson published a paper concerning the risks of gastric aspiration when an anaesthetic is required during an obstetric procedure. This resulted in both policy and practice changes, where food and fluids were restricted in labour for women deemed high risk. There were subsequent knock-on effects when the line between high- and low-risk labour became blurred. Anaesthetic procedures have advanced over time and, alongside this, the use of regional anaesthesia where possible is favoured and therefore has resulted in a decline in use of general anaesthesia within obstetrics.

There is no evidence to suggest that with increased volumes of oral intake in labour there is a correlating increase in emesis. Within the literature, women who have suffered from emesis in labour did not necessarily consider this to be an adverse experience.

Fluid replacement

If oral intake is restricted in labour there is the potential for dehydration to occur, affecting the body's fluid balance. Where the body is working hard in labour, the woman's respiratory rate increases and her basal metabolic rate increases, and if this is not compensated by adequate hydration then she will become dehydrated. One of the signs of dehydration is thirst, although it is important to recognise that a woman's thirst might be quenched prior to sufficient fluids being consumed so other signs of dehydration, such as oliguria, should be considered.

Intravenous therapy has been used as an alternative to oral fluids as a method of hydration and as a means of treating ketonuria. This has potential coexisting iatrogenic risks such as extravasation, phlebitis and sepsis. An intravenous infusion has an impact on a woman's mobility, positions in labour and her belief that labour is a normal life event, not a medical illness (Figure 26.3).

Where food is restricted and a woman is experiencing a labour where general anaesthesia is a potential risk, oral antacids and H_2 blockers can be used. These reduce the amount of acid produced by the stomach lining cells, thereby reducing the damaging effects of high gastric acid levels (Chapter 89).

Food to eat in labour

The literature advises that women can eat a light diet in labour but does not identify the components of such a diet. In order to meet the energy requirements of labour, a woman needs to eat food that is rich in complex carbohydrates which will support and replenish glycogen storage and withstand concentrated muscle activity (uterine contractions).

Foods that incorporate complex carbohydrates include vegetables and fruit such as carrots, tomatoes, cucumber, strawberries, apples, pears, grapefruit and prunes. This list is not exhaustive; these could be eaten raw, as finger foods, rather than as main meals. Breads and pasta made with whole grains also offer the benefits of 'glycogen loading' and in pregnancy these could be used to prepare for labour, ensuring the woman has sufficient nutritional resilience (Figure 26.4).

With the majority of births in the UK taking place in hospital, it is important that women are informed of the foods that would be nutritionally beneficial for them to eat in labour. Maternity services need to be responsive to the needs of women and supply an appropriate nutritional diet across the 24-hour period required on the labour ward.

Giving women information about risks and benefits enables them to make decisions and when, what and if they want to eat and drink; supporting them in having choice and control and maintaining their autonomy. Further research into the most effective diet and fluid regimes for women in labour is required.

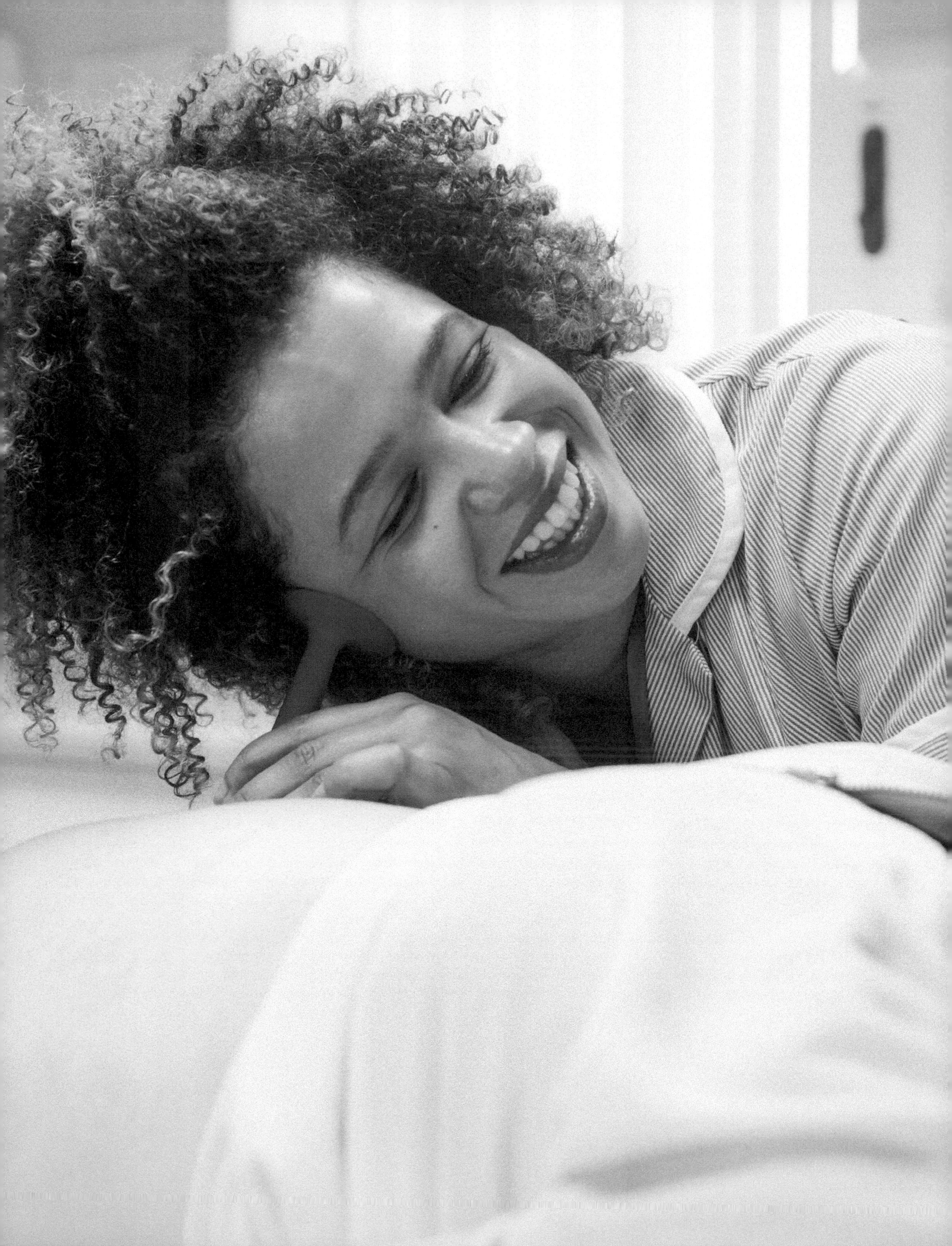

Postnatal care

Chapters

27 Immediate care: 0–6 hours

Figure 27.1 Postnatal recovery process.

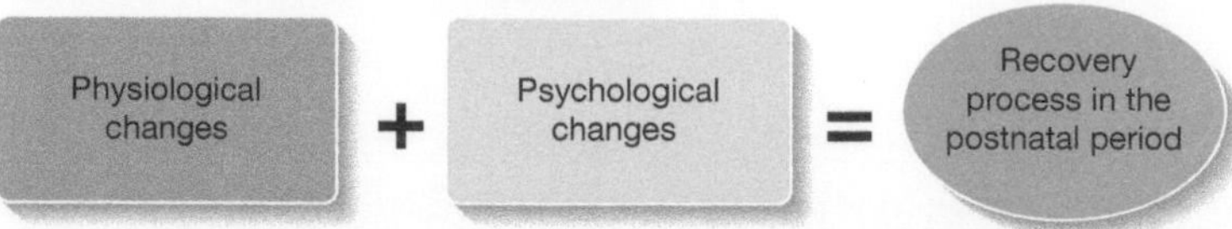

Table 27.1 Potential postnatal life-threatening conditions.

Action	Clinical signs	Condition
Emergency	• Fever, shivering, abdominal pain • Offensive vaginal loss • Repeat temperature in 4–6 hours if exceeds 38°C • If temperature still high or other signs & symptoms: evaluate further	Sepsis: genital tract infection
Emergency	Sudden or heavy blood loss; signs & symptoms of shock: hypotension, tachycardia, change in conscious level	Postpartum haemorrhage
Emergency	Chest pain; shortness of breath	Pulmonary embolism
Emergency	Calf pain in 1 leg; red or swollen	Deep vein thrombosis
Emergency	• Severe/on-going headache • Diastolic BP higher than 90 mmHg: with other sign of pre-eclampsia • Diastolic BP higher than 90 mmHg: no other sign of pre-eclampsia: repeat BP within 4 hours • Evaluate if diastolic BP remains higher than 90 mmHg after 4 hours	Pre-eclampsia or eclampsia
Urgent	• Tender abdomen • Offensive vaginal discharge • Excessive vaginal loss • Fever • Consider other causes if no obstetric cause found	Postpartum haemorrhage Sepsis Other causes

The postnatal period incorporates the time immediately following the end of labour until at least 10 days postnatal or longer, as deemed necessary by a midwife. This chapter will focus on the midwifery care of women in the first 6 hours following normal vaginal birth. Although most women will give birth in hospital, many will have a home birth. This should not alter the immediate care given to women and the principle of assessing individual need is applicable wherever the birth took place. Local and national guidelines must be considered to ensure basic care such as postnatal observations, and education regarding hygiene after birth is carried out according to best evidence. The purpose of conducting postnatal observations and examination is to risk assess for problems, detect problems early and to enable prompt, appropriate actions and to refer if problems arise. Immediate care of women following birth should take into consideration any relevant factors from the antenatal period, including any plans for the postnatal period and the co-ordinating healthcare professional for the woman, identified. It is important to ask how the woman feels as her response can be used as a guide to aid assessment of her physical wellbeing and can link into assessment of her psychological wellbeing (Chapter 65). Women should be informed of the recovery process after birth (Figure 27.1) and the signs and symptoms of life-threatening conditions (Table 27.1).

Recording of vital signs

Monitoring of vital signs provides an indication of the woman's wellbeing and an opportunity to observe skin colour, pallor and respiratory rate and to ascertain if in pain. It is recommended that recording of temperature, pulse and blood pressure occurs immediately after birth (Chapter 80). If normal, these should be repeated after an hour to ensure continuing normality. However, if there is no history of hypertension or signs of infection, these do not necessarily have to be repeated during this period, but will depend on local policy and procedure guidelines.

Blood loss

The cord, placenta and membranes must be examined to ensure they appear normal and complete. This will help the overall evaluation of the woman's wellbeing in conjunction with physical observations. It is normal for women to have blood loss (lochia) following childbirth as the uterus progressively involutes and the muscles of the myometrium contract. The amount, colour and duration of lochia varies between women, but is normally heaviest in the early days following birth and diminishes on average by about 21 days postnatal. Initially, the blood loss can be fresh red and must be observed for amount and clots to exclude a primary postpartum haemorrhage (PPH) (Chapter 53). Lochia should also be noted for odour, as an offensive odour may indicate infection.

Uterine palpation

Immediately following birth, the abdomen should be gently palpated to ascertain the height of the uterine fundus, usually around the level of the umbilicus and to ensure that the uterus is firmly contracted and in a central position, which indicates the start of the involution process. Care must be taken to avoid 'fiddling' and overstimulation of the uterus as this could cause bleeding. The uterine recordings should be taken in conjunction with the woman's blood loss.

Circulation

Where possible, women should be encouraged to mobilise gently to promote circulation, reduce ankle oedema and reduce the risk of deep vein thrombosis (DVT). Ankle oedema noted should be pain free and bilateral to exclude DVT. Pain, inflammation or swelling in the calves must be noted as this may indicate a DVT. Advise women about simple ankle rotation exercises and to elevate feet when at rest to reduce normal ankle or pretibial oedema.

Bladder and bowel function

Following childbirth it is common for women to pass large amounts of urine as the body adjusts to a change in fluid volume. However, many women may experience reduced bladder tone and require encouragement to pass urine. The midwife should ensure that women void within the first 6 hours of giving birth and document this. It is common for women's bowel function to not return to normal within the first 6 hours of giving birth; particularly so if a woman has not eaten during labour. She may be afraid to open her bowels, especially if she has stitches to her perineum. Advise women regarding diet and fluid intake and decide whether it requires monitoring or immediate action.

Breasts

Breast examination is not necessary within the first 6 hours of giving birth unless requested by the woman. Although it is not recommended that women be asked about how they intend to feed their baby until after the first skin-to-skin contact, breastfeeding should be commenced within the first hour of birth. To help initiate this, the woman should not be separated from her baby for procedures such as weighing or bathing unless specifically required or requested by the mother. Within the initial 24 hours following birth, the midwife can provide skilled breastfeeding support and give information regarding the particular benefits of colostrum and breastfeeding (Chapters 34 and 62).

Pain

Women may experience pain in the perineum or abdomen in the initial hours after giving birth. Pain in the perineal area following birth is common, regardless of whether the birth resulted in trauma or not. The perineum and vagina can feel bruised for several days following a normal birth; injury will result in a greater degree of pain and women should be offered analgesia and advice regarding immediate management within the first 6 hours. Afterpains are more commonly experienced by women following the birth of their second or subsequent babies. It is often associated with oxytocin and the let-down reflex when breastfeeding. Analgesia should be offered as required.

28 On-going care

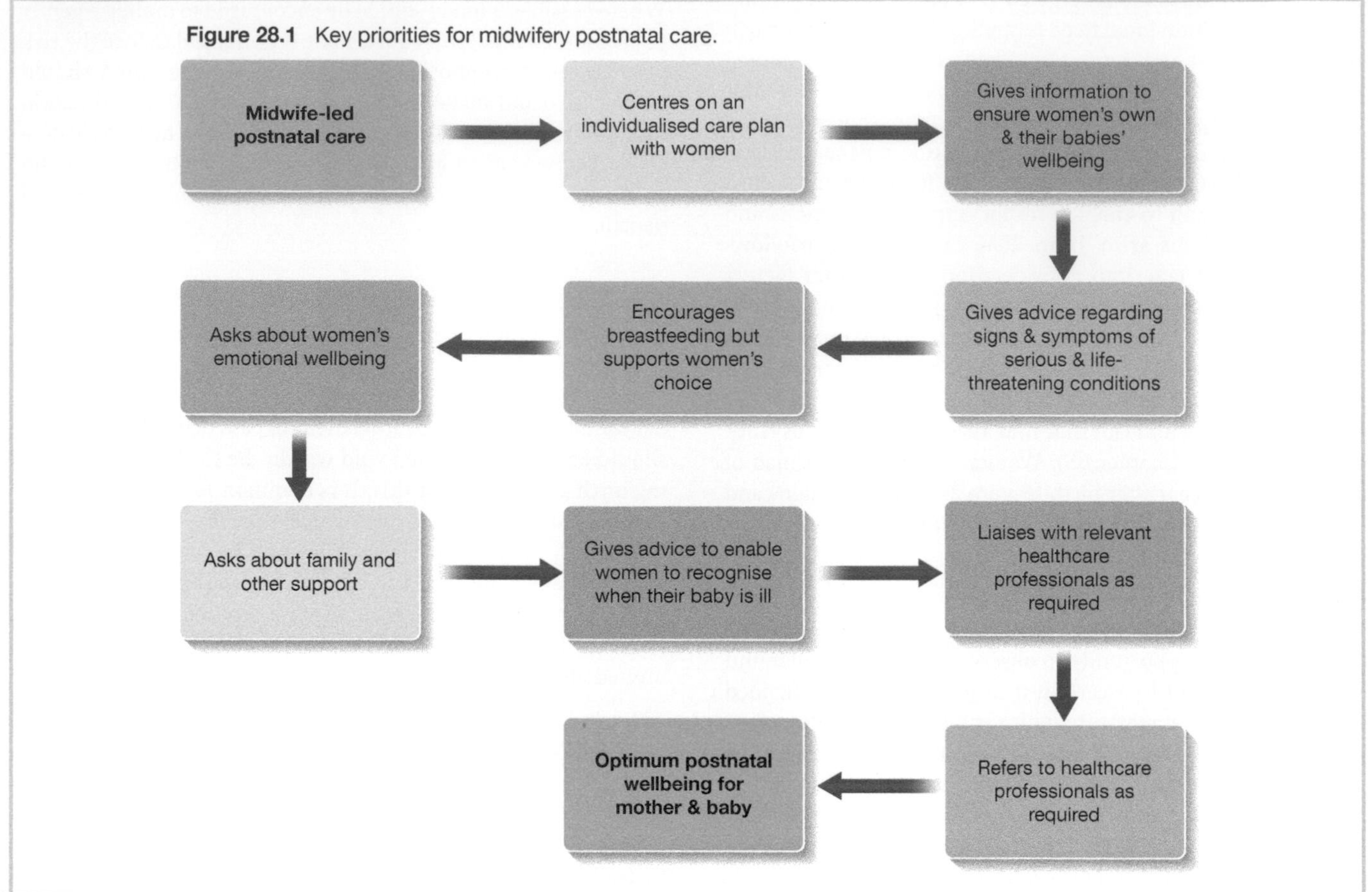

Figure 28.1 Key priorities for midwifery postnatal care.

Midwifery at a Glance, First Edition. Edited by Eleanor Forrest © 2019 John Wiley & Sons, Ltd. Published 2019 by John Wiley & Sons, Ltd.
Companion website: www.wiley.com/go/forrest/midwifery

This chapter addresses the on-going postnatal care provided by midwives for women having a normal vaginal birth, until discharge from midwifery care. After the 10th postnatal day the health visitor will usually also be involved in the care of the woman and her baby.

Postnatal care has changed over the years and there is a varied approach throughout the UK. Much has been written suggesting that postnatal care lacks the attention given at other times in the childbearing continuum. It has not always been clear what women or midwives want from this care, which may contribute to differences in approaches to the care offered. However, key elements for care focus on maternal and infant health, infant feeding and a framework for the content of postnatal care and its delivery (Figure 28.1).

Throughout the postnatal period, women should be involved in care planning, including when and where postnatal visits take place. The timing of discharge from hospital varies greatly and can be at the woman's request; therefore the number of on-going visits in the community will also vary. Following discharge, the midwife normally visits within a day and can ascertain if any problems have arisen and discuss an individual plan of care with the woman. Consideration should also be given to cultural aspects of care and additional needs such as disabilities. Being cognisant of these issues, midwives can show women respect and help forge a therapeutic relationship.

Observations

On-going recordings of vital signs do not necessarily have to be repeated if there is no history of hypertension, or signs of infection during this period. However this may depend on local policy and procedure guidelines (Chapter 80).

Blood loss and lochia should continue to be monitored and women must be asked about this at every visit as there can be a risk of a secondary postpartum haemorrhage (PPH) (Chapter 53), which includes bleeding up to 12 weeks postnatal. Lochia should also be noted for odour as an offensive odour may indicate infection. Perineal hygiene requires discussion, even in the absence of an episiotomy or tear. The perineum or vagina may remain bruised and sore for several weeks and advice can be given regarding pain relief, soothing packs or warm showers. There is no need to palpate the abdomen to ascertain the fundal height if the lochia is reducing and the woman has no abdominal pain or discomfort.

During the visit, the woman's mobility can be observed and a discussion about whether she is getting around in relation to reducing the risk of deep vein thrombosis (DVT). Normal ankle or pretibial oedema should reduce gradually but midwives can continue to advise women to do simple ankle rotation exercises and to elevate feet when at rest.

It is important to ask women about their appetite and diet as many neglect this as they are often too tired. Continued advice regarding diet and fluid intake must be given as constipation should be addressed within 3 days of giving birth. Bladder function should also have returned to normal, but women need to be asked to ensure there are no signs of infection or pelvic floor problems.

Advice

The importance of advising women to take time to rest and look after themselves is something that midwives can reinforce – even if it is just time to relax when the baby is sleeping between feeds. This is a good opportunity to discuss support at home and who is available to help with household chores. Support in the community can also be discussed as there may be local groups that the woman can attend; women should be advised of these ideally within 2–8 weeks. The emotional wellbeing of women during the postnatal period is of utmost importance and should not be overlooked. Information and advice on the normal emotional changes that can occur should be given to women and their partners within 3 days of giving birth (Chapter 65).

Some women may require immunisation: MMR (measles, mumps, rubella) to seronegative women should be offered before hospital discharge. Remember to advise women that following MMR immunisation, they can continue breastfeeding, but should avoid pregnancy for 1 month.

Infant feeding advice should continue during this period. If breastfeeding, the midwife should teach women how to hand express, store and heat milk.

Within the 2–6 weeks postnatal, advice should be given to women regarding resumption of sexual intercourse and contraception methods (Chapter 33).

Midwives can also provide information to women on common postnatal health problems such as dyspareunia, haemorrhoids, fatigue and urinary incontinence (Chapter 31) and issues such as jaundice, feeding and nappy rash in babies.

Safety issues should be discussed with the family, such as the correct use of infant car seats, smoke alarms and room temperature and infant positioning (Chapter 61).

Midwives should be aware of the signs of gender-based violence or child abuse (Chapter 67) and have knowledge of local guidance and local child protection policy.

By the 10th postnatal day or beyond, the midwife should assess if the woman and her baby have made a normal adjustment to the postnatal period and can make a final review of their physical, emotional and social care. It is normal practice that the health visitor and GP be involved in the on-going care of women and their babies from this point on to give advice on issues such as screening (Chapter 88), immunisation and feeding and weaning (Chapters 34 and 83).

29 Daily maternal examination

Table 29.1 Elements of maternal postnatal examination.

Postnatal examination	How	Why
Time	Discuss with the woman when would be convenient to conduct the examination	Allows the woman to plan infant feeding or attend to personal hygiene
Read notes		To ensure recent knowledge of her birth & postnatal recovery
Void urine	Ask the woman to pass urine just prior to the examination	To empty the bladder; correct fundal height & position and ensure comfort
Privacy	Draw curtains around woman's bed	To ensure privacy & dignity whilst conducting examination
Hand hygiene	Thoroughly wash hands	Reduce cross-infection
Observations	Temperature, pulse, blood pressure	To ensure within a normal range. Not generally required however in the absence of illness: check local policy
Discussion	Sit down at woman's level to discuss how she is feeling: sleep, appetite and mood	Shows interest in her wellbeing; shows giving time to listen to her
Breasts	Discuss how breasts & nipples feel	Can provide information about breast & nipple care, examination & signs of inflammation
Bladder	Ask if any problems passing urine	To ensure there is no infection & that pelvic floor exercises are being performed
Bowels	Ask if any problems opening her bowels	To asses if problems with constipation (should be asked within 3 days of giving birth); ascertain any problems with haemorrhoids; give advice regarding treatment & diet
Blood loss	Ask the woman about her lochia: amount, colour, odour, presence of clots	To assess if normal involution is taking place & advise normal pattern & what to do if bleeding increases or passing clots; advise what to do if any abdominal tenderness or pain – palpate abdomen & record temperature, pulse and respiration
Legs	Observe legs	Discuss leg comfort & give advice regarding any oedema – exercises & how to prevent DVT; signs of DVT
Perineum	Discuss perineal comfort	May have bruising or episiotomy wound; give advice regarding hygiene, healing & pain relief, such as cold pack; examine perineum as required
Exercises	Ask the woman if she is doing postnatal exercises	Give advice on postnatal exercises; abdominal, pelvic floor
Concerns	Ask the woman if she has any questions or concerns	Provides an opportunity to discuss any issues of concern or home circumstances
Wash hands	Thoroughly wash hand-held	Reduce cross-infection
Documentation	Record findings in hand held record & other notes	Ensure record & continuing plan of care; discuss findings with woman

Postnatal care involves midwives conducting an examination of the woman to ensure wellbeing and continued safe and healthy physical and psychological recovery from childbirth. The length of stay in a maternity unit varies but should be based on the individual woman's needs, the support she has at home and also take account of her health and wellbeing and that of her baby. Whilst in hospital, the maternal examination will be performed daily, however once at home in the community, the frequency of this will depend on the needs of the woman and subsequent number of visits from the community midwife. Midwives need to fully understand the processes involved in normal recovery at this time to enable them to detect any problems. This chapter focuses on the maternal postnatal examination of a woman following vaginal birth.

Communication with the woman is of utmost importance to ensure that she understands why the examination is being carried out and to inform her of the findings. The postnatal care plan can then be altered according to the findings and the woman's needs. The use of a hand-held maternity record can help promote such communication.

As women become more familiar with the examination, they will understand what to expect and become more familiar with the normal changes to their body during this time. However, women should be informed early in the postnatal period of the signs and symptoms of life-threatening conditions in order that they can alert midwifery or medical healthcare professionals if they have any concerns.

Some suggested aspects of a postnatal examination follow below and Table 29.1 illustrates these components.

Time

Having enough time to adequately care for women and their babies is an on-going issue for midwives and many feel pressure when trying to fulfil all their obligations to the required high standard. Despite this, the timing of the postnatal examination should be at a mutually convenient time for the midwife and the woman. The midwife should therefore discuss with the woman when it would be convenient to do the examination. For example, the woman may be just about to eat a meal, have a shower or be planning to feed her baby.

It is important that women feel they are being treated as individuals and as such should also not feel rushed. The midwife should sit down at the woman's level if possible to indicate that she has time and is ready to listen.

Time needs to be given to allow for discussion of the woman's general wellbeing, such as sleep pattern, appetite and how she is eating and her mood. This enables the midwife to give advice about rest, sleep and a nutritional diet. In addition, the postnatal examination provides a good opportunity for the midwife to discuss support at home and who will be there when the woman and her baby go home. The nature and quality of that support is important and the midwife can discreetly and sensitively enquire about whether the woman feels supported, or if there are any issues with gender-based violence at home.

Observations

Recording of temperature, pulse and blood pressure are only required in the first 24 hours following normal birth, unless otherwise indicated by previous history or current signs and symptoms of illness or infection. Local policy and procedure guidelines should be followed regarding this.

Breasts

Although it is not necessary to examine every woman's breasts, they should all be asked how their breasts feel. If a woman expresses concern about her breasts or nipples, or is experiencing pain, it may be necessary to examine them, with consent. The normal changes to the breast following the birth of a baby should be discussed in order that women know what to expect over the coming weeks. It is important that women recognise the signs of infection such as redness or lumps.

Blood loss and uterine involution

As the uterus involutes and gradually returns to be situated in the pelvis, this process is reflected in the amount and colour of the lochia. The value of fundal palpation to ascertain complications is currently being questioned and may not always be needed (check local policy and guidelines). There may be value in estimating fundal height if infection is suspected.

Blood loss will vary between each woman but generally diminishes by 21 days and for most women has gone by 42 days postnatal. Any changes to a woman's lochia, such as colour, odour or amount, should be noted and women should be advised about how to seek advice if concerned.

Perineum

The perineum is often bruised and sore following vaginal birth, even if intact, therefore women should be asked how it is feeling. It is not always necessary to assess the perineum, unless there are any indications of infection, odour or pain. The midwife should advise women on hygiene and pain relief as required, such as cleansing with warm water, oral analgesia and cooling gel packs.

Bladder and bowel

The bladder should be emptied prior to the examination to ensure comfort. Pelvic floor exercises can be discussed to help prevent incontinence problems. By about the third postnatal day, women should have managed to open their bowels. Midwives should provide advice regarding fluid intake, voiding regularly and high fibre diet and using some support for any stitches to help prevent constipation and haemorrhoids.

Legs

Women's legs should be examined for signs of redness, swelling or pain, which might indicate a deep vein thrombosis (DVT). Some ankle and pretibial oedema is normal following birth but the midwife can encourage women to do gentle rotation exercises.

Documentation

Remember to discuss your findings with the woman and to document accurately; discuss any concerns immediately with senior or medical staff.

30 Physiological changes

Figure 30.1 Uterine involution and vaginal fluid loss.

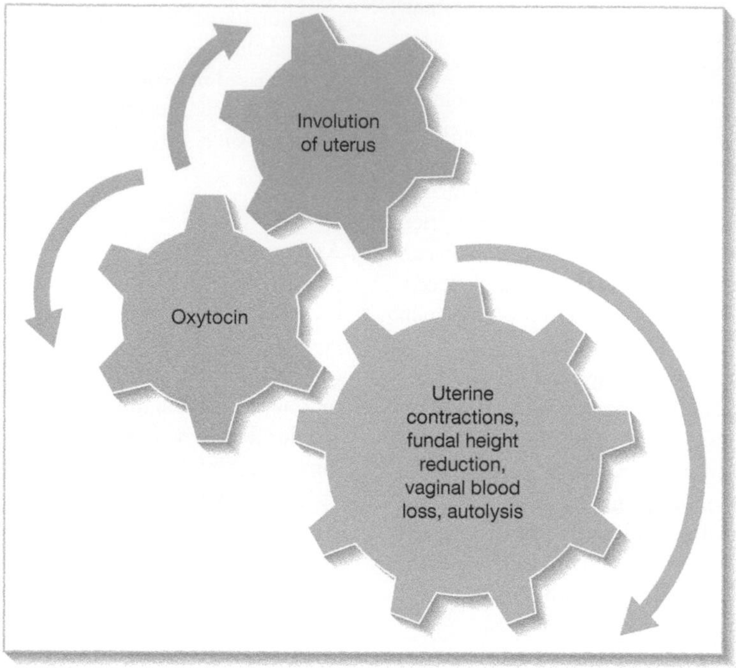

Involution of uterus

Oxytocin

Uterine contractions, fundal height reduction, vaginal blood loss, autolysis

Figure 30.2 Postnatal vaginal blood loss.

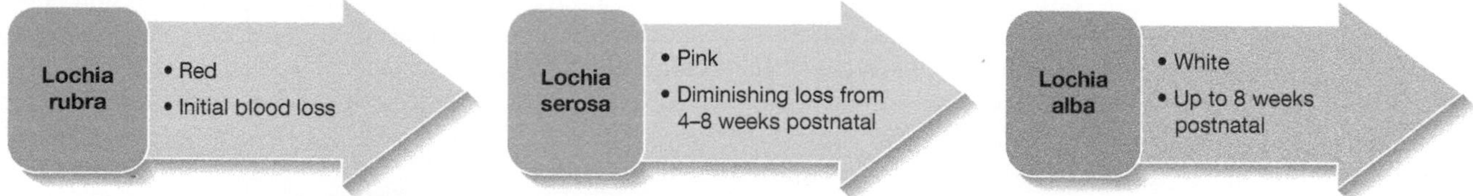

Figure 30.3 Changes to body systems.

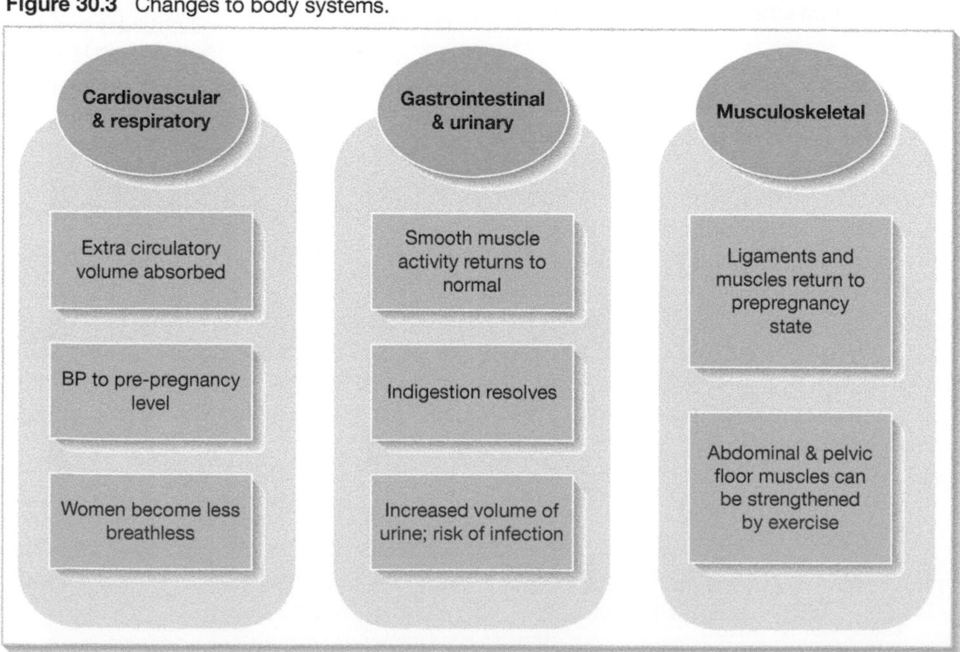

Following the birth of a baby, a woman's body undergoes many changes as it adapts to its prepregnant condition. This chapter will focus on the normal physiological changes during the puerperium. Although psychological and emotional changes in the postnatal period will be addressed in Part 10, these should be considered in conjunction with the physiological changes. This will enable midwifery care to be woman centred and adopt a holistic approach.

The puerperium is traditionally referred to as the time following birth to when the body and reproductive organs return as much as possible to their prepregnant state. Although there is no clear evidence to support the exact timing of this, it is widely accepted as being around a period of 6–8 weeks from the birth. From a midwifery perspective, the Nursing and Midwifery Council (NMC) rules and standards inform midwives' practices, and attendance of a midwife is required for at least 10 days, but can be longer as deemed necessary by the midwife. Therefore, the midwife must be knowledgeable of the expected normal physical changes that a woman will undergo during this time.

Uterine involution and vaginal fluid loss

Under the influence of the hormone oxytocin, the placenta is expelled from the uterus and the uterine walls start to collapse inwards, sealing off blood vessels to reduce blood loss. The muscle layers of the uterus contract further constricting blood vessels and blood flow to this area. Autolysis occurs and the epithelium starts to regenerate and proliferate. During this process of involution, the uterus reduces in size and returns to being situated in the pelvis, as do the ovaries and uterine tubes (Figure 30.1). Although much reduced in size, it still remains a larger cavity than normal; this requires on-going observations of uterine contractions, fundal height and vaginal blood loss (Chapters 27–29).

Abdominal cramps, commonly known as afterpains, can be experienced by women due to involuntary contractions. These are more usually experienced by multiparous women but can be triggered by breastfeeding, due to oxytocin production during let-down. Generally, afterpains can last around 2–3 days post birth and analgesia such as non-steroidal anti-inflammatory drugs (NSAIDs) can be prescribed to relieve discomfort.

The vaginal blood loss is known as lochia. This comprises the decidual lining of the uterus, which is being shed, blood and serum. From the 10th postnatal day, a new endometrium starts to develop and builds up until around 6 weeks. The duration of lochia differs for each woman; however, it generally lasts for around 4–8 weeks. During this time, the lochia changes in colour and decreases in amount: lochia rubra (red), lochia serosa (pink) and lochia alba (white) (Figure 30.2). Any oedema of the cervix gradually reabsorbs, with tears and bruises healing. The increased vascularity of the cervix and vagina decreases within several days of birth.

Perineum

Following vaginal birth, women are likely to experience some degree of swelling and discomfort to their vaginal tissues and perineum for a few days, regardless of presence of actual trauma. If trauma has occurred, healing will inevitably take longer and women are likely to experience more pain (Chapters 81 and 82).

Breasts

The breast is addressed more comprehensively in Chapters 7 and 34. However, as part of normal physiological adjustment following childbirth, the levels of oestrogen and progesterone fall rapidly following the delivery of the placenta, and prolactin levels increase. The latter stimulates the production of milk.

Body systems

Cardiovascular

Following birth, the body reabsorbs the additional circulatory volume which was required in pregnancy to ensure that the uterus and placenta were well perfused. This results in an increased volume of urine and oedema of the feet and ankles. Oedema should be bilateral and pain free; otherwise it may indicate a deep vein thrombosis (DVT). A decrease in circulatory blood volume results in cardiac output and blood pressure returning to prepregnancy levels. This normally occurs within 24 hours and in the absence of previous hypertension or morbidity, there is usually no requirement for routine blood pressure monitoring once a baseline recording has been established.

Respiratory

Following the birth of the baby, the uterus reduces in size and this takes pressure off the lungs. As full inflation of the basal lobes can be resumed women become less breathless. Within 1–3 weeks, normality of respiratory rate and tidal volume is restored.

Musculoskeletal

Within approximately 12 weeks of birth, ligaments and muscles return to their normal state due to reducing progesterone levels. This affects the uterine, abdominal and pelvic floor muscles and these can be strengthened by exercise.

Gastrointestinal and urinary

The smooth muscle of the alimentary tract gradually returns to normal due to reducing levels of progesterone. Constipation may continue but heartburn will resolve. Any dilatation of the urinary tract returns to normal; however infection risk can be increased if the woman had an indwelling catheter or operative delivery (Figure 30.3).

Role of the midwife

Midwives need to be aware of normal adaptation in order to recognise when problems arise. Many changes take place in women that alter depending on whether they have just given birth or are a few days postnatal. It is important to talk to women to ascertain lochia changes, pain experienced and sleeping patterns. Perineal care should include asking women how they feel and if necessary checking the perineal area after asking permission to do so. Pain relief should be offered and advice given about how to reduce inflammation and avoid infection. Perineal trauma and pain following childbirth is a major source of morbidity for many women and is a widespread health problem. Discussing breast care with women may prevent or elicit problems such as sore or cracked nipples, engorgement and mastitis or thrush infection.

31 Pelvic floor

Figure 31.1 Pelvic floor muscles.

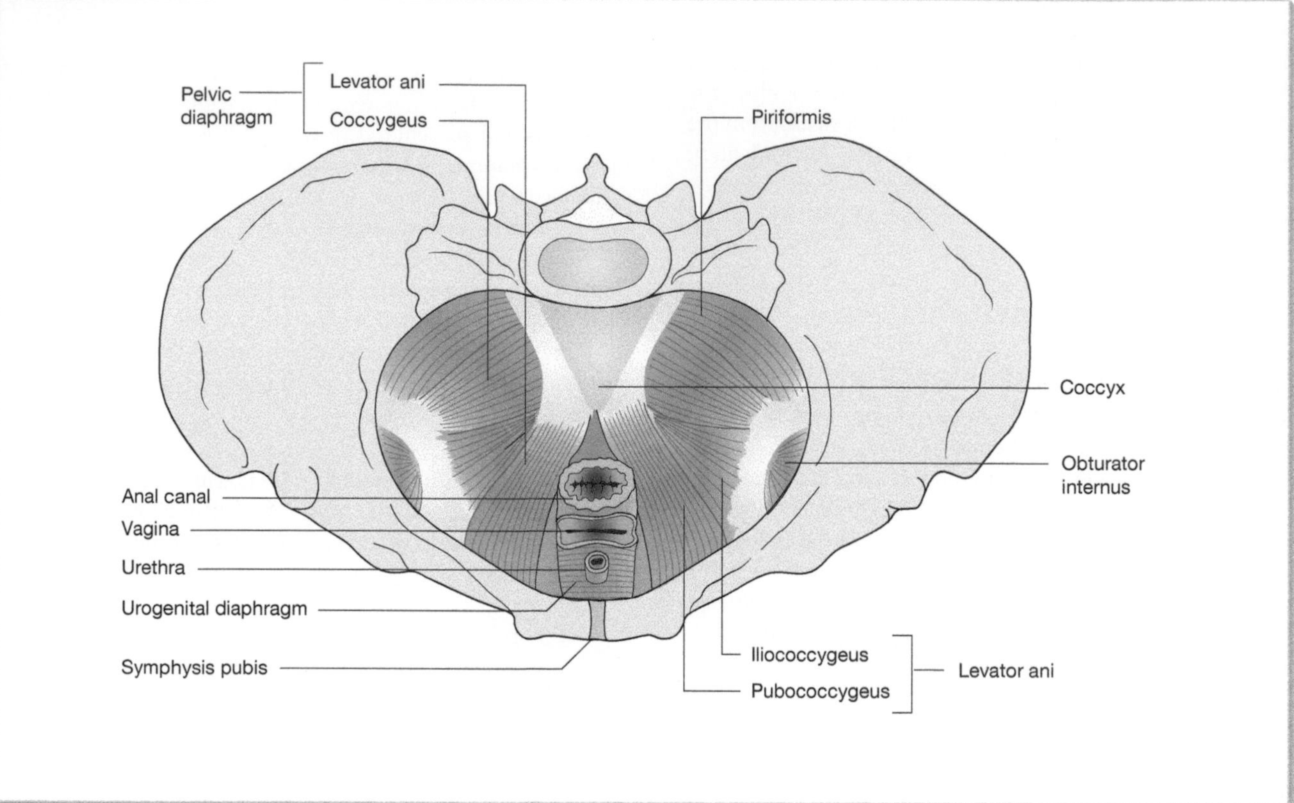

Figure 31.2 Stress urinary incontinence.

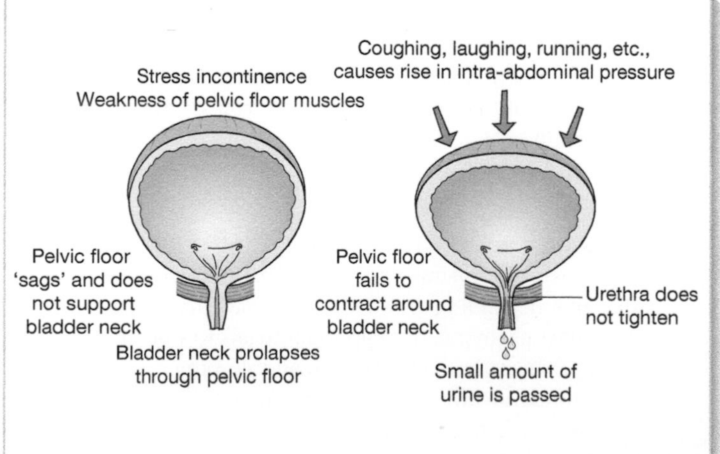

Figure 31.3 Pelvic organ prolapse.

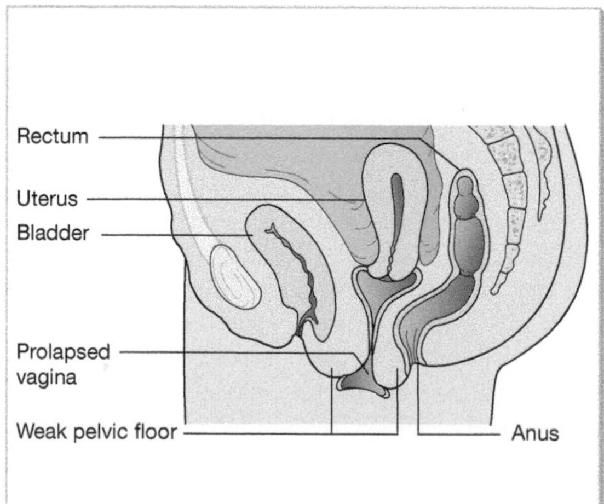

Box 31.1 Risk factors for incontinence.

- Large babies, prolonged second stage, forceps deliveries and third degree tears
- Heavy lifting such as car seats can also put extra strain on already weakened muscles
- For most of these conditions women will be referred to a specialist women's health physiotherapist for individual treatment & assessment. However it is important that the midwife is aware of basic pelvic floor exercises so she can teach any woman unable to access this service, or as a preventative measure

Childbirth is one of the main causes of pelvic floor muscle (PFM) trauma and in the absence of an obstetric physiotherapist it may fall to the midwife to educate women with regards to this. It is important to ensure that women have the knowledge and training to strengthen their pelvic floor muscles and thus prevent the complications that can arise from weakness in this area.

Muscles

The PFMs are located in the floor of the pelvis extending from the pubic bone at the front to the coccyx at the back. They provide a sling of support for the vagina, cervix, bladder and rectum and are extremely important in maintaining continence and preventing prolapse (Figure 31.1). The levator ani muscle is the most important of these and this can be divided into the pubococcygeal muscle and the iliococcygeal muscle.

The pubococcygeal muscle is a large muscle stretching from the pubic bones at the front, passing behind the rectum and attaching to the walls of the vagina, the perineal body and the anal sphincter. This provides a sling giving vital support within the pelvis, and the part of the muscle known as the pubovaginalis also lifts the urethra during a pelvic floor contraction. The puborectalis portion forms a sling around the rectum maintaining the anorectal angle and also forms part of the external anal sphincter, and thus is integral in maintaining anal continence. The iliococcygeus forms a more horizontal sheet across the pelvic opening, providing a support for the internal organs. The levator ani muscles are formed by striated muscle fibres, with 67% of the fibres being type 1 (slow twitch fibres) with a more supportive, postural role and 33% being type 2 (fast twitch fibres) providing a quick response contraction.

Nerve supply

The pelvic floor muscles are innervated by the pudendal nerve which arises from the lumbosacral plexus at the level of S2–S4. This nerve can be damaged during childbirth by traction injuries to the pelvic floor muscles, leading to PFM weakness.

Function

The PFMs promote bladder and bowel control, help prevent prolapse, have an effect on sexual function and help to provide stability to the lower back and pelvis. These muscles become stretched and weakened during childbirth and are also affected by the mechanical changes of pregnancy, leading to a loss of function, which can present in several different ways.

Stress urinary incontinence

The International Continence Society defines stress incontinence as 'the involuntary loss of urine occurring when, in the absence of a detrussor contraction, the intravesical pressure exceeds the maximum urethral pressure'. It is the most common form of female incontinence and often associated with activities such as coughing, sneezing and laughing. Some studies suggest that up 20% of all women between the ages of 18 and 49 years have urinary incontinence, with 83% of this being stress incontinence. Weak PFMs are incapable of providing sufficient counterpressure around the urethra at times of increased intra-abdominal pressure, leading to the involuntary loss of urine (Figure 31.2).

Faecal incontinence

This very distressing condition is much less frequently discussed than urinary incontinence yet some studies suggest that 4% of primagravida women have some form of faecal incontinence or faecal urgency. Faecal urgency can be related to the lack of voluntary control around the external anal sphincter. This is comprised mainly of the puborectalis muscle and is thus affected by any pelvic floor weakness. Passive soiling is more likely to be related to a defect in the internal sphincter which is not under voluntary control.

Pelvic organ prolapse

Damage to the pelvic floor and subsequent reduction of PFM strength can predispose women to pelvic organ prolapse as these muscles provide important support for the bladder, uterus and rectum (Figure 31.3).

Sexual function

Sexual function can also be affected by poor PFM strength. Vaginal gaping can decrease satisfaction for both parties, and some women are affected by incontinence during sexual intercourse itself. Women very rarely disclose this form of incontinence without prior questioning.

Pelvic stability

The PFMs also have a role in preventing back pain and pelvic pain. These muscles co-contract with the transverus abdominus to provide support for the lower back and pelvis. This is particularly important in the postnatal period as this area loses its stability due to the still present effects of relaxin and the weakened abdominal muscles.

Risk factors

There are certain intranatal and postnatal factors that suggest a higher risk of urinary or faecal incontinence (Box 31.1).

Pelvic floor muscle exercises

The following instructions should be given for PFM exercises:

Lie, sit or stand with your knees slightly apart. Imagine that you are trying to stop yourself passing wind and stopping yourself from passing urine at the same time. You then want to 'squeeze and lift', closing and drawing up the back and front passages. This squeeze and lift is called a pelvic floor contraction. Make sure you do not hold your breath, tighten your buttock cheeks or squeeze your legs together. Tighten your pelvic floor muscles as described above and hold for as many seconds as you can up to a count of 10. Repeat this as often as you can up to a maximum of 10 times. This becomes your starting point.

Perform this 3–4 times a day and gradually increase until you can hold for 10 seconds and repeat this 10 times. You also want to do short 1-second holds, building these up until you can repeat that 10 times as well. Once you can do this you want to perform this *at least* once a day for the rest of your life.

It is important to give sufficient time to teach pelvic floor exercises correctly, questioning about understanding and the appreciation of the pelvic floor contraction.

32 Sepsis

Box 32.1 Risk factors for sepsis in the postnatal period.

Pregnancy-related risk factors
- Amniocentesis
- Cervical cerclage
- Vaginal trauma
- Caesarean wound
- Wound haematoma
- Retained products of conception

Non-pregnancy-related risk factors
- GAS/throat infection in family/close contacts
- Obesity
- Black or minority ethnic group origin
- Diabetes
- Impaired immunity
- Anaemia
- History of pelvic infection

Figure 32.1 Signs and symptoms of sepsis.

Are any of these present?						
Temperature ≥38°C or ≤36°C Heart rate >100 bpm Respiratory rate ≥20 breaths/minute	Lower abdominal pain/uterine tenderness Offensive smelling lochia	Diarrhoea & or vomiting Urinary symptoms	Signs of caesearean wound infection	Breast engorgement or redness	Acutely altered mental state	Generalised rash Productive cough

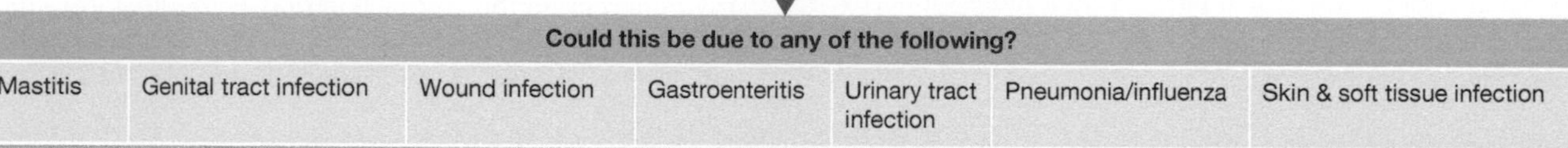

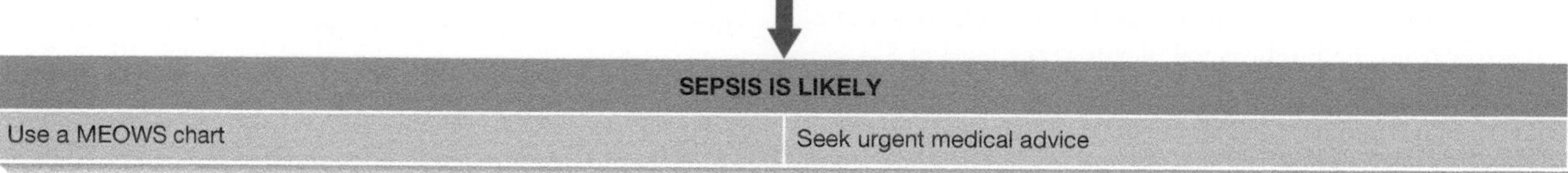

Figure 32.2 Prevention of postnatal sepsis.

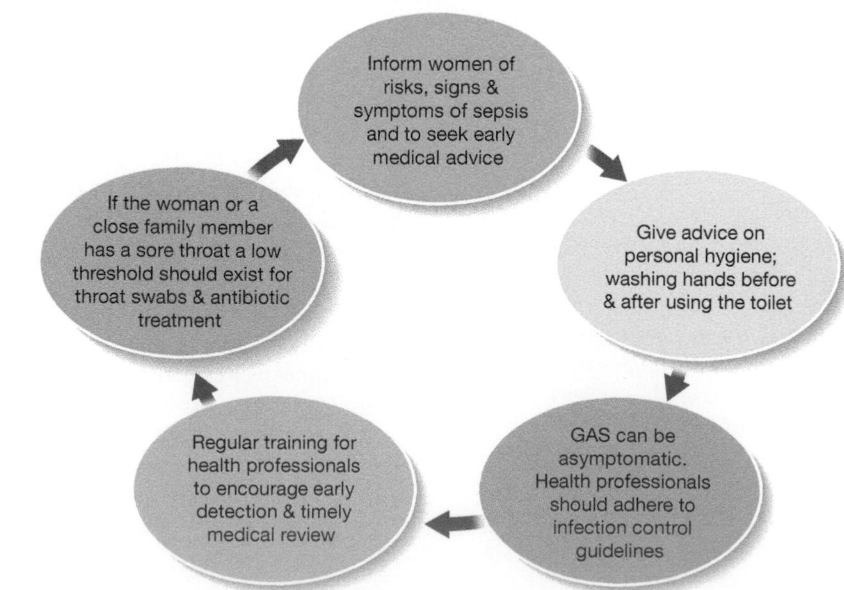

Sepsis that occurs after pregnancy and within 6 weeks of birth is called postpartum sepsis or puerperal sepsis. It may colloquially be referred to as blood poisoning but the medical definition for sepsis is an infection plus systemic manifestations of infection. It may further be graded into severe sepsis or septic shock. In severe sepsis, the immune system of the body goes into overdrive as it attempts to fight the infection and can result in multiple organ failure. Septic shock occurs when there is a persistent hypoperfusion (an inadequate perfusion and supply of oxygen and nutrients to the body tissues), despite adequate fluid replacement.

The onset of sepsis is often insidious but may progress very rapidly and is potentially a life-threatening condition. Sepsis can occur in the antenatal period. The majority of morbidity and mortality is, however, experienced in the postpartum period. In the latest MBRRACE review (Knight et al., 2015), sepsis was identified as one of the leading causes of maternal death, with an overall epidemiology of 1.56 per 100 000 maternities.

Sepsis is triggered by an infection and can develop as a result of a variety of complications. It can be viral in origin and may result from influenza and some types of pneumonia. However it has been identified that the bacterial organisms group A beta-haemolytic streptococci (GAS) have attributed to the majority of severe, life-threatening cases of maternal sepsis in the puerperium. Other bacterial organisms known to cause maternal sepsis include group B, C and G *Streptococcus*, *Staphylococcus aureus*, *Escherichia coli* and methicillin-resistant *S. auerus* (MRSA).

By far the most common site of sepsis is in the genital tract, usually within the uterus, resulting in endometritis. Outside of the genital tract, mastitis, urinary tract infection, gastroenteritis, pharyngitis and skin and soft-tissue infections are all likely causes of sepsis.

Who is most at risk of postpartum sepsis?

The known risks for sepsis are identified in Box 32.1. Risk factors related to childbirth include frequent vaginal examinations in labour, prolonged spontaneous rupture of the membranes, retained products of conception, any trauma to the vagina, wound haematoma or caesarean section. Poor personal or perineal hygiene in the postnatal period also increases risk of sepsis.

Recognition of sepsis

The symptoms of sepsis are wide ranging. Not all symptoms will feature and importantly women may present with extreme pain that seems disproportionate to the clinical signs of sepsis. This may indicate a deep and severe infection and should trigger urgent referral for senior review, or if in the community setting, urgent hospital admission via emergency ambulance. The clinical features of sepsis will include one or more of the following: pyrexia ≥ 38°C, tachycardia ≥ 100 beats per minute, tachypnoea, lower abdominal pain with possibly a sub-involuted uterus that has not returned to its normal size after giving birth, hypotension, diarrhoea, vomiting, heavy, purulent or offensive vaginal discharge, breast engorgement or redness, a generalised maculopapular rash and possible signs of infection/discharge in any wound (Figure 32.1).

How is postpartum sepsis diagnosed?

It is vitally important that midwives are aware of the symptoms and signs of sepsis and have a low threshold for suspicion of sepsis in the postnatal period. Figure 32.1 identifies how clinicians may initially diagnose sepsis/severe sepsis and septic shock. Importantly, sepsis should *always* be considered in women who have recently given birth and feel unwell, especially if they have pyrexia or hypothermia along with tachycardia. Such symptoms indicate the need for urgent intravenous antibiotics and senior review. If mastitis is suspected, it is important not to overlook the symptoms and to assume that they can be relieved by continued breastfeeding alone; senior review is required.

The use of a MEOWS (modified early obstetric warning system) chart may help midwives trigger a referral to senior medical colleagues. It is important that a general history is taken to try and determine the cause of sepsis. This should include asking about any illness in close family members, including children who may have had a sore throat. GAS is a common cause of infection in children and toddlers and may easily be transferred through coughs and sneezes.

Diagnostic tests will include urgent blood cultures. Other tests will be dependent on clinical suspicion of the source of infection and may include swabs of the throat, perineum, high vagina and any wound for culture and sensitivity, as well routine blood tests to include C-reactive protein and a midstream urine test.

How is it treated?

Any abscess of a breast, wound or pelvis will be drained. Uterine evacuation may be warranted if genital tract sepsis is suspected. Best practice recommends that intravenous broad-spectrum antibiotics are commenced within 1 hour of the initial suspicion of severe sepsis. It is important to consider advice from a consultant microbiologist with regard to the suitability of some antimicrobials if the mother is breastfeeding. If the mother has a GAS acquired infection it is important that baby is also treated with antibiotics.

How can postpartum sepsis be prevented?

Postpartum sepsis and its possible severity can be prevented or limited (Figure 32.2). It is fundamental that women are informed by midwives about the signs and symptoms of postpartum sepsis and know to seek early advice if they feel unwell. It is also important that information is provided with regard to good personal hygiene to include the importance of hand washing before and after using the toilet and changing sanitary pads. Because GAS has also been linked to healthcare professionals who may have no symptoms of infection, it is vital that infection control guidelines are adhered to.

33 Contraception

Table 33.1 Sex in pregnancy: giving information.

Situation	Explanation
Positions best for sex during pregnancy	Woman on top, rear entry and side to side are usually the best for comfort and accessibility. Avoidance of deep and weight-bearing positions Avoid the woman being on her back to prevent dizziness caused by central venous compression
Use of various forms of stimulation	Most forms of stimulation including intercourse are safe
To start labour when woman overdue	Stimulation of cervix releases of prostaglandins; also contained within seminal fluid which may stimulate uterine activity
Use of sex toys	As long as they are clean and used gently
Medical reason, e.g. placenta praevia, high blood pressure	Explain why and state a time limit if possible
Either partner has an STI	Use protection to reduce transmission (avoid sex for at least 7 days after treatment)
Sex hurts or causes bleeding, discharge or cramps	Seek the advice of a midwife or obstetrician for an explanation

Table 33.2 Classification of contraceptive methods and effectiveness.

Long-acting reversible contraception	Short-acting hormonal reversible contraception	Spontaneous reversible contraception
Implant (Nexplanon) >99% effective	Combined pill (COC) >99% effective	Condoms – male/female 98% (best use)/95%
Copper coils (IUD) >99% effective	Contraceptive patch/vaginal ring >99% effective	Diaphragms and caps 92–96% effective
Hormone coil Mirena/Jaydess (IUS) >99% effective	Progestogen only pill – (desogestrel 75 mg) 99% effective	Natural family planning, including lactational amenorrhoea 98% effective
Injectables (e.g Depo-Provera 150 mg i.m.; Sayana Press ® 104 mg s.c.) >99% effective	Progestogen only pills (POP-levenorgestrel or norithesterone in various doses) 98–99% effective	Withdrawal effectiveness unknown

Box 33.1 Summary of the menstrual cycle.

Before ovulation

- Follicle-stimulating hormone (FSH) produced from anterior pituitary in response to low oestrogen levels (negative feedback) prepares the 'dominant follicle' in the ovary
- The ovarian follicle increases and produces oestrogen. Increasing oestrogen levels are required to produce a positive feedback mechanism, which causes a surge in both FSH and lutenising hormone (LH) levels
- The LH surge causes the ovarian follicle to rupture, ovulation, which is usually followed by a rise in basal body temperature of between 0.2 and 0.5°C. Ovulation is of variable length in the cycle. The life span of an oocyte is a maximum of 24 hours

After ovulation

- Following ovulation the follicle shrinks to become the corpus luteum
- The corpus luteum produces oestrogen and progesterone which prepare the lining of the uterus to receive a fertilised ovum for implantation
- If fertilisation does not occur then progesterone and oestrogen levels decline and menstruation occurs. Ovulation to menstruation constant is a length of 14 days

Box 33.2 Resumption of sexual activity following childbirth.

- The time to resume sexual activity will vary between couples
- There is no set timeframe in which sexual activity should have resumed
- Both partners need to be physically and emotionally ready
- Some people may experience difficulties with sexual activity following the birth of their child
- Sexual desire or sex drive may be low in the first few months
- Any difficulties or concerns should be discussed with a health professional

Box 33.3 The ideal contraceptive.

- 100% reversible
- 100% effective
- 100% forgettable
- 100% convenient – not related to having sex
- 100% free from side effects
- 100% protective against STIs
- Possessing other non-contraceptive benefits
- 100% maintenance free
- Acceptable to every culture, religion and political view
- Cheap and easily available
- Not dependent upon healthcare practitioners to access

A midwife should provide advice on reproductive sexual health, with discussions regarding contraception following birth best initiated from the 36-week antenatal visit, to allow the woman and her partner time to contemplate and further discuss acceptable contraception. This allows time for further review in the postnatal period and initiation of their chosen method prior to return of fertility. Effective contraceptive is important as inter-pregnancy intervals of less than 6 months are associated with an increased risk of negative perinatal outcome and can pose increased risks to maternal health.

Menstruation may be regarded as the return of fertility; however some women may ovulate and therefore conceive if they have not started contraception prior to menstruation (Box 33.1 and Chapter 9). The earliest date of ovulation in non-breastfeeding women is day 28, menstruation returning by week 6. In breastfeeding women ovulation is suppressed, returning when the frequency and duration of suckling decreases. Menstruation occurs on average 28.4 weeks (range 15–48 weeks) after birth for women who are breastfeeding. The mean time to initiation of ovulation is 33.6 weeks (range 14–51 weeks). The first 'true period' is defined as any bleeding lasting at least 2 days, requiring the use of sanitary protection for at least 1 day, followed by a second bleeding episode within the next 21–70 days.

Women often require information regarding sex in pregnancy (Table 33.1) and this can link to discussions about resumption of sex and contraception needs for the postnatal period. The weeks following childbirth can be a time of significant change for women. Sex can be influenced by bio/psycho/social concerns, for example: lower circulating oestrogen levels while breastfeeding may cause vaginal dryness; orgasm may cause an oxytocin rise and stimulate milk leakage; fear of dyspareunia (painful sex) and pain from perineal or abdominal wounds; or concern that they will be interrupted by the baby crying. The midwife needs to convey information regarding resumption of sexual activity following birth with sensitivity and women should be reassured that it is a very individual matter and for some couples this may not be for some months, with a small proportion who have still not resumed sexual intercourse by 6 months. Evidence suggests that there is a possible association between sexual dysfunction and assisted vaginal delivery, however this is disputed by some research sources. Sexual activity may be resumed when both partners feel ready (Box 33.2).

However, following a few deaths from air embolism following sexual intercourse, the Centre for Maternal and Child Enquiries (CEMACE, 2011) advises recommending abstinence for 6 weeks, or gentle intercourse avoiding positions (for example, all fours) that might allow excess air to be forced into the vagina. Although there are many different types of contraceptive available, the ideal contraceptive still remains unavailable (Box 33.3).

Contraceptive decision-making can be complex and women may base their decisions on personal beliefs and reported concerns over side effects and risks rather than systematically weighing up the benefits and possible disadvantages of a method determined by safety, efficacy, ease of use, availability and accessibility. A midwife must have a good knowledge of all contraceptive methods, such as long- and short-acting reversible and spontaneous reversible contraception to fulfil the EC directive to be able to provide sound family planning advice. A midwife therefore must be able to give verbal and written/online access to information (e.g. from the Family Planning Association) on mode and duration of action, failure rate, side effects and risks, the benefits of the methods and when to seek advice and referral to specialist reproductive health services.

UK Medical Eligibility Criteria for Contraceptive Use (UKMEC) provides practitioners with evidence-based guidance using a numerical category of use for each of the main reversible methods of contraception for a range of conditions. However, it only considers one risk factor at a time, not multiple factors occurring at the same time. It is imperative that discharge information provides GPs with adequate information of all the risk factors for women postpartum. UKMEC also provides categories for the use of hormonal contraception in postnatal women. MBRRACE (2015) reports two late deaths where women had been prescribed the combined oral contraceptive pill. Women should not be prescribed oestrogen-based contraception until after 6 weeks to avoid the risk of venous thromboembolism (VTE).

While UKMEC guidance suggests that intrauterine contraception (for either the copper device (IUD) or hormonal system (IUS)) is category 1 within the first 48 hours following birth, few if any women will have a coil fitted at this time. Between 48 hours to 4 weeks post-birth, including caesarean section, intrauterine contraception is category 3 and therefore should be avoided. After 4 weeks an intrauterine device can be inserted (category 1) except in women who have postpartum sepsis (category 4).

Lactational amenorrhoea as a contraceptive method is 98% effective (similar to best use of condoms and greater than the typical use rate of 95%) in preventing pregnancy. However, this is dependent on the mother fully breastfeeding, the baby is less than 6 months old and the woman is not already menstruating. Regular night feeds maintain high prolactin levels which inhibit ovulation.

Contraception should be used from day 21 following delivery to prevent further pregnancy. Women may opt to use barrier methods such as condoms until a higher efficacy or long-acting method can be started.

34 Lactation

Figure 34.1 Pattern of a breastfeed. Source: Picture courtesy from UNICEF Baby Friendly Initiative.

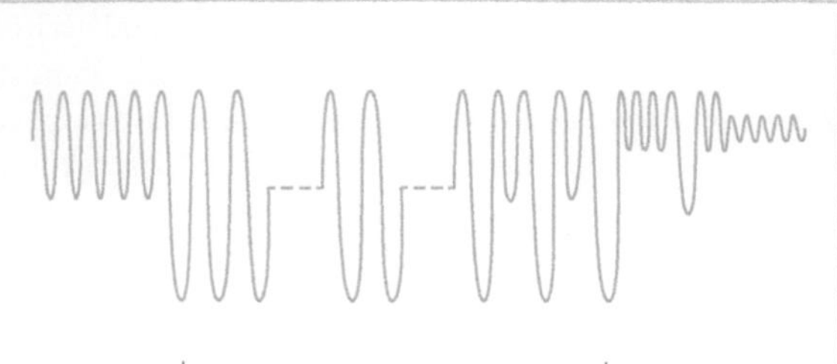

Figure 34.3 Positioning for breastfeeding – off to a good start.

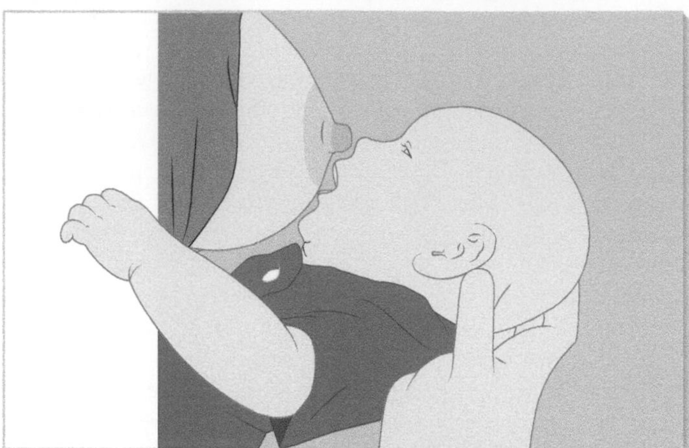

Figure 34.2 Advice to parents to prevent SUDI.

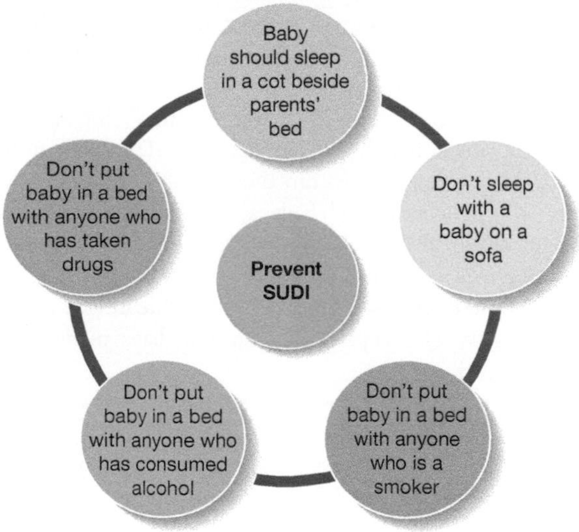

Prevent SUDI

- Baby should sleep in a cot beside parents' bed
- Don't sleep with a baby on a sofa
- Don't put baby in a bed with anyone who is a smoker
- Don't put baby in a bed with anyone who has consumed alcohol
- Don't put baby in a bed with anyone who has taken drugs

Figure 34.4 Principles of good positioning.

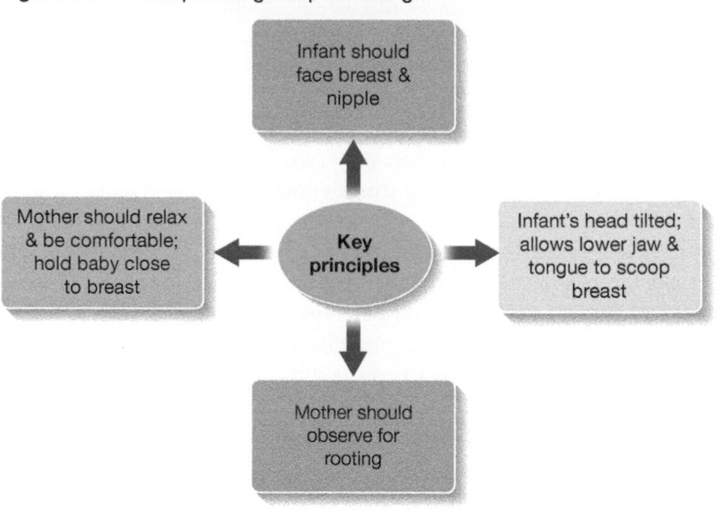

Midwifery at a Glance, First Edition. Edited by Eleanor Forrest © 2019 John Wiley & Sons, Ltd. Published 2019 by John Wiley & Sons, Ltd.
Companion website: www.wiley.com/go/forrest/midwifery

Responsive feeding

Healthy term babies are natural communicators – they are able to provide their primary care givers with cues about how they are feeling and what they need. Restlessness, eye flickering, finger knitting, rooting, hand to mouth movements and lip licking are just some of the ways an infant might communicate his/her needs. The symbiotic relationship between a mother and her infant enables her to interpret the infant's signal and to respond quickly and reciprocally to meet the infant's needs. Therefore, keeping her infant close by will provide a mother the best opportunity to recognise this sometimes subtle communication. Consistently responding to an infant's communication with an offer of a feed, a cuddle or a lullaby reassures the infant that their needs are recognised and will be met. This in turn reduces the level of the stress hormone, cortisol, in the infant's brain and helps the infant regulate his/her emotions.

A mother responding to her infant's feeding cues will ensure that there are frequent opportunities for breastfeeding. If the infant is well attached at the breast and is allowed to feed until satisfied this will ensure a good milk supply.

Pattern of infant sucking: effective breast feed

Following the maternal recognition of infant feeding cues, the infant accesses the breast offered by the mother and exhibits characteristic feeding behaviours. The way an infant sucks at the breast typically changes as the feed progresses. Initially the infant is hungry and displays concentrated vigorous sucking activity as he or her attaches to the breast. This is followed by a more organised, rhythmic, sucking pattern with deep sucks followed by pauses; swallowing may be heard at this time. As the feed progresses the pauses or resting phases between feeds will increase and the sucking becomes less forceful until the infant spontaneously releases the breast.

As the feed progresses the fat concentration increases while the volume of milk decreases. Allowing the infant to decide how long he or she sucks for at the breast is important in ensuring that the infant is satisfied. The infant should be offered the second breast at this stage. The sucking pattern of an effective breastfeed is illustrated in Figure 34.1.

Night feeds

Breastfeeding at night is important in establishing a good milk supply. Prolactin levels are highest during the night and reach their peak after each breastfeed to secure sufficient breast milk for the next feed (Chapter 7).

Heath professionals should discuss with parents how they will manage feeding their baby during the night. The UNICEF/UK Baby Friendly Initiative propose that the discussion with parents include the following key points to reduce the risk of sudden unexpected death of an infant (SUDI) (Figure 34.2):

- The safest place for babies to sleep is in a cot beside the parents' bed
- Sleeping with a baby on a sofa puts a baby at greatest risk
- Babies should not share a bed with anyone who:
  - Is a smoker
  - Has consumed alcohol
  - Has taken drugs (legal or illegal) that make them sleepy.

Attachment for breastfeeding

Attachment is best described as the way in which the infant takes the breast into his mouth to access milk (Figure 34.3). In order to access milk effectively, the infant requires scooping the underside of the breast with the tongue. The breast is then formed into a teat shape, with the nipple resting at the junction of the hard and soft palate. The nipple will not be damaged if an effective attachment is achieved as it is not dynamic in the feeding process.

Once the mouth is full of breast, the infant will instinctively compress the breast tissue and along with the negative pressure within the infant's mouth milk is transferred from the breast to the infant.

Signs of effective attachment

- Chin is indenting the breast
- Nose is free of the breast because held is extended
- Evidence of a gape > 90
- More areola is visible above the top lip than under the bottom lip
- Infant spontaneously sucks
- Cheeks are round and full due to large amount of breast within mouth
- Bottom lip may be seen to be curled outward, but usually not by the mother
- Mother has no pain within breast or nipple; oxytocin reflex may be felt as a tingling sensation within the breast
- Swallowing may be heard and pattern of a feed seen.

Positioning for breastfeeding

Positioning for breastfeeding is the way in which the mother holds her baby in order to achieve a good attachment at the breast (Figure 34.3). Effective positioning for breastfeeding can be achieved in many different positions. However, all positions should enable the baby to attach effectively at the breast. Effective positioning and attachment are essential for stimulating a good milk supply, to ensure adequate milk transfer to the infant and to prevent damage and pain to the mother.

Principles of good positioning

- Mother should be relaxed and comfortable. If a bra is worn, she should release the breast from it and allow the breast to fall in its natural lie. The infant should be held close at the level of the breast, with the head and body in alignment
- The infant should be facing the breast with the nipple pointing towards the nose
- The infant should be able to tilt the head to allow the lower jaw and tongue to scoop the breast into the mouth. The chin will lead as the infant is brought into the breast
- The mother should watch for the baby rooting and then showing a wide, gaping mouth (Figure 34.4). At the height of the gape the mother moves her infant to the breast with the chin leading and the head tilted back.

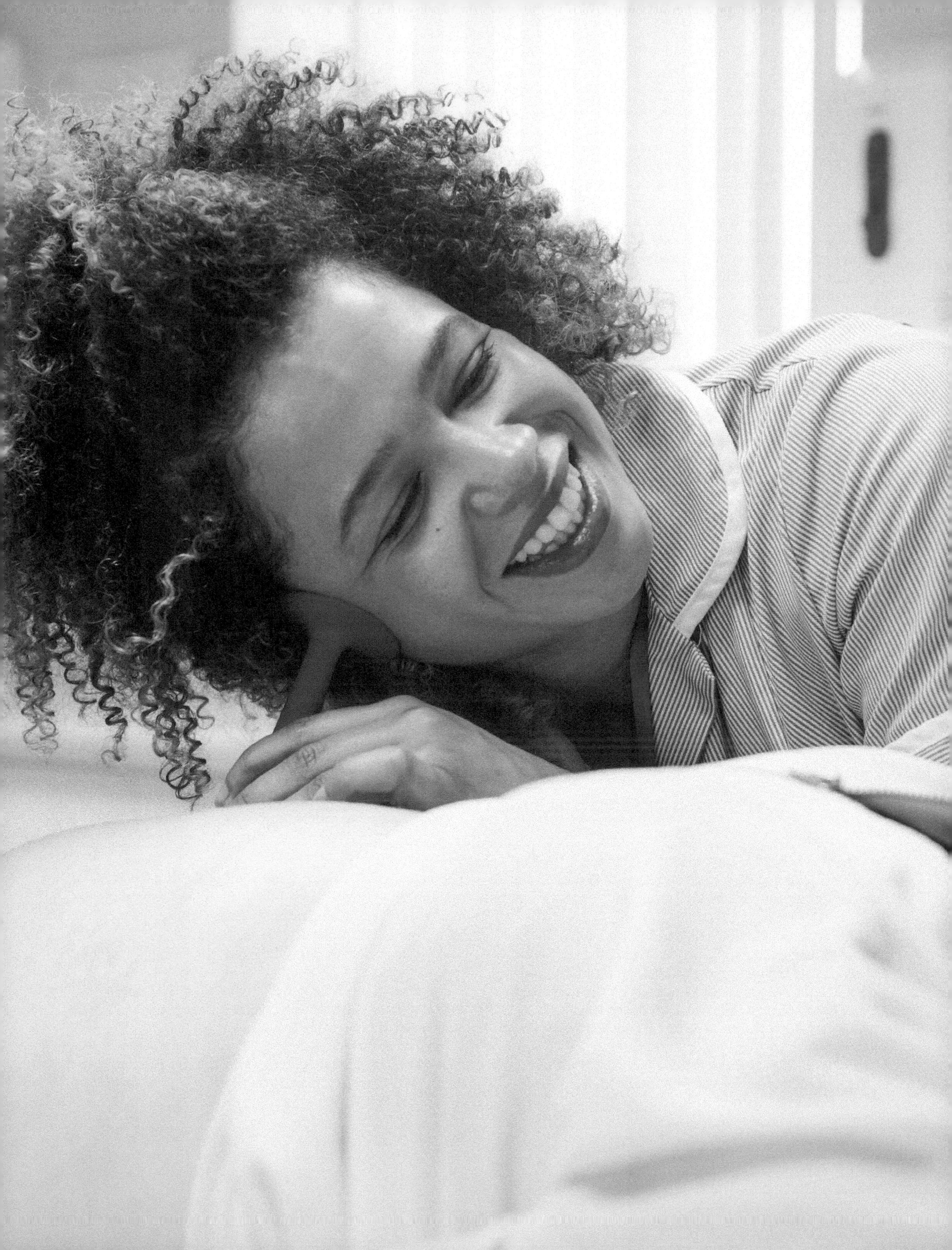

Common medical disorders

Chapters

35 Hypertensive disorders of pregnancy

Box 35.1 Complications of gestational and chronic hypertension.

- Worsening hypertension which increases the maternal risk of complications, e.g. stroke
- Pre-eclampsia superimposed on existing hypertensive state
- Placental abruption
- Intrauterine growth restriction

Box 35.2 Management of gestational and chronic hypertension.

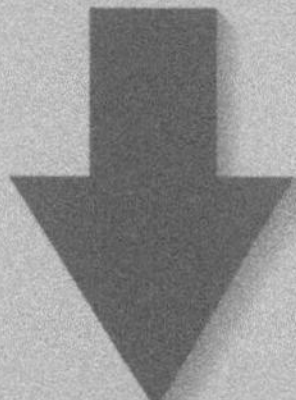

Chronic hypertension
Book for consultant obstetric unit

Review at clinics already attending

Review medication: discontinue ACE inhibitors/angiotensin receptor blockers (ARBs) and prescribe alternative or reduce/cease in 1st trimester depending on physiological drop in BP sufficient

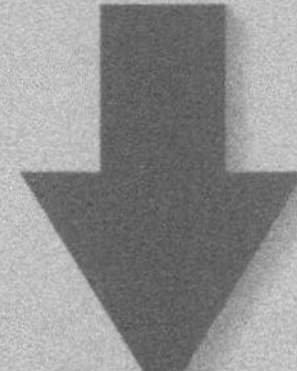

Gestational hypertension

Book for consultant obstetric unit

Refer to maternal medicine clinic

- Midwife/doctor antenatal appointments at 16, 25, 28, 31, 34, 36 & 38 weeks, gestation with additional medical clinic appointments as needed
- At every visit monitor BP and fetal growth using symphysis pubis height and analyse urine for proteinuria. Observe for signs of PE
- Drugs: 75 mg aspirin daily from 12 weeks. Adjust antihypertensive therapy to maintain BP <150/100 mmHg
- Continued assessment and management of coexisting conditions throughout pregnancy and following birth
- Diet: advise low sodium intake
- Additional fetal assessment: arrange ultrasound assessment of fetal growth & amniotic fluid volume, plus Doppler assessment of umbilical artery velocimetry at 28–30 weeks' and 32–34 weeks' gestation. Do not repeat unless clinical indication

- Labour: Induce at 37 weeks or earlier if BP remains elevated, fetal compromise is detected or other antenatal complications develop
  Monitoring: hourly maternal BP and continuous fetal monitoring
  Drugs: adjust antihypertensive medication to maintain safe BP. Consider use of epidural
  Birth: normal if possible. Intervention to shorten length of 2nd stage only if severe hypertension develops. Use oxytocin for management of 3rd stage
- Postpartum: encourage breastfeeding. Monitor BP daily for first 3 days and then on day 5. Adjust medication to maintain BP below 140/90. Medical review prior to discharge to resume prepregnant drug therapy and midwifery visits at home should continue until BP appears acceptable. Medical review at 2 & 6 weeks following birth. Appropriate contraception should be discussed and advice on lifestyle factors given

Box 35.3 Risk factors for developing pre-eclampsia.

- Extremes of maternal age <20 & >40 years
- First pregnancy or first pregnancy with current partner
- Family history of pre-eclampsia
- Previous history of pre-eclampsia
- Maternal obesity
- Pre-existing medical condition, e.g. hypertension, diabetes, renal disease
- Medical condition that develops in pregnancy, e.g. gestational hypertension, diabetes
- Multiple pregnancy
- Assisted conception

Box 35.4 Investigations following diagnosis of PE.

Urine: Following a positive result for protein using a dipstix:
- A midstream specimen of urine should be obtained to exclude a urinary tract infection
- Test to quantify the amount of protein present in urine, e.g. 24-hour collection. A significant level of protein is >300 mg of protein/total urine output in 24 hours. Alternatively a urinary protein: creatinine ratio of 30 mg/mmol is considered significant

Blood:
- Full blood count – haemoglobin level may appear raised in comparison to what might be expected from previous readings as a result of haemo-concentration. Normally haemoglobin levels appear to drop during pregnancy as a result of the haemodilution that occurs due to the expansion of the plasma volume being greater than the increase in red blood cells; this occurs as a normal physiological change in pregnancy
- Urea and electrolytes – these provides some indication of renal function
- Liver enzymes to assess hepatic function

Ultrasound:
- Assessment of fetal growth and liquor volume
- Doppler velocimetry of the umbilical arteries

A systolic blood pressure of ≥140 mmHg and/or a diastolic blood pressure of ≥90 mmHg are indicative of hypertension in pregnancy. Elevation of blood pressure is a frequently encountered problem within midwifery practice and is likely to be due to one of the following hypertensive conditions:

- Chronic hypertension (CHT)
- Gestational hypertension (GH)
- Pre-eclampsia (PE).

Hypertensive disorders in pregnancy are associated with poorer outcomes for both mothers and babies. Hypertension in pregnancy continues to be one of the main causes of maternal death in the UK and is also associated with increased maternal morbidity, such as antepartum haemorrhage, eclampsia and HELLP syndrome (haemolysis, elevated liver enzymes and low platelet count), with women often requiring admission to intensive care units. Maternal hypertension, particularly CHT, is associated with an increased risk of cardiovascular disease in later life. Hypertension in pregnancy, and PE in particular, are associated with increased risk of stillbirth, prematurity and restricted fetal growth (Part 9).

Chronic hypertension

CHT will have existed prior to the pregnancy but may have gone unrecognised. For the majority of women with CHT there will be no obvious cause and their hypertension will be classified as essential hypertension. This form of hypertension is more common amongst older women and is linked to risk factors including family history and obesity (Chapter 38). If women are aware that they have CHT prior to pregnancy they may have had a preconceptual referral to assess their condition and any comorbidity such as renal disease. Any antihypertensive medication should be reviewed and modified prior to conception as some drugs, particularly angiotensin-converting enzyme (ACE) inhibitors and angiotensin-11 receptor blockers, are associated with an increased risk of congenital abnormalities. Some women presenting for antenatal care will be unaware that they suffer from CHT and the normal fall in blood pressure that occurs in pregnancy may make these women appear normotensive at the time of booking. Hypertension occurring later in pregnancy may then be attributed wrongly to gestational hypertension.

Gestational hypertension

Hypertension presenting after 20 weeks' gestation without proteinuria is classified as gestational hypertension. Both CHT and GH share the same complications (Box 35.1) and with the exception of initial management are likely to be managed similarly (Box 35.2).

Pre-eclampsia

Hypertension presenting after 20 weeks' gestation with significant proteinuria is classified as PE. The aetiology is unclear but abnormalities in early placental development appear to be associated with the development of the condition. The overall incidence is 3% of all pregnancies with the majority of cases occurring in either first time mothers or mothers having a first pregnancy with a new partner (Box 35.3). The likelihood of it reoccurring in a subsequent pregnancy relates to the severity of the condition and the gestation at which delivery occurred. In women with a history of severe PE requiring delivery before 28 weeks' gestation, the incidence of reoccurrence may be as high as 55%. In addition to women with a history of PE in a previous pregnancy, women with a history of CHT, chronic renal disease, diabetes (type 1 or 2) (Chapter 36) or an autoimmune disease, in particular systemic lupus erythematosus (Chapter 40) or antiphospholipid syndrome, are considered to be at particular risk of developing PE. Underlying medical disorders should be considered in these high-risk women and as with women diagnosed with CHT or GH the use of low-dose aspirin: 75 mg per day should be advised from the 12th week of gestation. Not all women who develop PE will be high risk and the midwife must be vigilant to the clinical features. In the early stages women tend to feel well so the onset is usually recognised from the following signs:

- A raised diastolic blood pressure >90 mmHg or a raised systolic blood pressure >140 mmHg
- Proteinuria
- Oedema.

Many women experience ankle oedema but the oedema of PE tends to be more generalised, affecting the face, fingers, abdomen, sacrum and pretibial area. Tightening of rings, a ring mark left on the abdomen following auscultation with a Pinard stethoscope and pitting oedema over the lower legs are frequently observed and should be taken seriously, particularly if the onset is sudden. Women presenting with the above signs should be referred urgently to a consultant obstetrician for investigations (Box 35.4). Following diagnosis a continuous programme of maternal and fetal monitoring and drug therapy will be instigated with women being involved in decisions regarding their care. Depending on the severity of PE, labour is likely to be induced at 37 weeks or earlier. When preterm delivery is required, maturation of the fetal lungs through the use of corticosteroid therapy is recommended.

Antihypertensive drug therapy should continue throughout labour. The use of an epidural is often helpful in controlling blood pressure during labour but a platelet count should be performed before this is done. With the exception of women with severe PE that has not responded to treatment there is no need to limit the length of the second stage of labour. Following birth, regular blood pressure measurement and review of antihypertensive medication should continue (Box 35.2).

Sometimes PE may become severe with a blood pressure of ≥160/110 being noted on two occasions accompanied by significant levels of proteinuria. Additional features such as epigastric pain, severe headache, visual disturbance, vomiting and papilloedema may be noted. A low platelet count of $< 100 \times 10^6$/l and elevated liver enzymes may be seen. Urgent treatment with i.v. antihypertensive drugs and magnesium sulphate is usually required to prevent eclamptic convulsions occurring. It should be noted that whilst the incidence of eclamptic seizures is quite low it has an associated morbidity and can occur up to 6 weeks after birth, even one without a history of PE. Eclampsia requires emergency management to maintain the airway and the administration of anticonvulsant drugs. Another significant complication of severe PE that may occur in the last trimester or postnatal period is the HELLP syndrome. This is a multisystem disorder that is associated with high maternal and perinatal morbidity.

36 Diabetes

Box 36.1 Risk factors for gestational diabetes.

- Body mass index above 30 kg/m^2
- Previous macrosomic baby weighing 4.5 kg or above
- Previous gestational diabetes
- Family history of diabetes (first-degree relative with diabetes)
- Family origin with a high prevalence of diabetes:
  - South Asian (specifically women whose country of family origin is India, Pakistan or Bangladesh)
  - Black Caribbean
  - Middle Eastern (specifically women whose country of family origin is Saudi Arabia, United Arab Emirates, Iraq, Jordan, Syria, Oman, Qatar, Kuwait, Lebanon or Egypt)

Box 36.2 Information on gestational diabetes testing.

- In most women, gestational diabetes will respond to changes in diet and exercise
- Some women (between 10% and 20%) will need oral hypoglycaemic agents or insulin therapy if diet and exercise are not effective
- If gestational diabetes is not detected and controlled there is a small risk of birth
- Complications such as shoulder dystocia
- A diagnosis of gestational diabetes may lead to increased monitoring and interventions during both pregnancy and labour

Box 36.3 Information on how diabetes can affect pregnancy and how pregnancy can affect diabetes.

- The role of diet, body weight and exercise
- The risks of hypoglycaemia and hypoglycaemia during pregnancy
- How nausea and vomiting in pregnancy can affect glycaemic control
- The increased risk of having a baby who is large for gestational age, which increases the likelihood of birth trauma, induction of labour and caesarean section
- The need for assessment of diabetic retinopathy before and during pregnancy
- The need for assessment of diabetic nephropathy before pregnancy
- The importance of maternal glycaemic control during labour and birth and early feeding of the baby in order to reduce the risk of neonatal hypoglycaemia
- The possibility of transient morbidity in the baby during the neonatal period, which may require admission to the neonatal unit
- The risk of the baby developing obesity and/or diabetes in later life

Diabetes refers to a medical disorder of the metabolism of carbohydrates. Carbohydrate metabolism and glucose homeostasis are complex processes that need to be understood in order to provide best care for childbearing women. Energy metabolism requires the interplay of several hormones: insulin, glucagon, adrenaline, growth hormone and glucocorticoid. The actions of insulin and glucagon maintain the blood glucose level within a small range (3–5 mmol/l), but in diabetes the metabolism of carbohydrates does not work in this way, often requiring insulin therapy.

Diabetes is a significant health problem for childbearing women. Pregnancy is a challenge for women with diabetes irrespective of when it developed, but advances in medical science have resulted in better outcomes, allowing women to conceive and have a healthy pregnancy.

Pre-existing diabetes

Women with pre-existing diabetes who are planning to become pregnant need to establish good glycaemic control before conception and continue this throughout pregnancy; therefore individualised dietary advice should be offered. This will reduce but not eliminate the risk of miscarriage, congenital malformation, stillbirth and neonatal death.

In conjunction with routine antenatal care of the healthy pregnant woman, those with diabetes need individualised targets for self-monitoring of blood glucose which should be agreed with the woman, taking into account the risk of hypoglycaemia. Women should aim to keep fasting blood glucose between 3.5 and 5.9 mmol/l and 1-hour postprandial blood glucose below 7.8 mmol/l during pregnancy to be safe.

Specialised intrapartum care for women with diabetes should be given in conjunction with care given to healthy women and their babies during childbirth. Pregnant women with diabetes who have a normally grown fetus should be offered elective birth through induction of labour, or by elective caesarean section if indicated, after 38 completed weeks. However, diabetes should not be considered a contraindication to a vaginal birth after a previous caesarean section. Pregnant women with diabetes who have an ultrasound-diagnosed macrocosmic fetus should be informed of the risks and benefits of vaginal birth, induction of labour and caesarean section. Women with comorbidities such as obesity or autonomic neuropathy should be offered an anaesthetic assessment in the third trimester of pregnancy. If general anaesthesia is used for the birth, blood glucose should be monitored regularly (every 30 minutes) from induction of general anaesthesia until after the baby is born and the woman is fully conscious. During labour and birth, capillary blood glucose should be monitored on an hourly basis and maintained at between 4 and 7 mmol/l.

Women with diabetes or women whose blood glucose is not maintained at between 4 and 7 mmol/l should be considered for intravenous dextrose and insulin infusion from the onset of established labour.

It is important to reduce women's insulin immediately after birth and their blood glucose levels should be monitored carefully to establish the appropriate dose. Additionally, women should be informed that they are at increased risk of hypoglycaemia in the postnatal period, especially when breastfeeding and are therefore advised to have a meal or snack available before or during feeds. Women with pre-existing type 2 diabetes who are breastfeeding can resume or continue to take metformin and glibenclamide immediately following birth but other oral hypoglycaemic agents should be avoided while breastfeeding. It is advised that breastfeeding women continue to avoid any drugs for the treatment of diabetes complications that were discontinued for safety reasons in the preconception period. Referral back to their routine diabetes care arrangements should be made. Babies of women with diabetes should be kept with their mothers unless there is a clinical complication or abnormal clinical signs that require admission for intensive or special care. Blood glucose testing should be carried out routinely in babies of women with diabetes at 2–4 hours after birth.

Gestational diabetes

Midwives need to be aware of the risk factors for gestational diabetes (GD) (Box 36.1), and when screening for risk during routine antenatal care, offer those women at increased risk testing for GD. In order to make an informed decision about screening and testing for GD, women need to be provided with all the relevant information available (Box 36.2). When screening for GD the 2-hour 75 g oral glucose tolerance test (OGTT) should be used and diagnosis made using the criteria defined by the World Health Organisation. Women who have had GD in a previous pregnancy should be offered early self-monitoring of blood glucose or an OGTT at 16–18 weeks, and a further OGTT at 28 weeks if the results are normal. Women with any of the other risk factors for GD (Box 36.1) should be offered an OGTT at 24–28 weeks.

It is beneficial to demonstrate to women how to self-monitor blood glucose and for them to understand targets for blood glucose control in the same way as for women with pre-existing diabetes. Additionally, women with GD should be informed that good glycaemic control throughout pregnancy will reduce the risk of fetal macrosomia, trauma during birth (to themselves and the baby), induction of labour or caesarean section, neonatal hypoglycaemia and perinatal death. As such, it is important to inform women about the possibility of transient morbidity in the baby during the neonatal period requiring an admission to the neonatal unit and the risk of the baby developing obesity and/or diabetes in later life. Women with GD require advice on diet, calorie intake and possibly hypoglycaemic therapy. This therapy may include regular insulin, rapid-acting insulin analogues and/or oral hypoglycaemic agents tailored to the glycaemic profile of, and acceptability to, the individual woman (Box 36.3). Women diagnosed with GD should discontinue hypoglycaemic treatment immediately after birth and they require having their blood glucose tested to exclude persisting hyperglycaemia before they are transferred to community care.

37 Thromboembolic disease

Figure 37.1 Virchow's triad and contributing factors to thromboembolism in childbearing women.

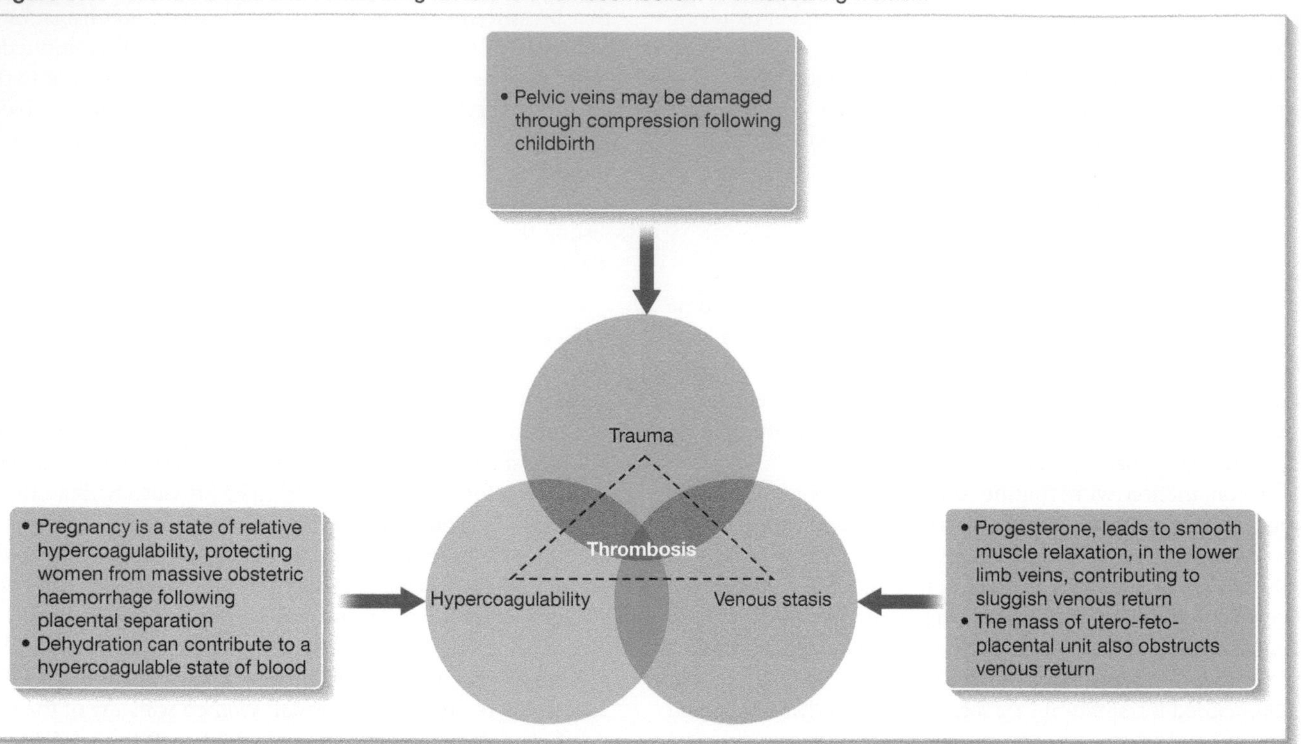

Table 37.1 Additional risk factors for VTE.

Non-pregnancy related	Pregnancy related
Personal or family history of VTE	Caesarean section
Obesity (BMI >30 kg/m^2)	Maternal age >35 years
Prolonged bed rest/reduced mobility	Multiparous women
Surgery	Multiple pregnancies
Present major illness (cardiac, pulmonary, cancer)	Sepsis
Inherited thrombophilias (e.g. factor V Leiden)	Pre-eclampsia
Sickle cell disease	Reduced mobility
Long haul flights	Dehydration (secondary to hyperemesis and diarrhoea and vomiting for example)
Smoking	Surgical procedures during pregnancy
Combined oral contraceptive pill	Massive obstetric haemorrhage

Venous thromboembolism (VTE) is a collective term for a group of inter-related coagulation disorders (coagulopathies) including deep vein thrombosis (DVT), pulmonary embolism (PE) and cerebral and venous thrombosis (CVT) (Bothamley & Boyle, 2009; Meetoo, 2010; Moatti et al., 2014).

Pathophysiology

The development of VTE was shown by German physician, Rudolph Virchow, in the 19th century to be provoked by three factors, known collectively as Virchows. The triad consists of hypercoagulability, trauma and venous stasis (Figure 37.1). Childbearing women are at 10 times' greater risk of developing VTE than their non-pregnant counterparts of the same age; their highest risk of developing VTE is during the puerperium. This is because pregnancy is characterised by haematological adaptations including a reduction of naturally occurring anticoagulants in the maternal circulation and decreased fibrinolysis. These haemostatic changes of pregnancy produce a low-grade, continuous activation of the coagulation system from the end of the first trimester in the uteroplacental circulation. This prevents massive obstetric haemorrhage following the third stage of labour.

Increased secretion of progesterone during pregnancy causes smooth muscle relaxation, with consequent sluggish venous return from the lower limbs, leading to venous stasis. The mass of the gravid uterus, as well as the turbulence produced by the vascular feto-utero-placental unit, also further disrupts venous return and contributes to venous stasis. Whilst voluntary muscle contraction in physically active individuals helps to encourage venous return from the limbs, increasing immobility towards the end of pregnancy contributes to venous stasis.

Vaginal birth and operative delivery can lead to endothelial damage in the maternal pelvic vessels. Childbearing women may also experience additional risk factors for VTE (Table 37.1).

Classification of VTE

A blood clot or thrombus consists of erythrocytes and platelets enmeshed within polymerised strands of the plasma protein fibrin. DVT, also known as phlebothrombosis, is an obstruction of one of the deep veins with a thrombus. In around half of cases, people with DVTs experience symptoms such as unilateral swelling of the affected calf to a circumference more than 2 cm greater than the unaffected calf, localised deep muscle pain, erythema (tissue redness), pitting oedema, low-grade pyrexia, groin pain or lower abdominal pain. However, around half of cases are asymptomatic.

An embolus is a thrombus that has become detached by the continued, sheer forces of blood flowing past it. It becomes a PE once it reaches the lungs and occludes the pulmonary artery, or one of its branches. This may lead to collapse and hypotension, or even death, providing the embolus is sufficiently large. However, smaller PEs can express much less specific symptoms and become difficult to diagnose.

CVT is the formation of thrombi in the cerebral sinuses. Although rare, affecting 11.6 per 100 000 deliveries, it is three times more common in women than men, particularly in childbearing women or those taking the oral contraceptive. Symptoms of CVT vary based on site of occurrence. Where the cerebral cortical vein is affected patients may experience intracranial hypertension and impaired cerebrospinal fluid absorption which leads to headache vomiting and swelling of the optic disc. A CVT in the cavernous sinus may cause eye pain and exophthalmos.

Identification

Thrombosis and thromboembolism have been documented as leading causes of direct maternal deaths. Therefore, it is imperative that midwives, obstetricians and GPs recognise symptoms, facilitate accurate diagnosis and initiate prompt treatment. This will involve undertaking a thorough patient history and performing a physical examination. It is recommended that 'Any woman with symptoms and/or signs suggestive of VTE should have objective testing performed expeditiously and treatment with low-molecular-weight heparin (LMWH) given … until the diagnosis is excluded by objective testing…' (RCOG, 2015). This objective diagnosis of VTE should also be subject to an agreed protocol in the maternity units, including appropriate referral pathways and professional involvement.

Objective testing for DVT consists of compression duplex ultrasonography of the proximal limb veins. If the ultrasound is negative, but there is still a high level of clinical suspicion of a DVT, treatment with LMWH should persist until after a repeat ultrasound can be carried out on days 3 and 7.

Women who show symptoms and signs of acute PE should first have an electrocardiogram (ECG) administered and then a chest X-ray. If they also have signs and symptoms of DVT, objective testing by compression ultrasound should occur. If positive for a DVT, then continue to treat for VTE. If the woman has no symptoms of DVT, then a ventilation/perfusion scan of the lungs (V/Q) or a computerised tomography pulmonary angiogram (CTPA) should be performed. If there is no sign of a DVT, in the presence of symptoms of PE and abnormal chest X-ray, a CTPA should be performed. CT venography and magnetic resonance imaging (MRI) are used to confirm CVT.

Prevention and thromboprophylaxis

Midwifery must include awareness of childbearing women's increased risks of developing VTE and being vigilant in identifying additional risk factors (Table 37.1). The Royal College of Obstetricians and Gynaecologists (RCOG) recommend that every pregnant women, or even those actively planning pregnancy (or having fertility treatment), should receive a document risk assessment for VTE during early pregnancy or prepregnancy. Their risk status should be reviewed whenever the woman is admitted to hospital and if she develops an illness or complication during the intrapartum periods or in the early postpartum period. Thromboprophylaxis includes the use of graduated compressions stockings, and the administration of LMWH. Health promotion on mobilisation and hydration and self-administration of LMWH is also part of the midwife's role.

38 Obesity

Box 38.1 Prepregnancy counselling.

- Women with obesity have an increased risk of having a baby with congenital malformations, including neural tube defects
- Accurate weight and height measurement
- Information about the risks of obesity in pregnancy and childbirth
- Advice and support to lose weight
- Advice on appropriate supplementation prior to conception (5 mg folic acid and 10 μg vitamin D)

Box 38.2 Folic acid supplementation and vitamin D.

- 5 mg folic acid at least 1 month before conception
- Current recommendations all women to have 10 μm of vitamin D daily

Table 38.1 Weight gain in pregnancy for different BMI categories.

Weight category	BMI	Recommended weight gain during pregnancy	Mean kg/week
Underweight	<18.5	12.5–18 kg	0.5
Normal weight	18.5–24.9	11.5–16 kg	0.4
Overweight	25–29.9	7.0–11.5 kg	0.3
Obese	>30	5.0–9.0 kg	0.2

Tackling obesity is a major public health issue in the UK as levels of obesity have grown by 400% in last 25 years. For example, since 1980, figures have risen in England from 8% of women being obese to 21% of women in 1998. More current figures show that around 26% of all women in the UK are classified as obese. Predictions are that by 2050, 50% of women, 60% of men and 25% of children will be obese.

Obesity occurs when energy intake (food and drink) is greater than expenditure (such as exercise and metabolism), causing a build-up of fat cells which are stored as additional body fat. Food and drink energy is measured in kilocalories (kcal) and the recommended intake changes throughout life, but 2000 kcal daily is generally recommended for women of childbearing age. In pregnancy, expected weight gain differs for the various body mass index (BMI) categories (a classification to define weight risk) (Table 38.1).

Weight, height and calculating BMI

- At booking record BMI in hand-held notes and electronic patient system
- Discuss health lifestyle if BMI >30 – offer patient information leaflet (Chapter 74)
- Discuss weight gain
- Anaesthetist referral if BMI >40 or 100 kg
- Weigh at 36 weeks to make appropriate plans for equipment and delivery
- Weigh on admission to delivery suite – calculation of drugs required during labour.

As a disease, obesity can affect many organs in the body, causing chronic problems. For example, excessive fat around the abdominal area is known to be associated with an increased risk of diabetes and cardiovascular problems. Recommendations from the Confidential Enquiry into Child and Maternal Health (CEMACH), Centre for Maternal and Child Enquiries (CMACE) and National Institute for Health and Care Excellence (NICE) reports advise that obesity is also related to health risks which can be further compounded by pregnancy.

Risks of obesity to childbearing women

- Spontaneous first trimester and recurrent miscarriage
- Increased likelihood of caesarean section (37%) and post-caesarean wound infection
- Pre-eclampsia – BMI >35 doubles the risk
- Gestational diabetes – BMI >30 = threefold increase
- Increased likelihood of induction of labour (33%)
- Thromboembolism
- Increased risk of postpartum haemorrhage (38%)
- Maternal death or severe morbidity
- Low breastfeeding rates (56%).

Risks of maternal obesity to fetus/infant

- Stillbirth – increase × 4.7
- Prematurity due to maternal medical conditions not spontaneous delivery
- Neonatal death – increase × 2.6
- Congenital anomalies – increase × 2
- Fetal origins of adult disease
- Life course of infant.

Obesity is therefore an issue that midwives could help address throughout the preconception, pregnancy and postnatal periods by providing advice and support. For example, midwives can help provide advice regarding healthy eating and encourage weight loss preconception, where necessary (Box 38.1), and discuss the need for folic acid supplementation and vitamin D (Box 38.2).

Information to give during pregnancy

- Risks of obesity
- Poor ultrasound visualisation
- Increased risk of induction of labour and C section
- Fetal monitoring, anaesthesia and C section require senior obstetric and anaesthetic involvement
- Prioritise safety of mother at all times
- Importance of healthy eating and exercise (30 min/day)
- Importance of breastfeeding.

Surveillance and screening in pregnancy

- BMI >30 – glucose tolerance at 24–28 weeks
- BMI ≥35 – risk factors for pre-eclampsia
- Commence aspirin 75 mg daily from 12 weeks.

Thromboembolism and thromboprophylaxis

- Women with booking BMI ≥30 should be assessed at first antenatal visit and throughout pregnancy for risk of thromboembolism
- Antenatal and post-delivery thromboprophylaxis should be considered
- Women with BMI ≥30 should mobilise as early as possible following childbirth
- All women with BMI ≥40 should be offered postnatal thromboprophylaxis regardless of mode of delivery.

Place and mode of birth

- BMI ≥35 – consultant-led obstetric unit
- BMI ≥30–34.9 – individual risk assessment
- BMI ≥40 – assessed to identify any extra staff, equipment and facilities required during childbirth.

Challenges for the midwife

- Feeling confident in raising the subject
- Moving and handling issues
- Equipment sourcing: scales; correct size BP cuffs
- Difficulty in accurate palpation
- Monitoring fetal wellbeing
- Reducing choices for birth: place, position
- More time needed – increased appointments; length of time at appointments; increased number of visits.

39 The thyroid gland and thyroid disorders

Figure 39.1 Thyroid gland location and internal structure.

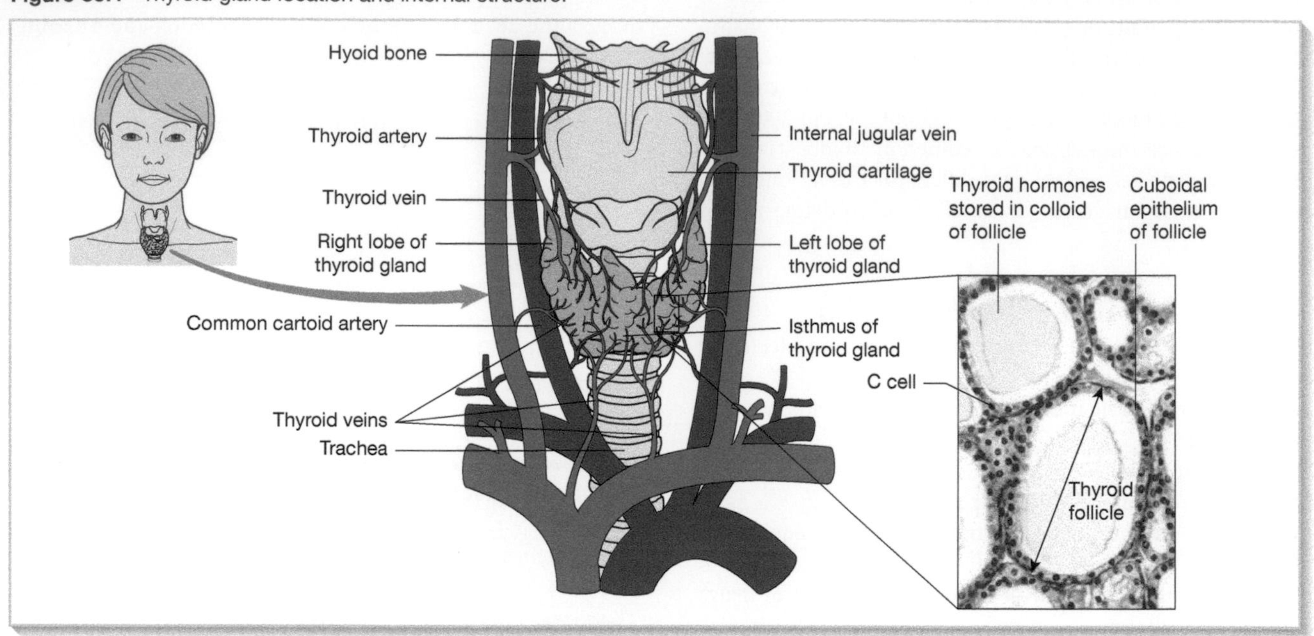

Figure 39.2 The thyroid hormones.

The thyroid gland secretes two metabolically active thyroid hormones. One contains four iodine (I) atoms, tetra-iodothyronine (thyroxine or T_4) and the other contains three iodine atoms, tri-iodothyronine (T_3)

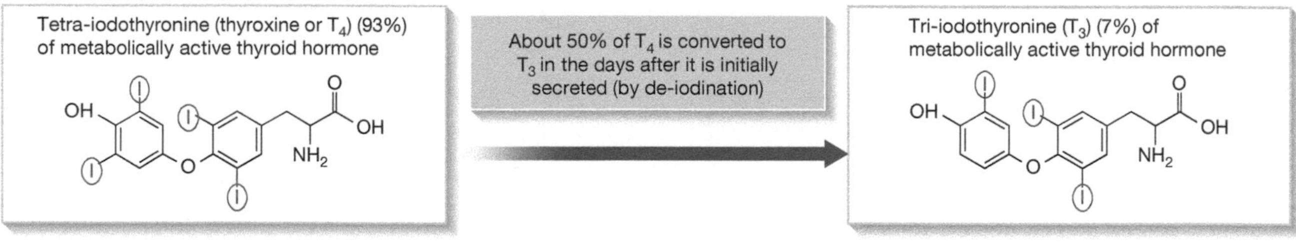

Figure 39.3 Thyroid hormone production is controlled by negative feedback.

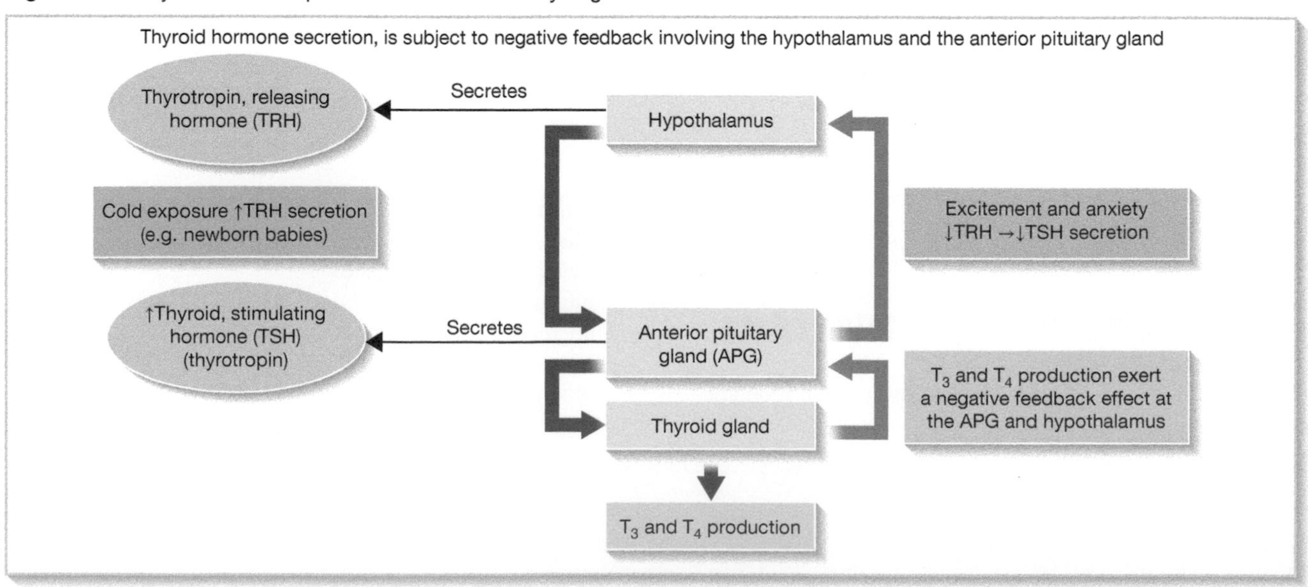

Thyroid gland

The thyroid gland is an important endocrine gland that has widespread effects on bodily metabolism, growth and development. It lies immediately inferior to the thyroid cartilage of the larynx. It consists of two lobes connected by a narrow stalk of tissue – the isthmus, giving it its characteristic butterfly shape (Figure 39.1). The thyroid gland is surrounded by a capsule of connective tissue and has the capacity to store large quantities of the hormones it secretes for around 3 months. Follicles within the thyroid gland contain colloid – mainly consisting of a glycoprotein called thyroglobulin, which is a macromolecular precursor for the two metabolically active thyroid hormones. Thyroglobulin consists of 140 molecules of the amino acid tyrosine. The thyroid hormones are produced by the follicular cells of the thyroid gland, in a stepwise fashion, with the rate-limiting step being the energy-dependent process of iodide trapping. Iodine is obtained from the diet. In the follicular cells this is bound to tyrosine molecules forming thyroid prohormones and eventually the two metabolically active thyroid hormones thyroxine (tetra-iodothyronine or T_4 with four iodine ions) and tri-iodothyronine (T_3 with three iodine atoms) (Figure 39.2). Only T_4 and T_3 are released into the bloodstream from the thyroid gland. T_4 accounts for about 90% and T_3 about 10% of the thyroid hormones released into the circulation, although probably only T_3 is metabolically active. About 80% of T_3 is derived from the de-iodination of T_4, in the kidneys and the liver. T_4 and T_3 are bound to plasma proteins, for transport, including thyroxine-binding globulin (TBG) and albumin. The secretion of T_4 and T_3 is controlled through negative feedback from the hypothalamic–pituitary–thyroid axis (Figure 39.3). Thyrotropin-releasing hormone (TRH) from the hypothalamus acts on the anterior pituitary gland (APG) to activate the secretion of thyroid-stimulating hormone (TSH), also called thyrotropin. TSH then initiates the breakdown of thyroglobulin into the active thyroid hormones, and their release into the bloodstream, from the thyroid follicles.

T_4 and T_3 stimulate the production of numerous proteins – enzymes, structural or transport proteins – as well as many other substances, in almost all body cells. Thyroid hormones increase the basal metabolic rate and protein synthesis in most tissues of the body (except the spleen, retinas and lungs). Their effects include increased heat production in the cells, tissues and organs – a calorigenic effect – and increased oxygen consumption. They accelerate catabolism of glucose, lipids and proteins and increase glucose absorption from the gastrointestinal tract. T_4 and T_3 are essential for normal growth, development and maturation, including skeletal and neurological development during fetal life and childhood. Cardiovascular effects include increased heart rate and cardiac contractility and decreased peripheral resistance, which relate partly to increased tissue responsiveness to catecholamines. Thyroid hormones increase wakefulness, memory and alertness, as well as reflex responsiveness. Thyroid hormones are also essential for allowing normal reproductive function.

During pregnancy, free T_4 and T_3 levels increase transiently in the first trimester, corresponding with increased levels of human chorionic gonadotropin (HCG). Concurrently, the first trimester embryo and fetus receives its supply of thyroid hormones exclusively via the placenta. From 10 to 12 weeks' gestation the fetal thyroid begins to concentrate iodine and synthesise thyroid hormones.

Thyroid disorders

Thyroid disorders are more prevalent in women than in men; and are the second most common endocrine disorder of pregnancy in women of childbearing age. It is estimated that 0.3–0.5% of women have overt hypothyroidism (an underactive thyroid gland) during pregnancy, and 2–3% have subclinical hypothyroidism. About 5–15% of women of childbearing age are found to have thyroid autoantibodies. Chronic autoimmune thyroiditis is the main contributing factor to hypothyroidism during pregnancy. Maternity care is normally with the multidisciplinary team: obstetric, medical and midwifery.

Hypothyroidism reduces the basal metabolic rate, leads to myxoedematous features (dry, firm waxy skin), non-pitting oedema of the mucous membranes and a deep voice. There is decreased responsiveness to catecholamine stimulus; women may experience mental and physical sluggishness, and increased somnolence (sleepiness). The heart rate and cardiac output are also reduced. The gastrointestinal system becomes sluggish, leading to constipation and reduced appetite. Muscle tone and reflexes are suppressed. Metabolically, the patient experiences hypoventilation (reduced respiration rate and depth) and cold intolerance. Hair texture becomes coarse and dry, as does the skin. Weight gain is another consequence. Treatment involves oral levothyroxine sodium (50–100 μg once daily), and iodine supplementation of the diet.

Dietary iodine intake is essential for optimal thyroid hormone production; pregnancy and lactation increase bodily iodine demands for the production of thyroid hormones. Severe iodine deficiency in pregnancy is associated with congenital disorders related to poor fetal brain development and severe mental retardation. Studies have shown that women of childbearing age in the UK are an at-risk group for suboptimal intake of dietary iodine and thus hypothyroidism goitre, a swelling of the thyroid gland, can occur in response to iodine deficiency as the thyroid gland grows to increase thyroid hormone production. Poorly controlled hypothyroidism during pregnancy can also result in pregnancy-induced hypertension, intrauterine growth restriction (IUGR) (Chapters 55 and 56) and fetal death.

Hyperthyroidism affects about 0.05–2% of women. It is most commonly caused by Graves' disease and autoimmune disorder affecting 5–10-fold more women than men, with its highest prevalence during reproductive years, in countries with plentiful dietary iodine intake. Its symptoms include exophthalmos, fatigue, heat intolerance, emotional lability, insomnia, polyphagia, sweating, tachypnoea, palpitations, ankle oedema and widening of pulse pressure; many of which mimic pregnancy symptoms. Increased free T_4 levels have been implicated in the nausea and vomiting of pregnancy and hyperemesis and correlate with increased HCG levels. Treatment involves antithyroid drugs (thioamides), surgical removal or thyroid destruction with the radioisotope ^{131}I. Propylthiouracil is less likely to cross the placenta than carbimazole and is usually considered the preferred antithyroid drug. Symptomatic relief can be given through beta-blockers, such as propranolol.

40 Systemic lupus erythematosus

Box 40.1 Symptoms of SLE.

- Fatigue
- Headaches
- Arthralgia/joint pains
- Fever/flu-like symptoms
- Weight loss
- Butterfly facial/cheek rash

Box 40.2 Diagnosis of SLE.

- **Full blood count (FBC):** May show neutropenia, thrombocytopenia and normochromic normocytic anaemia
- **Erythrocyte sedimentation rate (ESR):** Raised due to high immunoglobulin levels
- **CRP (C-reactive protein):** Normal
- **Antibodies:** Most common is antinuclear antibody (ANA). However, anti-Ro and anti-La are present in about 30% of women and anticardiolipin antibodies (aCLs) are present in about 40% of women and are of particular relevance to pregnancy

Box 40.3 Preconception considerations.

- Counselling
- Referral: obstetrician and rheumatologist
- Conception: advise during remission period
- Active lupus nephritis: awareness of additional pregnancy complications

Box 40.4 Complications in pregnancy.

- Increased risk of flares
- Identification and management of flares
- Pre-eclampsia
- Miscarriage
- IUGR
- Fetal loss
- Premature birth

Box 40.5 Postnatal.

- Increased risk of flare
- Differentiate between neuropsychiatric state and postnatal depression
- Prepregnancy drugs may need to be recommenced
- Lactation may be suppressed

Box 40.6 Midwifery care.

- Establish combined care
- Full history of disease and medications at booking
- Discuss risk of miscarriage or preterm birth
- Listen to the woman and address any concerns
- Antenatal monitoring of BP and urinalysis
- Promote diet rich in iron
- Encourage gentle exercise

Lupus erythematosus is an autoimmune condition whereby antibodies are produced against the body's own connective tissues. Often known as lupus, there are two common types: discoid lupus erythematosus (DLE) and systemic lupus erythematosus (SLE). This chapter is concerned with SLE, being the most common type affecting the whole body and including joints, skin, kidneys and serous membranes. Symptoms of SLE can be (Box 40.1):

- Fatigue
- Headaches
- Arthralgia
- Fever
- Weight loss
- Butterfly facial rash.

The immune system comprises a complex link of tissue, cells, chemicals and organs to provide a defence against organisms that cause disease. During pregnancy changes occur to the immune system and there is a balance between the body tolerating the fetus and protecting the mother and fetus from pathogens. In SLE antibodies which are normally produced to defend the body against viral and bacterial infections, attack the body's tissues. It is more commonly found in women of childbearing age, perhaps due to oestrogens promoting disease, with a high prevalence noted amongst the Afro-Caribbean population in the UK. It often appears for the first time in pregnancy or within the first 3 months postnatal. The exact cause of SLE is not entirely known but is thought to be connected to environmental issues and a genetic predisposition. SLE is of particular concern in pregnancy as it often worsens then; the presence of antiphospholipid antibodies increases the associated risks of miscarriage, intrauterine growth restriction (IUGR) (Chapters 55 and 56) and fetal loss. In addition, if there is associated kidney damage, there is an increased likelihood of morbidity and mortality.

Diagnosis

Diagnosis generally begins with clinical symptoms (Box 40.2) and approximately 90% of women with SLE have arthralgia and joint swelling. Diagnosis can be made more difficult in pregnancy due to additional pregnancy symptoms. Confirmation of the condition is by blood tests to detect circulating autoantibodies. See Box 40.2 for a more complete description of these.

Preconception

In order to facilitate assessment of a woman with SLE, preconception counselling is deemed essential (Box 40.3). This enables discussion and an accurate assessment of her current health to help prepare for pregnancy and reduce complications such as pre-eclampsia (Chapter 50), IUGR (Chapters 55 and 56) and preterm labour and birth (Chapter 49). Some additional considerations for advice are:

- Well balanced diet
- Avoid infections
- Avoid stressful situations
- Drugs as required for pain and disease flares
- Monitor bloods and urinalysis.

Pregnancy and birth

A multidisciplinary approach to antenatal care is recommended to improve the outcome of pregnancy for mother and baby. Combined care by midwives, obstetricians and physicians should include maternal disease monitoring and fetal growth such as examination of uterine artery Doppler blood flow (20–24 weeks) and umbilical artery blood flow (from 24 weeks) if the fetus is at risk. Maternal baseline values of full blood count (FBC), urea and electrolytes (U&E), serum creatinine and liver function tests (LFTs) should be established and serial measurements taken depending on disease progression. Disease flare rate in pregnancy differs between studies; however a general consensus is that it increases. Women who have discontinued maintenance medication or have had several episodes prepregnancy are more prone to flares in pregnancy (Box 40.4). However, flare symptoms can be confused with those of pregnancy and vice versa; for example, hair loss, erythema, fatigue, oedema, anaemia and a raised erythrocyte sedimentation rate (ESR) can occur. Care must be taken to ensure adequate function of the kidney, heart and central nervous system.

Complications in pregnancy depend on the level of disease and presence of lupus nephritis, hypertension and anti-Ro/La and antiphospholipid antibodies. Therefore, if the lupus is stable preconception, pregnancy complications are reduced. Overall, there is an increased risk of hypertensive problems in pregnancy and it can be challenging to differentiate between eclampsia and a lupus flare. However, lupus nephritis increases the risk of pre-eclampsia and preterm birth (Chapters 49 and 50). Fetal loss is increased with a raised antiphospholipid antibody titre, with the presence of lupus anticoagulant having the greatest association with recurrent fetal loss. However, for those women in remission with no hypertension or renal problems, the risk of pre-eclampsia and pregnancy loss is thought to be no higher than in the general population.

Although deemed as high risk, women with SLE in labour should be able to give birth vaginally if there are no obstetric complications. Continuous external fetal monitoring is required throughout labour, but can be midwife led.

Postnatal

There is an increased likelihood of a lupus flare during the postnatal period. If this occurs, it may be necessary for prepregnancy drugs to be recommenced. These pass into breast milk and discussions regarding suitability of some drugs for breastfeeding are required and adjustments made. Lactation can be suppressed due to corticosteroids and the disease process, whereas prolactin may add to an exacerbation of the condition. Lupus causes fatigue and following the birth of their baby women often become inordinately tired. It is important to differentiate between a neuropsychiatric state and the baby blues or postnatal depression (Box 40.5).

If a woman is anti-Ro/La positive, the neonate is at risk of being affected by neonatal lupus or congenital heart block.

Midwifery care

It is important for the midwife to be involved as part of the multidisciplinary team and ensure that combined care is established for women with SLE. At the booking visit a history of the condition and any medications should be noted. Pregnancy, postnatal risks and infant feeding need to be discussed and the woman notified of communication channels if she requires support or has any concerns (Box 40.6).

Obstetric cholestasis

Table 41.1 Normal serum bilirubin levels. Source: Adapted from NELSON-PIERCY, C. 2015, *Handbook of Obstetric Medicine*, 5th ed., London: CRC Press.

			Trimesters		
LFTs	**Non-pregnant**	**Pregnant**	**1**	**2**	**3**
Bilirubin (μmol/l)	0–17		4–16	3–13	3–14
Total protein (g/l)	64–86	48–64			
Albumin (g/l)	35–46	28–37			
AST (IU/l)	7–40		10–28	11–29	11–30
ALT (IU/l)	0–40	6–32			
GGT (IU/l)	11–50		5–37	5–43	3–41
ALP (IU/l)	30–130		32–100	43–135	133–418
Bile acids (μmol/l)	0–14	0–14			

Key: ALP, alkaline phosphatase; ALT, alanine aminotransferase; ASP, aspartate aminotransferase; GGT, gamma-glutamyl transpeptidase

Obstetric cholestasis (OC), also known as intrahepatic cholestasis of pregnancy, is one of several hepatic conditions that are peculiar to pregnancy. The main presenting features of OC are an extreme itch without a skin rash and abnormal liver function tests (LFTs) which have no apparent alternative explanation. Both resolve spontaneously postpartum. The aetiology of the condition appears complex with genetic, hormonal and environmental factors being implicated. The incidence appears to vary between populations. It occurs in 0.5–1.5% of pregnancies amongst European women; and is more common amongst Scandinavian and Polish populations. Globally, higher incidences are seen in women from South America, China, India and Pakistan. Many women developing OC have a family history of the condition. OC is associated with multiple pregnancies and also a history of pruritus before pregnancy in relation to combined oral contraception. This supports that view that increasing levels of reproductive hormones are linked to the development of OC. The presence of gall stones, selenium deficiency or a history of hepatitis C are also thought to be significant. Occurrence is said to be more common during the winter months.

The word stasis is indicative of a restricted flow. Cholestasis occurs when the flow of bile from the liver to the intestine is compromised, probably in connection with increasing levels of pregnancy hormones. Failure to excrete bile results in a build-up of bile salts in the blood. Left untreated hepatic failure may occur.

The condition usually presents after the 28th week of pregnancy; the first symptom is usually a severe generalised itch which appears on the palms and soles of the feet. Itching may also be experienced on the chest, back, face and in the ears and mouth. There is no accompanying rash although excoriation of the skin from scratching may be evident. The itching is particularly noticeable at night, resulting in sleep deprivation. Tiredness is therefore a common complaint. Women may complain of nausea and a poor appetite. Occasionally mild jaundice, pale stools and dark urine may be noted.

Diagnosis is made on the basis of presentation and elevated levels of bile acids and abnormal LFTs, although levels of serum bilirubin are usually normal (Table 41.1). Abnormal liver biochemistry may not become apparent for some time following the onset of symptoms. Monitoring of liver biochemistry should be repeated every 1–2 weeks if the pruritus continues and other possible causes for the pruritus such as hepatitis or eczema have been excluded. It is important that pregnancy-adjusted values are used in assessing liver function.

Women diagnosed with OC should be managed within a consultant-led unit as the potential for complications with this condition is considerable, particularly for the fetus. The incidence of fetal demise is increased and is usually sudden and difficult to predict with traditional monitoring methods such as estimation of growth and liquor volumes. Evidence for a relationship between elevated maternal liver enzymes and fetal death remains inconclusive although there is some evidence to suggest that elevated levels of maternal bile acids may be a more reliable predictor of fetal demise. The decision to deliver the pregnancy early to prevent stillbirth has to be balanced against the risks associated with early delivery. From the mother's perspective the main complications relate to discomfort and sleep deprivation. This combined with the possibility of stillbirth often has a negative impact on the mother's mental health. In addition, it has been suggested that women with OC may become deficient in fat-soluble vitamin K as a consequence of poor fat absorption resulting from reduced bile salts being available within the gut. As vitamin K is required for the generation of several clotting factors within the blood, OC is traditionally linked with an increased risk of postpartum haemorrhage for the mother and neonatal bleeding in the baby. Whilst the quality of evidence for the prophylactic use of water-soluble vitamin K is limited, it is considered prudent to discuss possible administration of vitamin K if a prolonged prothrombin time is evident.

Birth of the baby is the only effective way of reversing OC. Topical treatments to reduce itching, such as the use of emollients and calamine lotion, are safe to use in pregnancy and may provide relief for some women. The use of antihistamines may also provide a sedative effect to aid sleep. The use of ursodeoxycolic acid may be used to reduce pruritus and improve liver function but there is a lack of robust evidence to suggest it enhances the outcome for the fetus.

The incidence of spontaneous premature birth is probably not much higher amongst women with OC, however the decision to induce labour between 37 and38 weeks' gestation may be made. The evidence to support this intervention remains problematic, with the need to consider the risks associated with early delivery against the difficulties in predicting possible stillbirth if the pregnancy continues. Justification for induction is probably strengthened in cases of severe biochemical abnormality (bile acids > 40 μmol/l). The mother should be involved in the decision-making process regarding the timing and type of delivery. As there is an increased likelihood of the baby requiring care in a neonatal unit the mother and her partner may benefit from visiting the unit prior to delivery. As OC is associated with increased rates of fetal distress and the passage of meconium, continuous fetal monitoring throughout labour is recommended. The incidence of caesarean section associated with OC is high but it is difficult to differentiate OC as the cause of this from other factors such as other obstetric indications or patient anxiety. Following the birth of the baby, the mother should be followed up to ensure that the pruritus has resolved and LFTs have returned to normal. Symptoms normally resolve within 2 days of the birth but LFTs may remain elevated for over a week postpartum. Consequently follow-up should be deferred for 10 days following birth.

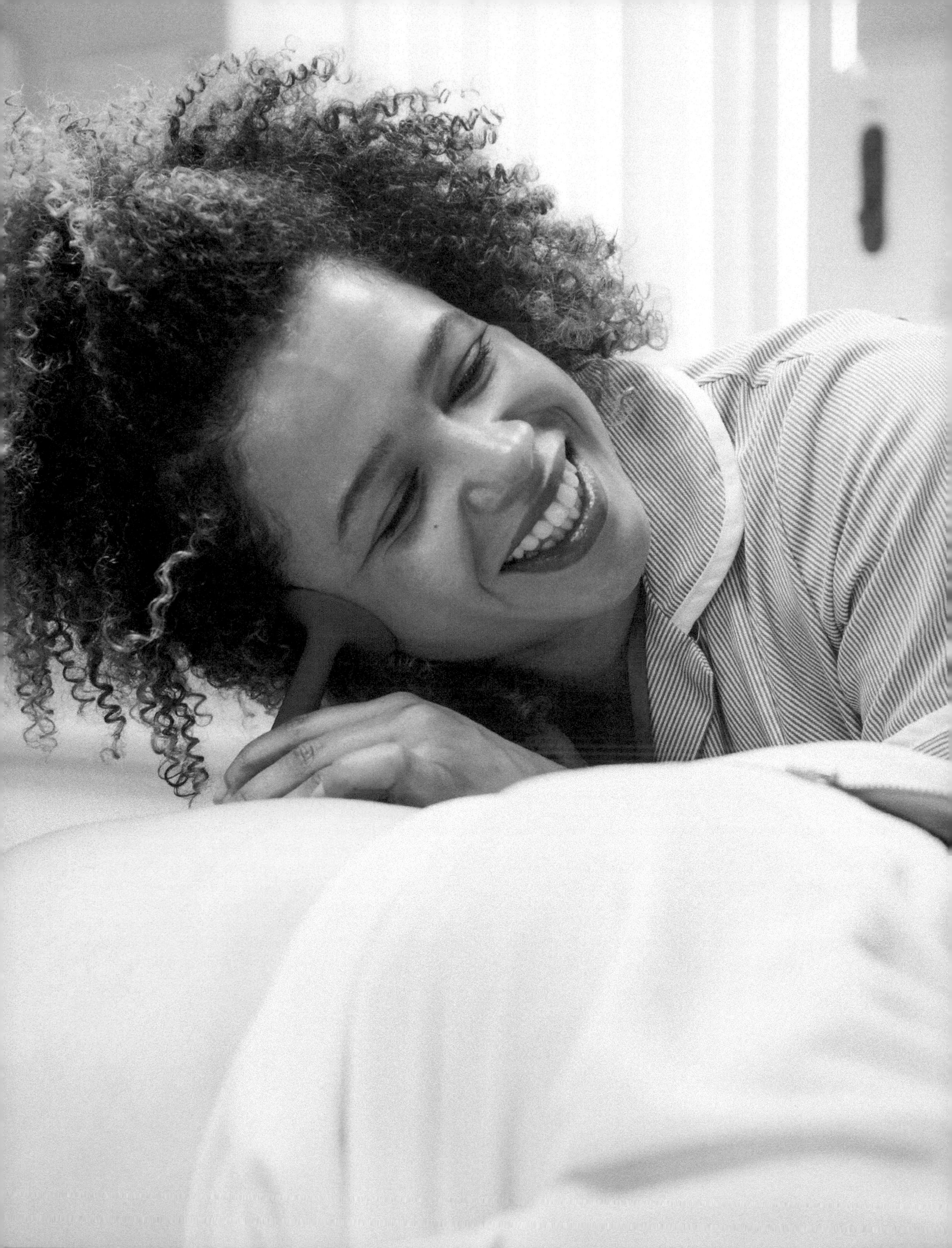

Obstetric complications

Chapters

42 Antepartum haemorrhage

Figure 42.1 Concealed placental abruption (20%).

Figure 42.2 Placenta praevia.

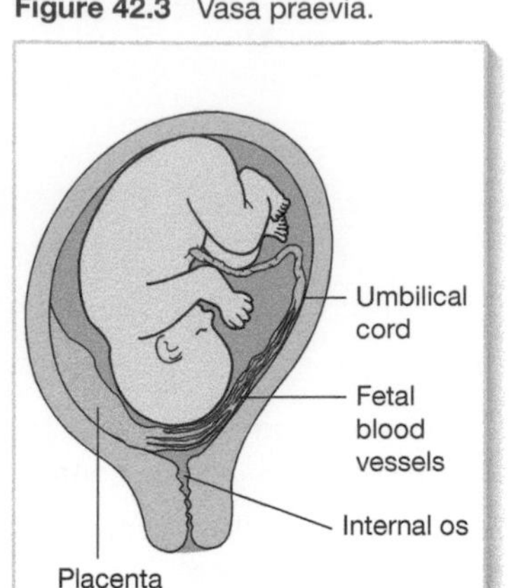

Figure 42.3 Vasa praevia.

Figure 42.4 Presentation of APH.

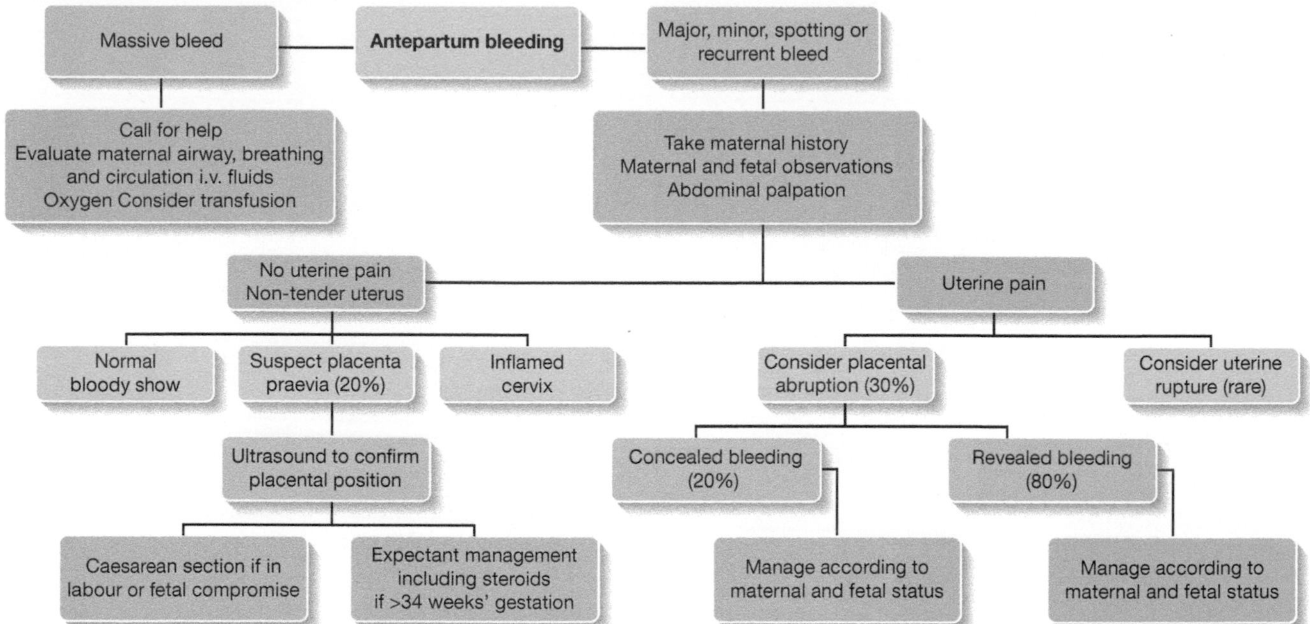

Table 42.1 Risk factors for placental abruption.

Maternal	Pregnancy	Social
Advanced maternal age	Polyhydramnios	Abdominal trauma (accidental & domestic violence)
Multiparity	Pre-eclampsia	Smoking & drug misuse (cocaine & amphetamines) during pregnancy
Low body mass index (BMI)	Fetal growth restriction	
Pregnancy following assisted reproductive techniques	Non-vertex presentations	
Previous placental abruption	Intrauterine infection	
	Premature rupture of membranes	
	First trimester bleeding associated with abruption	

Table 42.2 Risk factors for placenta praevia.

Maternal	Pregnancy	Social
Previous caesarean sections – risk increases with each caesarean birth	Multiple pregnancy	Smoking
Multiparity		
Advanced maternal age		
Previous termination of pregnancy		
Assisted conception		
Endometrial problems (endometriosis or fibroids)		
Previous placenta praevia		

An antepartum haemorrhage (APH) is vaginal bleeding in pregnancy after 24 gestational weeks and before the birth of the fetus. The epidemiology is 3–5% of all pregnancies and it is more common in multiparous than primiparous women.

The causes of APH include placental factors (placenta praevia (20%) and placental abruption (30%)), local bleeding from the vulva, vagina or cervix and commonly unexplained APH (40%) or a show (early labour).

A postpartum haemorrhage has a defined volume of blood loss (> 500 ml), but an APH does not have a volume. The blood loss may not all be revealed (concealed) and the estimation of the blood loss is frequently underestimated. Therefore, clinical signs and symptoms of the mother and fetus are vitally important. The following are terms often used to define the volume or frequency of an APH:

- Spotting (volume noted on a sanitary pad)
- Minor (< 50 ml)
- Major (50–1000 ml with no clinical shock)
- Massive (> 1000 ml or any amount with signs of clinical shock)
- Recurrent (happens on more than one occasion).

Placental abruption

Placental abruption is the premature separation of the placenta from the uterine wall. The cause is unknown. A haemorrhage in the deciduas layer of the placenta causes a haematoma (retroplacental clot); this haematoma can be small and self-limiting (partial abruption), or can continue and become larger (complete). Separation exceeding 50% of the placenta raises the stillbirth rate. Placental abruption can also present as pain without bleeding (concealed) (Figure 42.1) from the genital tract (20%) and is often more severe compared with (revealed) bleeding (80%). Concealed bleeds are not always identified.

Risk factors

Placental abruption is more common in women who have had a previous pregnancy affected by an abruption (see Table 42.1 for other risk factors). Abruption is a sudden and unexpected obstetric emergency and while there may be risk factors present, this is not always the case and 70% occur in low-risk pregnancies.

Placenta praevia

Placenta praevia is the implantation of the placenta over the cervical os (Figure 42.2). Placenta praevia is classified from 1 to 4, with grade 4 being the most severe.

Risk factors

Placenta praevia is more common in women who have had a pregnancy affected previously with this condition (see Table 42.2 for further risk factors). One very rare cause of an APH is vasa praevia (Figure 42.3). Bleeding from the umbilical cord is the first presention.

Presentation

The presentation of an APH can be bleeding accompanied by abdominal pain (associated with abruption) or without pain (associated with placenta praevia) (Figure 42.3). There may be uterine tenderness and/or contractions, non-engagement of the fetal head or malpresentation (due to gestation or placenta praevia), non reassuring fetal heart rate patterns or maternal signs of shock. The presence of a compromised mother or fetus is indicative of an obstetric emergency and imminent delivery (by caesarean section) of the baby and resuscitation of the mother is appropriate. This and all other case presentations are preceded, where time allows, with the following management.

Management

Maternal and fetal observations are essential to asses their condition (maternal blood pressure, pulse, temperature and fetal heart rate). A full medical and obstetric history should be taken, if possible (including cervical smear history as this is indicative of bleeding from the cervix, especially postcoital bleeds). The presence of pain is an important consideration. If the pain is continuous it is indicative of abruption, if intermittent of labour. An abdominal palpation, assessment of fetal position and presence of uterine tenderness or contractions are all clinical signs to be aware of.

As the midwife caring for this woman, you would refer to an obstetrician as the presence of an APH is outside your scope of practice. The obstetrician will assess the woman and perform a speculum examination, as digital vaginal examination is not recommended if placenta praevia is suspected, and this cannot be ruled out yet. The speculum examination may show cervical dilatation or bleeding from a cause in the lower genital tract.

Blood tests will usually be ordered to check full blood count, coagulation screening and in the case of major or massive haemorrhage order 4 units of cross-matched blood for transfusion. The initial haemoglobin level may not be accurate so clinical signs are important. Women who are rhesus-D negative need a Kleihaur test to assess the extent of the fetal maternal haemorrhage and prescribed sufficient anti-D.

An ultrasound is usually performed.

Women usually know whether their placenta was low lying at their 20-week anomaly scan and will have another scan booked for 34 weeks to reassess this. The position of the placenta can be determined by ultrasound but placental abruptions are poorly recognised on ultrasound (75% are missed). Therefore, the presence of an abruption cannot be excluded on ultrasound.

Corticosteroids are recommended for pregnancies less than 34 + 6 weeks' gestation.

The decision to manage the APH conservatively or expediently is determined by the gestation and compromise of mother or fetus.

Complications

Maternal complications from APH include: anaemia, infection, shock, consequences such as prolonged hospital stay, complications from blood transfusion and psychological trauma. Fetal complications include: hypoxia, small for gestational age and growth restriction (insufficient placental functioning due to poor blood supply), prematurity or fetal death.

Complications are more likely with placental causes of APH, a larger volume of bleeding and earlier gestations.

43 Shoulder dystocia

Figure 43.1 Maternal pelvis.

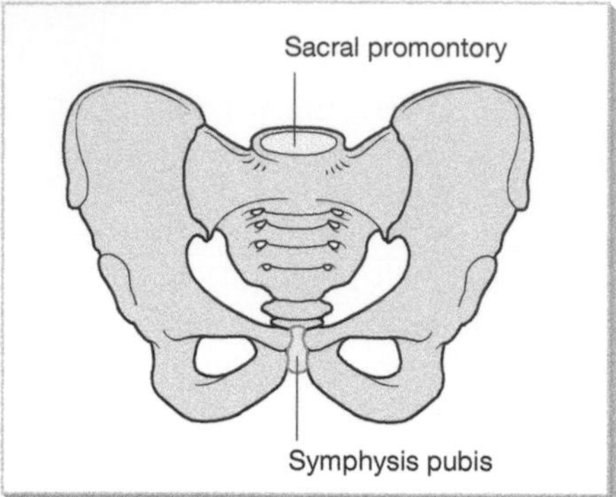

Figure 43.2 McRoberts manoeuvre.

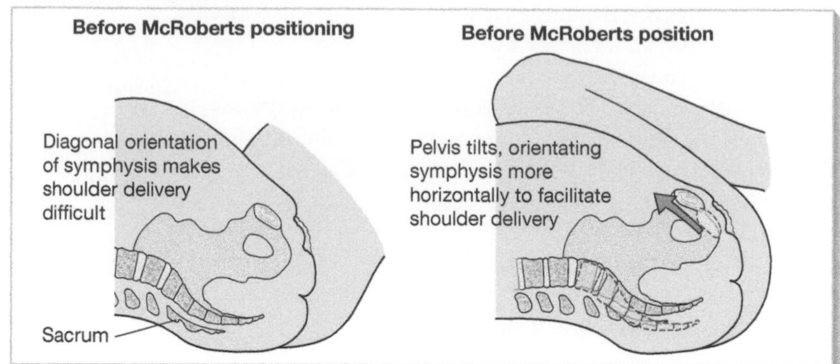

Figure 43.3 Shoulder dystocia and application of suprapubic pressure.

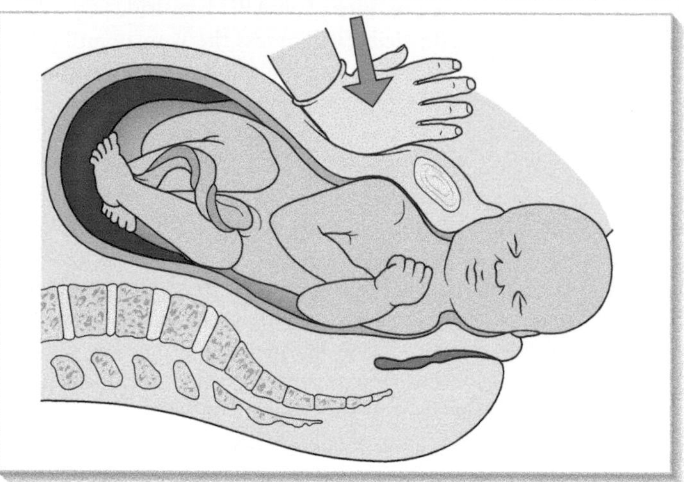

Figure 43.4 Maternal all fours position.

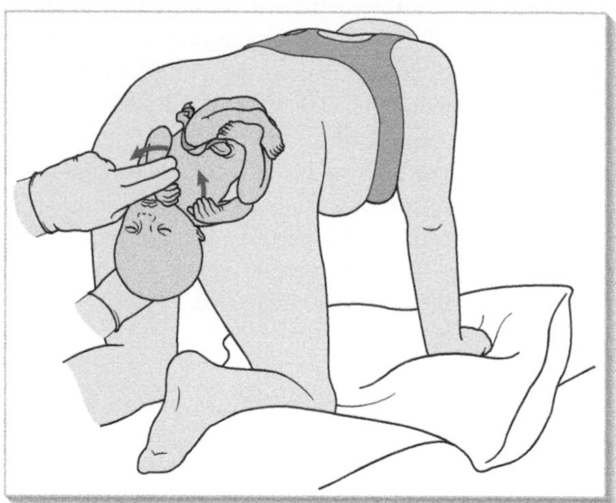

Figure 43.5 Internal manoeuvres.

The enter maneuvres for shoulder dystocia clarified (using **LOT** position as an example)

Rubin II

If ROT, insert fingers of left hand at 7 o'clock

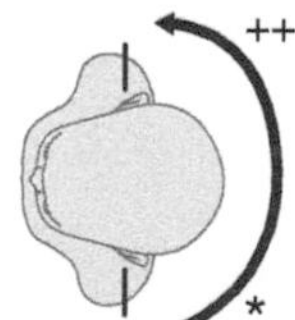

- If LOT, insert index & middle fingers of right hand through introitus at 5 o'clock*
- Swing fingers up & apply pressure with fingertips from **behind** the anterior shoulder ++
- If shoulders move into the oblique diameter – attempt delivery

Rubin II + wood screw

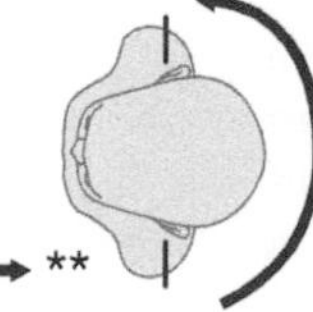

- If no rotation occurs, continue rubin II and **add** wood screw
- Use fingers of the opposite hand to apply pressure to the **front** of the posterior shoulder**
- This can help rotation in the **same direction** as Rubin II
- If shoulders now move into the oblique – attempt delivery
- If unsuccessful try to rotate through 180° to deliver

Reverse wood screw

Remove hand on side of fetal face

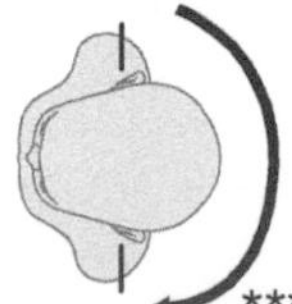

- If rotation in that direction cannot be achieved **change** to reverse wood screw
- Slide fingers down to the **back** of the posterior shoulder***
- Apply pressure to rotate in the opposite direction
- Attempt delivery if shoulders move into the oblique
- If unsuccessful, continue rotation through 180° to deliver

All attempts at rotation should be completed within 1–2 minutes
If unsuccessful - move on to other maneuvers

A shoulder dystocia is an obstetric emergency. The midwife needs to recognise the emergency, call for help and undertake the necessary measures to relieve the impacted fetal anterior shoulder from behind the maternal symphysis pubis (most common), although the posterior fetal shoulder can impact upon the maternal sacral promontory as well (Figure 43.1) (Chapter 10).

The incidence varies from 0.5% to 0.7% of births (approximately one in 200 births). The effects of shoulder dystocia can be brachial plexus injury (2–16%); this may resolve or in more difficult births can lead to fetal or neonatal death. For the mother, there is an increased risk of postpartum haemorrhage and third or fourth degree tears as well as anxiety for the baby's condition.

Predisposing factors

Several factors seem to increase the chance of shoulder dystocia but have low predictive value (even with one or two risk factors some births will be easy, for others without risk factors a shoulder dystocia will occur). The best predictor is a diabetic mother (twice as likely to have shoulder dystocia). She is more likely to have a macrosomic baby, defined as over 4.5 kg, but this alone is not a good predictor. Other pre-labour risks include previous shoulder dystocia, maternal BMI greater than 30 kg/m^2 and induction of labour. During labour a prolonged first or second stage, instrumental birth and oxytocin augmentation are associated.

Recognising and managing

All birth attendants should be able to recognise and manage shoulder dystocia. Timely management improves the outcome for the mother and baby. Signs to look for are: difficulty birthing of the fetal head and chin, the head remaining tightly applied to the vulva or retract (turtle sign), and the fetal head not restituting or descending on the next contraction.

As soon as it is evident that a shoulder dystocia is occurring, the midwife should call for help, stating the problem. The help required is usually another midwife, often the co-ordinating midwife, an obstetrician, paediatrician and anaesthetist. Each has a different role in the emergency. Stating the nature of the emergency helps those involved orientate themselves towards their roles and the management.

Maternal pushing is discouraged as this can further impact the shoulders. The first line of management is to alter the maternal position to open the pelvic outlet to enable to shoulders to be born. The maternal hips are flexed and abducted. This straightens the lumbosacral angle, rotates the pelvis and increases the anterior-posterior diameter (McRoberts manoeuvre) (Figure 42.2). It is the most effective intervention, enabling approximately 90% of babies to be born, and is the least invasive.

To help position the woman the midwife must communicate the need to her and her partner. She is then laid flat. One person on either side should lift the woman's legs simultaneously into the hyperflexed position. This should enable the attending midwife to deliver the baby with routine axial traction – that is, traction in line with the fetal spine. There should be no lateral or downward traction as this can exacerbate the injury to the brachial plexus.

If McRoberts manoeuvreand routine axial traction do not release the shoulder another manoeuvre is added with the woman in the same position. Suprapubic pressure (Figure 43.3) should be commenced. Ideally, the fetal position should be known so the pressure can be applied to its back. This intervention aims to reduce the bisacromial diameter – the diameter between the shoulders. The pressure can be continuous or rocking and intermittent. Routine axial traction along with the above manoeuvres can be tried again but if this does not birth the fetus another intervention needs to be considered. An all fours position can be tried to enable the birth. As the least invasive method is changing the maternal position, this will be offered first.

Maternal all fours position

Asking a woman to move into the all fours position (Figure 43.4) will depend on the woman and whether she has had any regional anaesthesia. The mechanism for freeing the shoulder is thought to be in the action of moving the woman as this may dislodge the shoulder but it also frees the sacrum from the pressure of the bed and may enable greater room for the fetus to move.

Internal manoeuvres

If none of the above work, the woman may be asked to return to her original position, although internal manoeuvres may be undertaken in the all fours position. An episiotomy may be performed to enable to attendant to undertake the internal manoeuvres.

The two internal manoeuvres are the wood screw and Rubins 11 (Figure 43.5). The arrows show you where to place fingers and the direction shows which way to rotate the fetal shoulders. The intention is to rotate the shoulders into the wider oblique diameter. If these do not work, the posterior fetal arm can be delivered.

Care after birth

The condition of the baby at birth will determine whether the baby can stay with the mother or is transferred to a neonatal unit. Resuscitation may be necessary, the longer the interval from birth of the fetal head to the rest of the baby, the greater the risk of trauma. Trauma includes brachial plexus injury, fractures to the clavicle or humerus, hypoxic brain damage and even death. The baby needs to be examined for injury.

The mother should also be examined carefully after birth for signs of perineal trauma. She and her birth partner will need to have an explanation of the events of the birth. The midwife and attending professionals need to document the events carefully, including time from birth of the head to the body, manoeuvres performed, their timing and sequence, condition of the baby, Apgars, cord bloods and mother's perineal and vaginal inspection and blood loss. A risk management form is usually required too.

Cord presentation and prolapse

Figure 44.1 Cord presentation and prolapse.

Cord presentation
Membranes intact

Cord prolapse
Membranes ruptured

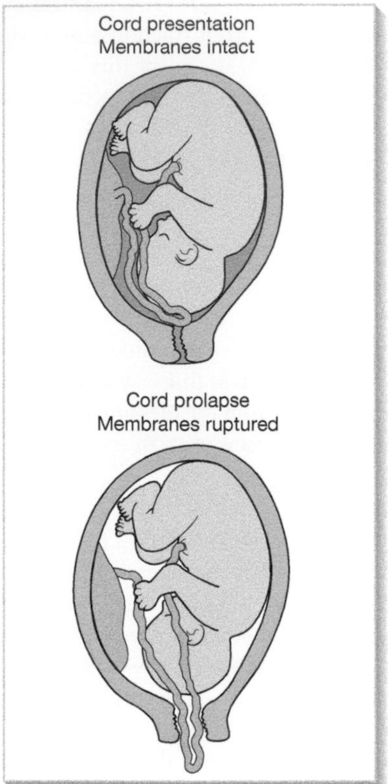

Figure 44.2 Types of cord prolapse.

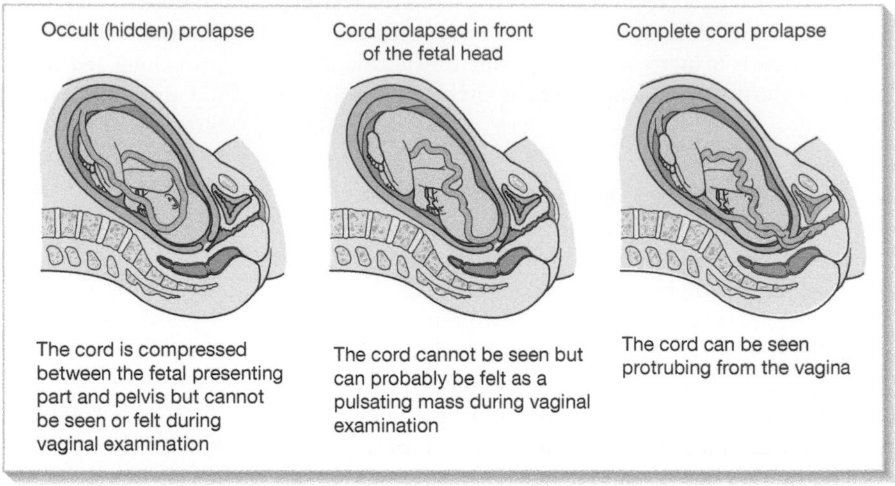

Occult (hidden) prolapse

The cord is compressed between the fetal presenting part and pelvis but cannot be seen or felt during vaginal examination

Cord prolapsed in front of the fetal head

The cord cannot be seen but can probably be felt as a pulsating mass during vaginal examination

Complete cord prolapse

The cord can be seen protrubing from the vagina

Figure 44.3 Maternal knee chest position.

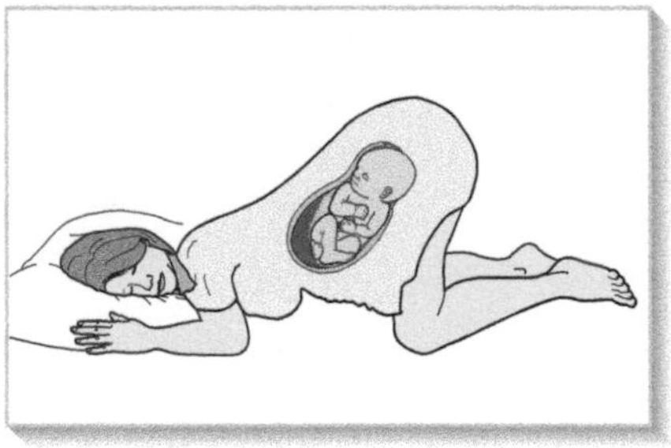

Figure 44.4 Digital elevation of the fetal head.

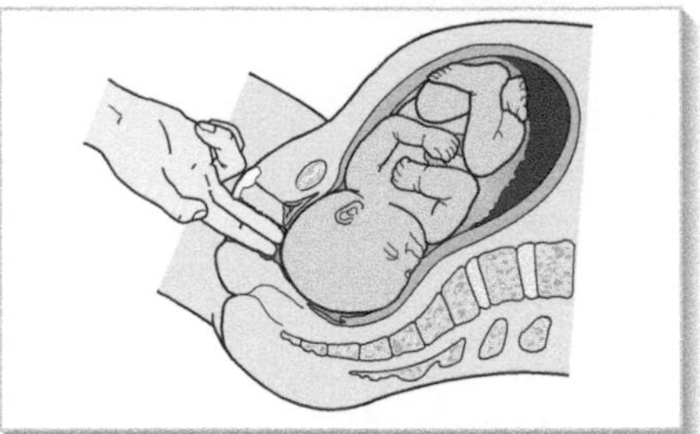

Figure 44.5 Management algorithm.

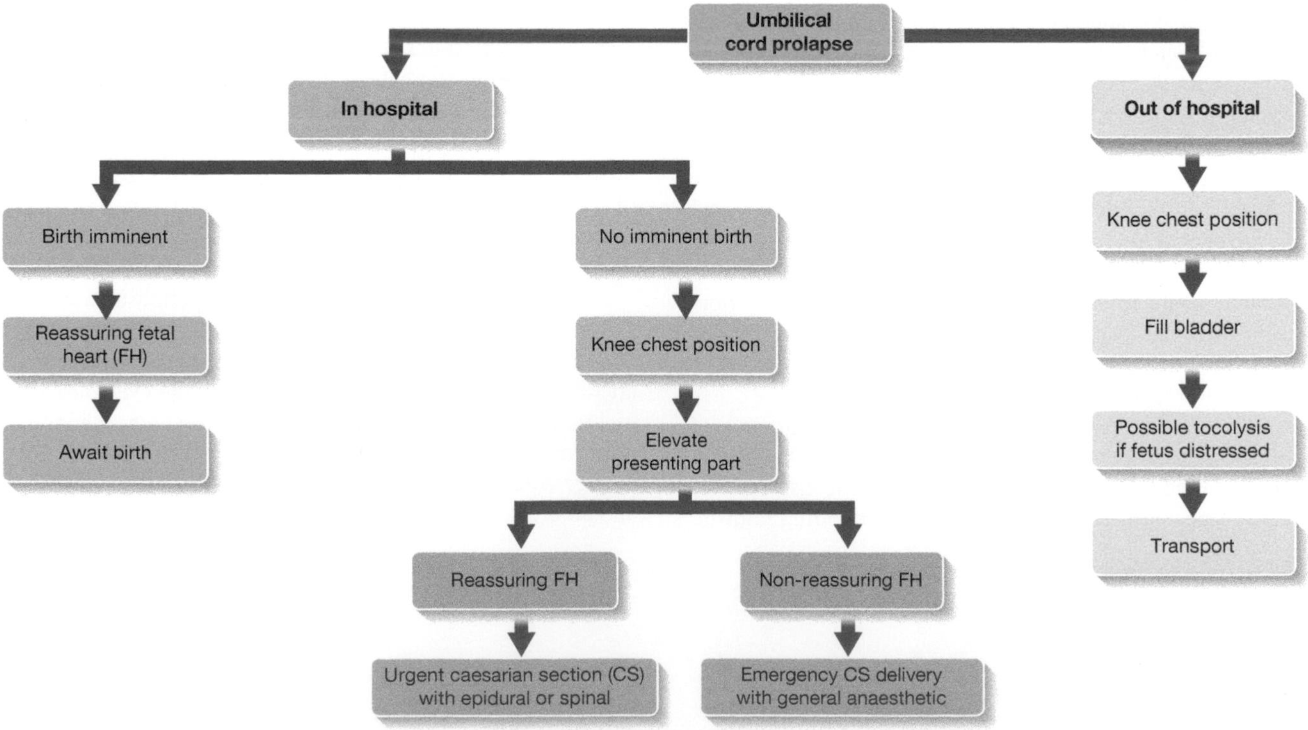

Umbilical cord prolapse

In hospital

Birth imminent

Reassuring fetal heart (FH)

Await birth

No imminent birth

Knee chest position

Elevate presenting part

Reassuring FH

Urgent caesarian section (CS) with epidural or spinal

Non-reassuring FH

Emergency CS delivery with general anaesthetic

Out of hospital

Knee chest position

Fill bladder

Possible tocolysis if fetus distressed

Transport

Midwifery at a Glance, First Edition. Edited by Eleanor Forrest © 2019 John Wiley & Sons, Ltd. Published 2019 by John Wiley & Sons, Ltd.
Companion website: www.wiley.com/go/forrest/midwifery

Definitions

Cord presentation is defined as the umbilical cord presenting adjacent to, in front of, or below the fetal presenting part, with intact membranes (Figure 44.1). It occurs most frequently when the presenting part is poorly applied to the lower segment or in malpresentations.

Cord prolapse occurs when the membranes have ruptured (Figure 44.1). It can be overt (complete), occult (hidden) or in between these two states (Figure 44.2). When the membranes have ruptured they are no longer able to protect the cord presentation from pressure and flow of blood from the placenta to the fetus can be occluded. This is an obstetric emergency and something a midwife should be able to recognise, appropriately call for help and manage.

As with most obstetric emergencies, there are predisposing factors, such as multiparity, low birth weight, breech presentation, low-lying placenta, artificial rupture of the membranes or vaginal manipulation of the fetus with ruptured membranes.

Prevention

When cord presentation is detected in labour, artificial rupture of the membranes is inappropriate and a caesarean section is indicated.

While cord prolapse in itself cannot be prevented with a mobile presenting part, artificial rupture of membranes should only be undertaken where there are facilities for immediate caesarean section.

Suspecting cord prolapse

Because the cord prolapse can be occult, there are clinical indications which may alert the midwife to suspect compression of the cord. These indications are abnormal or suspicious fetal heart rate patterns, including bradycardia or variable decelerations, especially if these occur following spontaneous rupture of membranes or amniotomy. Prompt vaginal examination is indicated here to diagnose cord prolapse and for optimal management.

Management

Depending on the place, stage of labour and parity there are differences in the management of cord prolapse. In essence, if the cord prolapses before full cervical dilatation preparations for immediate delivery in theatre are recommended.

For community midwives caring for women at home, the likelihood of a cord prolapse is likely to be reduced as there should be fewer predisposing risk factors. HoIf cord prolapse does occur and the birth is not imminent, transfer to an obstetric unit is recommended. Elevation of the presenting part for the duration of the transfer is recommended. For women awaiting an ambulance, the knee chest position is preferred (Figure 44.3). For transfer in the ambulance this is not safe, so the left lateral position is better.

The midwifery care options include performing a vaginal examination to digitally elevate the fetal head (Figure 44.4) or filling the maternal bladder. Insert a Foley's catheter into the bladder and fill it with 500–750 ml of fluid to elevate the fetal presenting part and prevent further compression of the cord; the catheter is then clamped to maintain a full bladder (refer to Part 2 for the female genitourinary system to refresh your anatomy and physiology if required, to enable you to understand how this might work). As with all management of cord prolapse, minimal handling of the cord is recommended to prevent vasospasm and further constriction of the fetal blood flow.

Hospital management

A caesarean section is the probable mode of birth for this mother and baby. However, a multiparous woman at full dilatation will vaginally birth her baby more quickly and it is probably safer than a surgical procedure with midwifery support; the adrenaline produced when the cord prolapse implications are communicated to her will aid this. The key word is imminent. For primiparous women at full dilatation an instrumental birth can be attempted, as this is favourable to a caesarean section. This is often performed in theatre in case the birth is not easily performed and the decision to revert to a caesarean is necessary. Similarly, for breech presentation at full dilatation, a breech extraction can be undertaken with appropriately trained medical staff.

For births that are not imminent a category 1 caesarean section should be performed within 30 minutes if the fetal heart rate is suspicious or pathological. Some hospitals use tocolysis to relax the uterus to prevent further contractions and compression of the fetal umbilical cord. If there is no fetal compromise a category 2 caesarean under regional anaesthesia is as safe. If the woman's bladder has been filled, this needs to be drained prior to the surgery. For the management algorithm see Figure 44.5. Verbal consent for the operation is sufficient.

After birth

A paediatrician should be at each birth as the need for neonatal resuscitation is likely. Cord gasses are usually undertaken to assess neonatal wellbeing.

The woman and her partner should be debriefed, explaining the events and management and giving them an opportunity for questions to enable them to understand the birth.

Staff training

Staff, especially midwives, are required to undertake annual updates which pertain to this emergency. These include cardiotocography interpretation, and skills and drills regarding management of cord prolapse. A clinical incident form and meticulous documentation of the birth events, as always, are required.

45 Embolism

Figure 45.1 (a) Pulmonary embolism, and (b) thrombus and embolus.

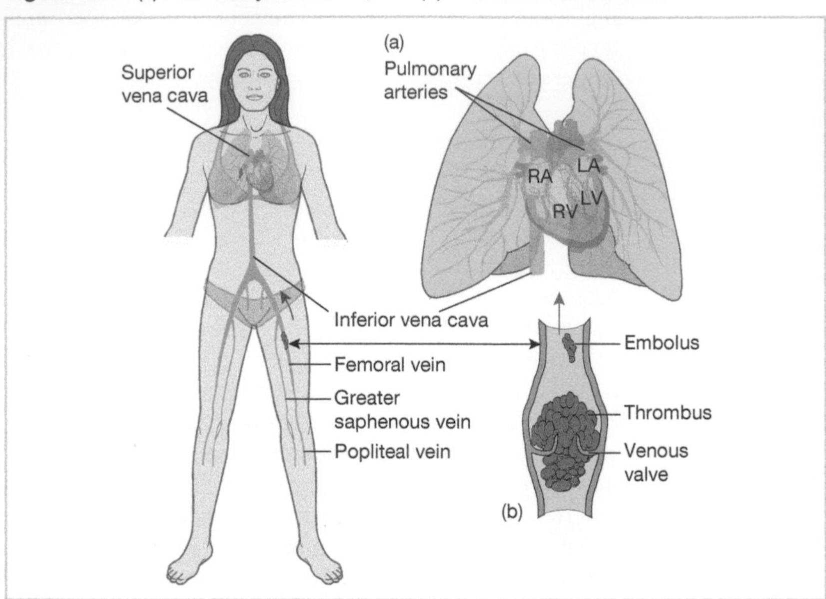

Figure 45.2 Amniotic fluid embolism.

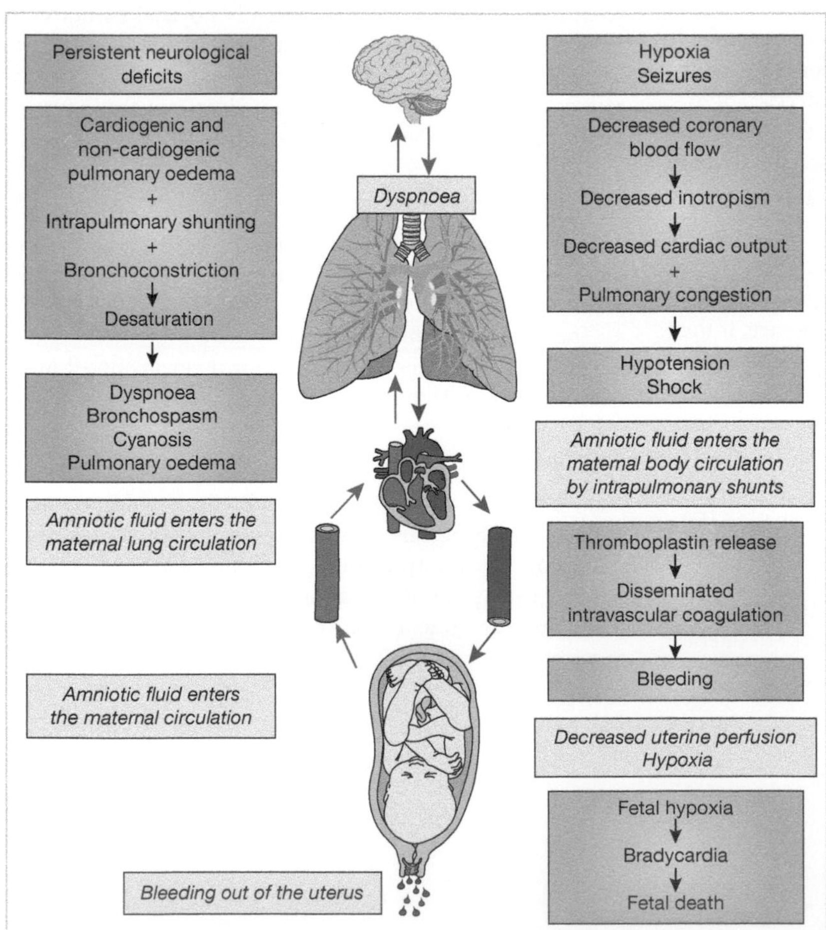

Box 45.1 Risk factors for amniotic fluid embolism.

- High intra-amniotic pressures
- Hypertonic uterine action – spontaneous or induced by oxytocic drugs
- Older multiparous women with rapid labours
- Multiple pregnancies
- Polyhydramnious
- Uterine trauma such as caesarean section, ruptured uterus or manual removal of placenta

Table 45.1 VTE contributory factors.

Cause	Result/details
Hypercoagulability with a decrease in the amount of natural anticoagulants	Increased levels of coagulation factors in the blood Increase in resistance to C reactive protein Decrease in antithrombin to prevent maternal haemorrhage
Increased venous stasis	Smooth muscles of the veins relax under influence of pregnancy hormones so venous return of blood slower
Vascular damage	Especially caesarean section when blood vessels are surgically cut but also following vessel damage after vaginal birth

Terminology

The term embolism comes from Greek meaning to block. It is related to the term thrombus, which is a clot (Figure 45.1). A clot or thrombus forms due to abnormal blood clotting. When a clot is formed and remains in the area in which it was made, whether this is a vein or artery, it is called a thrombus. Arterial thrombi are usually a result of cardiovascular disease; whereas venous thrombi are an obstetric complication.

The most common veins for thrombi are the deep veins of the legs or pelvis – deep vein thrombosis (DVT). An embolus is when all or some of the thrombus (clot) breaks away from its manufactured site and travels to another part of the body. This condition is called embolism. A pulmonary embolus is a clot made in the deep veins that travels to the lungs, causing a blockage in the pulmonary arteries (Figure 45.1). Because thrombus and embolus are related and the former frequently cause the latter, the term thromboembolitic disorders or thromboembolism are used.

Type

There are three types of thromboembolic events women are most at risk of in pregnancy and the postnatal period:

1 Venous thromboembolic events (VTEs) are the most common form, such as a pulmonary embolus preceded by a DVT (Table 45.1).

2 Arterial thromboembolitic events are rare, such as Type section aboveischaemic stroke and heart attack and are usually associated with pre-eclampsia and pre-existing cardiac disease, respectively.

3 Amniotic fluid embolisms are rare (Figure 45.2 and Box 45.1).

Causes of VTEs

A thrombus is caused by disturbed flow of blood, hypercoagulability and injury to the vessel wall (Table 45.1).

Importance of recognition

Thromboembolic events have been the leading cause of maternal mortality for many years. Venous thromboembolitic events are unpredictable – women may have risk factors but some present without any. Recognising a DVT reduces the risk of pulmonary embolus from 15–25% to 4–5% as effective treatment is administered.

Thirteen women in the latest maternal death statistics died of an amniotic fluid embolism. Whilst its incidence is rare, its mortality is high, especially in the first hour, so rapid recognition and treatment is the only way to improve survival rates. Recognition and treatment of obstetric emergencies are presented here; see Chapter 37 for further information on thromboembolic disease.

Symptoms

The symptoms of VTE are dependent upon the size and location of the blood clot. Some women present with no symptoms so recognition is a problem. Often women have no, or very minor, symptoms and have a sudden catastrophic event.

DVT symptoms

DVT symptoms are red, hot, swollen and painful unilateral swelling. It is common in pregnancy and usually attributed to oedema.

Pulmonary and amniotic fluid embolism symptoms

- Breathlessness with cyanosis
- Tightness in the chest or chest pain
- Cough or cough with blood (haemoptysis)
- Feeling unwell
- Sudden collapse
- Tachycardia
- Hypotension.

Breathlessness during pregnancy is common (experienced by 75% of woman), as the physiological changes and growing uterus decrease the available lung capacity. It usually presents gradually so a sudden onset should be investigated. After birth, breathlessness is not common and should always be investigated.

Timing of the emergency

Amniotic fluid embolism usually occurs at or near term or during delivery. It is often a sudden, unexpected collapse. If the collapse happens in a well-equipped hospital this is now considered a treatable and survivable event.

VTEs can occur at any time during pregnancy, however most occur in very early pregnancy or postnatally.

Treatment

Treatment can be conservative or an obstetric emergency depending on the event.

DVT management is conservative and includes: therapeutic doses of low-molecular-weight heparin (LMWH) which is administered subcutaneously. LMWH is safer than unfractionated heparin, can be administered in one or two doses as opposed to continuously and does not cross the placental barrier (oral anticoagulation treatments do). A balance between preventing further clot formation and increasing the woman's risk of bleeding is required. Treatment with LMWH should be stopped 24 hours prior to a planned birth or if labour is suspected or confirmed. Regional analgesia should not be administered for 24 hours after the last therapeutic dose of LMWH. Good hydration antenatally and postnatally is essential. Elevating the woman's legs, applying graduated compression stockings and remaining active also form the treatment plan, with pain relief as required.

Recognition of obstetric emergencies such as a collapse, whether attributed to thromboembolitic or amniotic fluid embolism, should initially be treated with resuscitative measures. For amniotic fluid collapses emptying of the uterus is paramount, so an emergency caesarean section is performed. Oxygen therapy and cardiopulmonary resuscitation of the mother and baby are likely. The amniotic fluid alters the blood clotting mechanisms so haemorrhage and disseminating intravascular coagulation are also likely.

For a pulmonary embolism, an obstetric team will manage the collapse, and treatment is usually oxygen therapy and continuous intravenous unfractionated heparin. Surgical embolectomy, removal of the clot, is rare. On-going anticoagulation with LMWH is usual and lasts for several months following the birth. The risk of reoccurrence is high in a subsequent pregnancy.

46 Obstructed labour

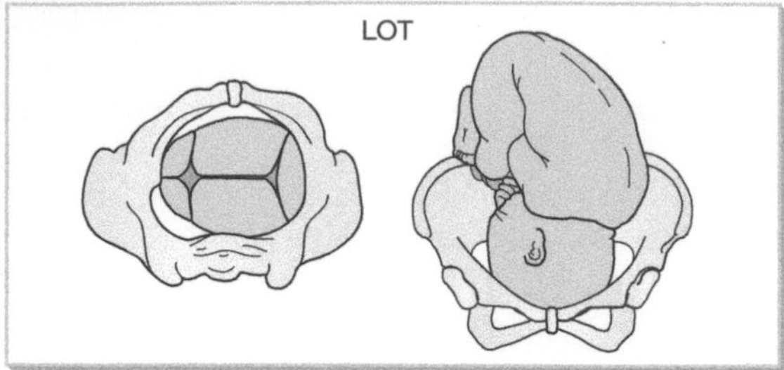

Figure 46.1 Deep transverse arrest.

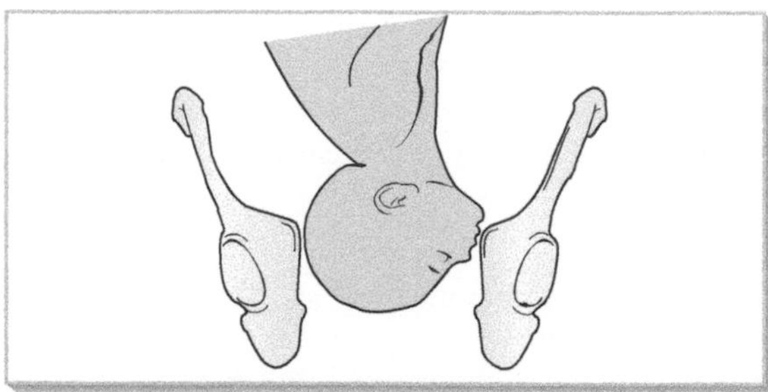

Figure 46.3 Brow presentation.

Table 46.1 Aetiology of obstructed labour.

Fetal	Maternal
Pelvic disproportion Malpresentations Face Brow Shoulder or arm presentation – transverse lie Breech Compound presentation	Small pelvis Childhood malnutrition Contracted or deformed bony pelvis
Malposition Persistent occipitoposterior Persistent occipitotransverse	Soft tissue tumours of the pelvis Uterine fibroids Ovarian tumours Rectal tumours
Malformations Hydrocephalus Abdominal tumours (e.g. Wilms' tumor) Cystic hygroma Conjoined twins	

Table 46.2 Maternal and fetal observations.

Maternal signs of obstructed labour	Fetal signs of obstructed labour
Pyrexia	Fetal tachycardia
Tachycardia	Fetal bradycardia – decelerations which become slow to recover
Pain	No accelerations
Anxiety	Meconium
Poor urine output – ketones	
Vagina hot and dry	

Figure 46.2 Face presentation – posterior not able to be born vaginally.

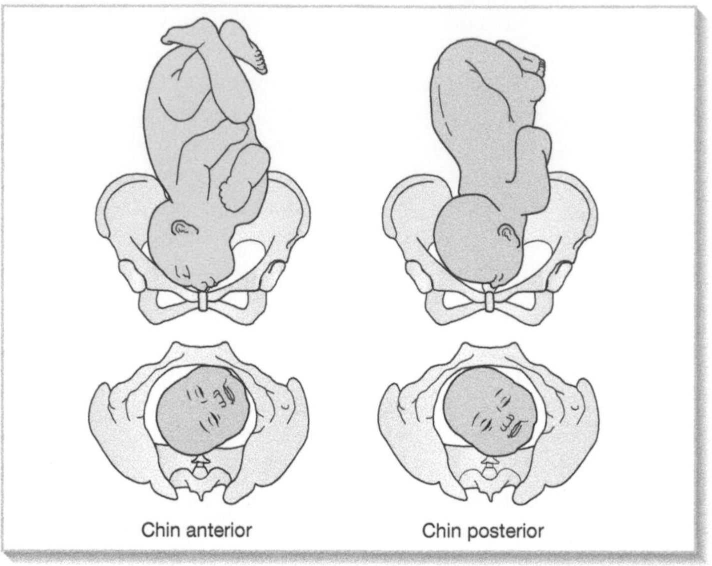

Figure 46.4 Bandl's ring.

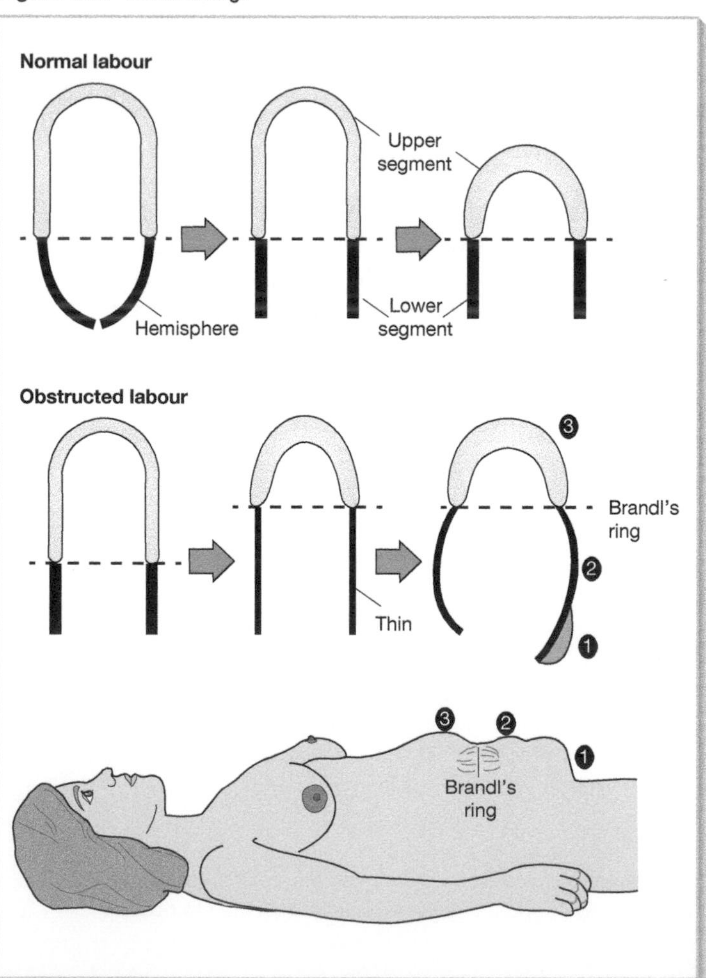

Midwifery at a Glance, First Edition. Edited by Eleanor Forrest © 2019 John Wiley & Sons, Ltd. Published 2019 by John Wiley & Sons, Ltd.
Companion website: www.wiley.com/go/forrest/midwifery

There are three 'P's that affect progress in labour:
1 The power of the uterine contractions.
2 The passenger's presentation and position.
3 The pelvis.

Obstructed labour is when there is no advance of the presenting part despite strong uterine contractions. In developing countries obstructed labour is a major cause of maternal and fetal morbidity and mortality. While this is not so in the UK it still needs recognising and managing.

Diagnosis and presumptive signs in early labour

On abdominal palpation the midwife will assess for fetal presentation. Signs that indicate obstructed labour are:

- Shoulder presentation/oblique or transverse lie – refer to an obstetrician for ultrasound and management plan, probably operative delivery
- Non-engaged fetal presenting part (i.e. three-fifths of the fetal head are palpable above the symphysis pubis), especially in a nulliparous woman – whilst not diagnostic it should be noted
- Occipitoposterior (OP) fetal positions – not diagnostic but due to the longer rotation from OP to occipitoanterior for birth, the likelihood of a deep transverse arrest is increased (Figure 46.1).

On vaginal examination (VE), face (Figure 46.2) presentation (mentoposterior cannot deliver) or brow presentation (Figure 46.3) may be found. These are hard to diagnose on abdominal palpation, and are sometimes missed on VE (depending on the cervical dilatation). However, using all clinical skills such as the engagement (both positions are likely to be non-engaged), application of the presenting part to the cervix (both are likely to be loosely applied) and whether there are early spontaneous ruptured membranes, the midwife can make a more informed assessment of fetal position.

Causes

Cephalopelvic disproportion (CPD) occurs when the presenting diameters of the fetal head are larger than the diameters of the pelvis. This can be due to: a maternal pelvis shape anomaly caused by bony conditions, rickets or osteomalacia; spinal deformities such as scoliosis; or pelvic trauma and fractures that have altered the shape of the pelvis. This often presents as an obstruction at the pelvic brim.

Obstructions may occur at the pelvic outlet such as in deep transverse arrest; or they may be due to other maternal or fetal factors. For example, there may be an obstruction in the uterus such as maternal tumours or fibroids which prevent progress in labour (see Table 46.1 for a fuller list). The fetus also may be the cause of the CPD: a large fetus, fetal abnormalities such as hydrocephalus as well as malposition (brow/face) and malpresentation (persistent OP or lateral positions which become deep transverse arrests).

Signs and symptoms as labour progresses

There is slow or little progress in labour despite efficient uterine contractions. If there is no cervical dilatation for 3–4 hours and the diagnosis of labour was made at 3–4 cm cervical dilatation, consider whether this woman was in active labour on the first VE and whether the contractions are effective. If she was in active labour refer to an obstetrician to consider whether the labour needs augmentation, with parental understanding and consent.

The presenting part, whether it is a chin (mento) or occiput, remains high. Caput or excessive moulding may be felt. Refer back to Chapter 20 for mechanisms of normal labour; descent is a vital component of an active labour.

If these early signs are missed the woman often becomes tachycardic, pyrexial and dehydrated. She will probably become anxious as to why, despite the time and contractions, her labour has not progressed. On examination the vagina feels hot and dry and the presenting part is still high. Urinary output is often reduced, frequently with ketones. Fetal heart monitoring, whether with intermittent auscultation or cardiotocography, depending on risk factors, is likely to become non-reassuring (Table 46.2). The fetus may pass meconium. Although rare in the UK, there may be a palpable pathological retraction ring (Figure 46.4).

Management

Reassure the woman and explain the situation. Refer to an obstetrician as obstructed labour is outside the role of the midwife. Depending on the stage of labour and fetal wellbeing, management may be conservative or active.

Conservative management includes discussing the possibility of oxytocin augmentation with the woman and her partner to increase the uterine contractions. This may enable to fetus to rotate and descent. The augmentation would require an i.v. cannula to be sited. When this is sited maternal bloods are taken for full blood count (FBC) and group and save in case an operative birth is under taken later. Continuous fetal monitoring will be started, if not already in progress. Analgesia may be requested by the mother for the increase in painful uterine contractions.

Active management may include an instrumental birth if the woman is in the second stage of labour. This is often performed in theatre so a caesarean section may be performed if the instrumental delivery is unsuccessful. If labour is in the first stage and the fetus (or woman) is showing signs of distress, an emergency caesarean section may be necessary. Often if the woman is symptomatic an i.v. infusion may be required in addition to the augmentation to correct the dehydration. If the woman is pyrexial, i.v. antibiotics are administered, with consent, as a prophylaxis for the fetus and to treat any potential infection.

After birth

A paediatrician and neonatal resuscitative equipment should be present at the birth. Depending on the clinical situation, whether the fetus was tachycardic, passed meconium or had a traumatic birth or suspected infection, he or she may be transferred to the neonatal unit for treatment or observations. Similarly, the mother may experience trauma or haemorrhage following the birth and need further antibiotics.

47 Uterine rupture

Figure 47.1 Myometrium, and peritoneum (or perimetrium).

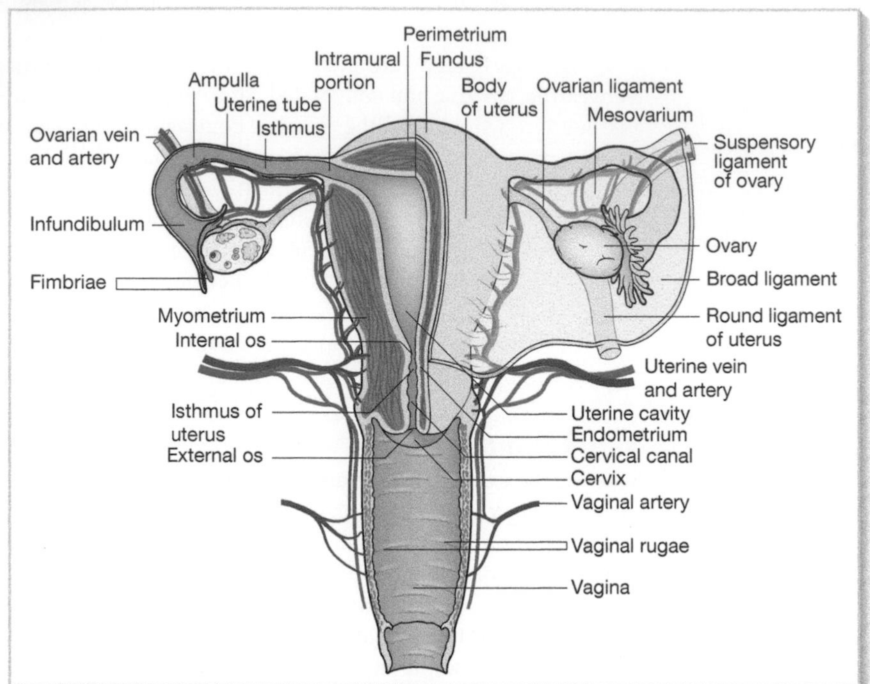

Figure 47.3 Incomplete rupture.

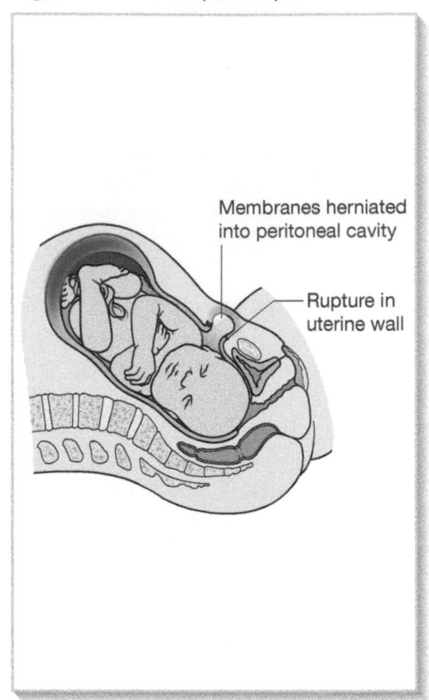

Figure 47.2 Complete uterine rupture and expulsion of fetus into abdominal cavity.

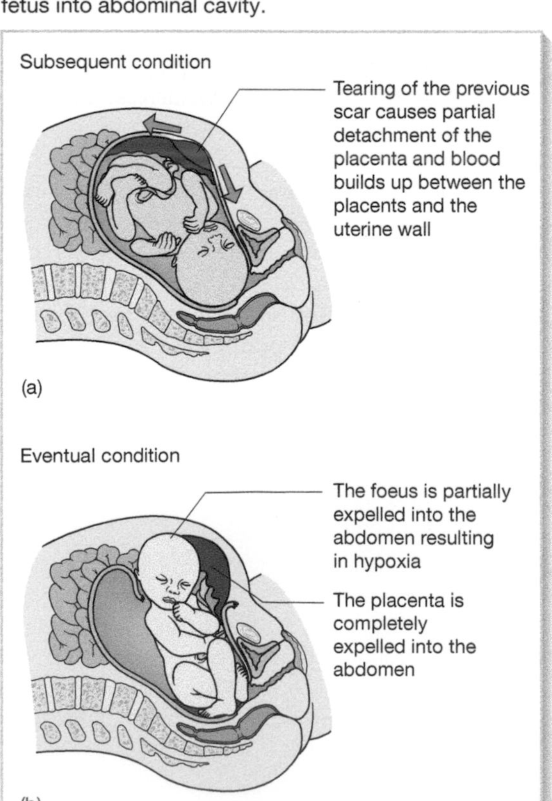

Figure 47.4 Forces that contribute to uterine rupture.

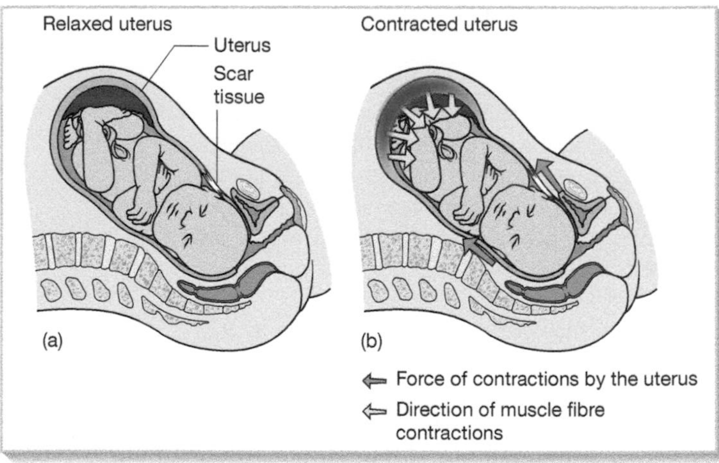

Table 47.1 Risk factors.

Antenatal	Intrapartum
Previous caesarean section, especially three or more, or high vertical classical incision	Strong contractions, with or without oxytocic
Misuse of oxytocin or prostaglandin	Intrauterine manipulations
	Shoulder dystocia
	Fundal pressure
	Unrecognised obstructed labour
	Instrumental birth, particularly high or rotational forceps deliveries
	Manual removal of placenta

Uterine rupture is a rare complication of pregnancy or labour which may cause maternal or fetal death. There are differing definitions and types of rupture.

Classification

Complete uterine rupture involves a full-thickness tear through the myometrium (middle layer of the uterine muscle) and peritoneum (a membrane that lines the abdominal cavity, sometimes called the perimetrium or outer wall of uterine muscle) (Figure 47.1). The fetus is normally partially or wholly expelled through the tear into the peritoneal cavity (Figure 47.2). This often leads to placenta abruption and fetal death.

A partial or incomplete uterine rupture involves the myometrium but not the peritoneum (Figure 47.3).

Types of rupture

Scar rupture is reported to be the most common type of rupture. This occurs where the uterine muscles have previously been operated on, most commonly a caesarean section. The chance of a scar rupture is dependent upon the type of previous C section, with lower segment caesareans considered the safest and high vertical classical incisions considered the most risky. Three previous C sections also increase the risk. There is limited evidence that other uterine operations such as myomectomy (removal of fibroids) or hysterotomy (any surgical incision in the uterus) increase the risk of uterine rupture.

Traumatic rupture may be caused by obstetric instruments such as forceps delivery or during a termination of pregnancy, internal uterine manoeuvres such as internal podalic version (turning a fetus by gripping its feet) or inappropriate oxytocic drug usage. Trauma may also be due to road traffic of other accidents.

Spontaneous rupture is associated with strong uterine contractions, often in multiparous women, with obstructed labours (Chapter 46).

Risk factors for uterine rupture are listed in Table 47.1.

Prevention

Women with a history of previous C sections should be counselled regarding vaginal birth after caesarean section (VBAC). The chance of a successful VBAC with an uncomplicated pregnancy is 72–76%. VBAC is usually safer than a C section for the mother and fetus, however the risks should also be explained and minimised. If a woman has had a previous ruptured uterus, classical incision or three previous C sections she will be counselled to have a repeat C section. Planned VBAC carries a uterine rupture risk of 22–74/10 000 compared with an unscarred uterus of 0.5–2/10 000 deliveries. Induction and augmentation of labour in these women should be prescribed by a consultant or registrar, respectively, and administered with care. Administration of oxytocics can increase the forces exerted on the scar (Figure 47.4). Progress in labour should be observed and any deviation in progress or maternal and fetal observations reported to the obstetrician.

Presentation

- Continuous pain – contractions are intermittent
- Cessation of previously efficient contractions
- Change in maternal expression of pain – 'I felt something give/strange'
- Tender on abdominal palpation, easily palpable fetal parts
- Scar tenderness
- Chest pain and shortness of breath
- Woman feels faint, pale
- Vaginal blood loss, variable
- Fetal compromise – atypical variable decelerations, bradycardia
- Maternal tachycardia, which, depending on severity, can develop into maternal collapse and haemorrhage.

Management

Recognition of the obstetric emergency is paramount. This is outside the scope of midwifery practice, so emergency help must be sought. The immediate help includes a senior obstetrician, anaesthetist, midwives and paediatrician. A theatre will be needed, along with the team to staff this. The obstetric consultant is usually called in. Often a haematologist will be consulted and blood is likely to be required.

For the midwife caring for this woman, communication with her and her partner is essential. Maternal observations, pulse, blood pressure and respirations will be recorded every 15 minutes. A MEOWS (modified early obstetric warning system) score is calculated to determine maternal compromise. Fetal monitoring, initially to establish whether he or she is alive, will then be continuous with cardiotocography. Contemporaneous records should be kept as far as is possible.

You can also gain i.v. access with a large-bore cannula and take baseline blood tests such as full blood count (FBC), clotting screen, urea and electrolytes and cross-match 4–6 units of bloods. Frequently, this task is undertaken by the anaesthetist. If the woman is bleeding significantly gaining i.v. access is often difficult as she will have peripheral shutdown of her veins to maximise the blood to her essential organs.

An i.v. fluid infusion is usually prescribed to help replace lost blood initially before cross-matched blood is available. Oxygen therapy may be ordered too, to perfuse the woman and fetus. If the woman continues to bleed, implement the major obstetric haemorrhage protocol.

This woman needs to be transferred to theatre, the quicker the transfer the greater the chance of fetal and maternal survival. An emergency C section will be performed with the paediatrician available for neonatal resuscitation if viable and the fetal heart was heard.

Depending on the severity of the rupture, the uterus will either be repaired, or uterine ligation used to control the major haemorrhage, or the uterus removed.

Postnatally

The woman will be transferred to a high dependency unit for postoperative recovery and management. Observations for the side effects of major haemorrhage such as renal failure or disseminated intravascular coagulation (Chapter 51) will be undertaken so appropriate care can be initiated and maintained. Fluid balance and oxygen saturation will be observed and antibiotics prescribed.

Psychological care will be required, to a greater or lesser degree depending on the maternal wellbeing and the condition of the baby. The experience will need to be explained in more detail and further emotional support is likely to be needed in the future.

48 Uterine inversion

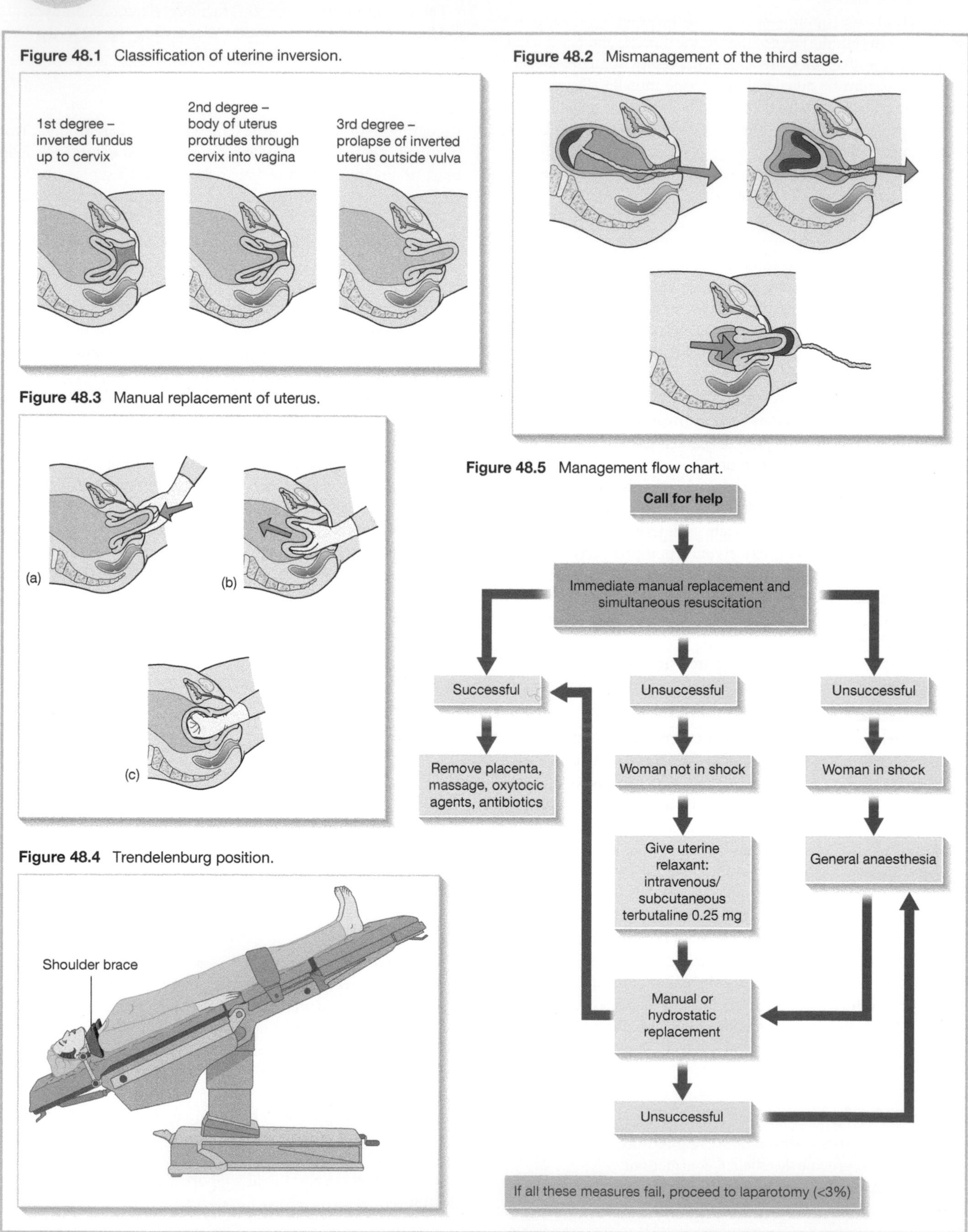

Figure 48.1 Classification of uterine inversion.

Figure 48.2 Mismanagement of the third stage.

Figure 48.3 Manual replacement of uterus.

Figure 48.4 Trendelenburg position.

Figure 48.5 Management flow chart.

Uterine inversion is a rare complication of labour, usually associated with the third stage. Often it is mismanagement of the third stage that causes the uterus to invert (turn inside out). Its incidence varies, with reports of 1:2500 to 1:100 000 cases.

Classification

There are two major classifications: incomplete and complete, which can be further divided into first, second and third degree (Figure 48.1). The definition of first degree (incomplete) inversion is that the fundus remains within the endometrial cavity. In second degree (complete) inversion the fundus protrudes through the cervical os but remains within the vagina, so is visible at the introitus. In third degree (complete or prolapsed) inversion the fundus is visible at the vulva.

It can also be classified in relation to the time of the inversion. Acute inversion occurs within 24 hours of birth and is most common. Subacute inversion occurs from 24 hours to 4 weeks after birth, and chronic inversion, which is rare, is after 4 weeks.

Causes and risk factors

The exact cause is not known, but 50% are estimated to be due to mismanagement of the third stage of labour (Figure 48.2). This includes: excessive controlled cord traction, omitting to guard the uterus at the symphysis pubis, and undertaking controlled cord traction on a relaxed uterus and without signs of separation of the placenta.

Spontaneous inversion can occur if the intra-abdominal pressure increases such as in coughing, sneezing or vomiting.

Other risks associated with uterine inversion are an abnormally adherent placenta, fundal placental attachment, a short umbilical cord, nulliparity and fetal macrosomia. Manual removal of the placenta is also a risk.

Recognition

The placenta may or may not be delivered. There is usually a haemorrhage whether or not the placenta is separated. The woman is likely to be showing signs of shock and severe pain, perhaps greater than you would anticipate, due to the nerves and ligaments of the uterus being overstretched. There may be a purple or bluish mass at the introitus, the internal side of the uterus (second and third degree). On abdominal palpation the fundus is not palpable (second and third degree) or a concave or hollow uterus may be felt (first degree).

Management

On recognising any of the symptoms above, call for help. Uterine inversion is an obstetric emergency and immediate action is required (Figure 48.5). While it is an obstetric emergency, midwives are trained and should revise manual replacement of the uterus at emergency study days. Manually replacing the uterus as soon as possible will reduce the woman's pain, and subsequent shock and haemorrhage. The uterus is easiest to replace before oedema and swelling occur in the organ and surrounding tissues. The fundus is pushed back into the vagina towards the posterior fornix (Figure 48.3). If the uterus is successfully replaced, keep your hand in the uterine cavity until a strong contraction is felt, this may be with the administration of an oxytocic. If the uterus is replaced successfully, the woman is likely to need an oxytocic infusion and close monitoring for several hours.

If the uterus is only partially replaced, raising the foot of the bed may reduce the traction on the uterine ligaments and structures (Figure 48.4). At this point more help should be arriving. If the placenta is in situ, no attempt should be made at removing it, as it will exacerbate the haemorrhage.

The midwife will communicate the situation to the woman and her family. She will ensure the baby is in a safe place, either with the partner or in the cot, not held by the mother. Undertake a set of maternal observations: blood pressure, pulse and respiratory rate. These will be recorded and a MEOWS (modified early obstetric warning system) score calculated, every 15 minutes, until the woman is stable. The woman is likely to need an indwelling urinary catheter to accurately monitor fluid balance and renal function.

The anaesthetist is likely to cannulate the woman, take bloods for a full blood picture, clotting screen and cross-match blood for transfusion (in case it is needed). They will administer analgesics, oxygen and fluids to replace the blood loss.

The obstetrician will assess the woman's condition; oxytocic drugs are not administered until after the uterus is replaced, and a uterine muscle relaxant such as terbutiline may be used to facilitate the manual replacement of the uterus. Prolonged manipulation of the uterus is not recommended, so if the woman is in too much pain for another attempt she will be transferred to theatre for anaesthesia and antibiotics prior to a further attempt.

If this is not successful a hydrostatic procedure can be attempted. This involves filling the uterine cavity with 2–3 litres of warm saline with the woman in the Trendelenburg position (Figure 48.4) for the fluid to infuse under gravity. The fluid fills and distends the uterus, which then repositions itself. Oxytocic drugs are administered to maintain uterine contractions once successful version has occurred. The placenta can also be removed.

If the above methods fail, there are surgical procedures that can be undertaken via a laparotomy. The worse case scenario is a hysterectomy.

Aftercare

Depending on management of the inversion and the woman's condition, a high dependency unit (HDU) may be required to monitor this woman's post-theatre recovery. If the inversion was managed in the birthing room and the woman's condition is stable she will not necessarily needs transferring to an HDU.

The woman and her family will need a full explanation of the events to make sense of their experience. Antibiotics for 5 days are required and a longer postnatal stay of 2–3 days is offered.

49 Preterm labour

Figure 49.1 Maternal and fetal risk factors.

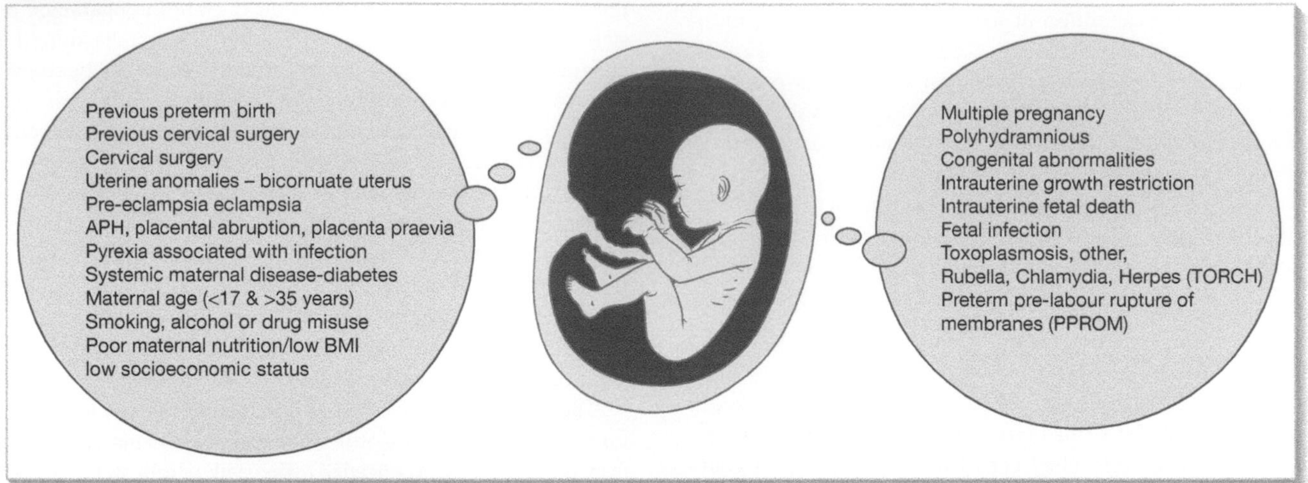

Figure 49.2 Gestation and birth weight.

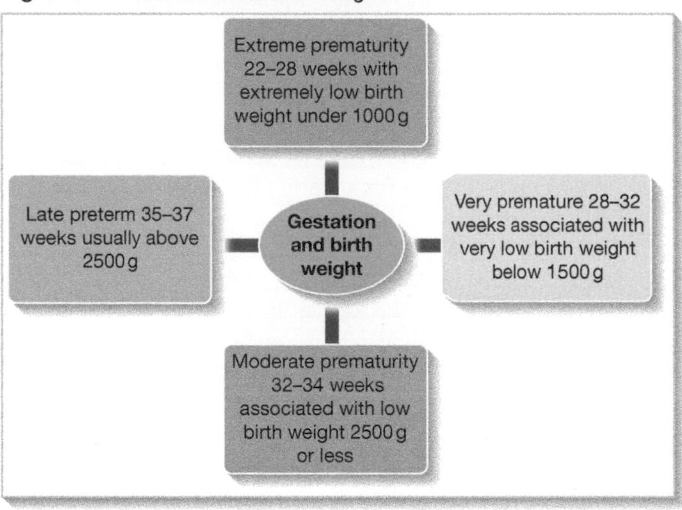

Figure 49.3 Care for the preterm baby.

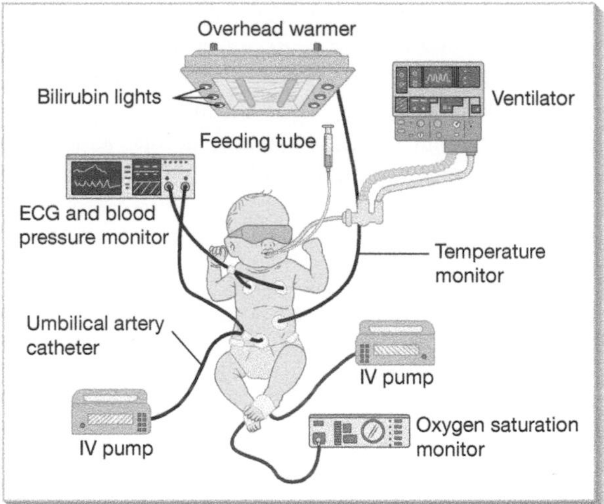

Figure 49.4 Characteristic signs of chorioamnionitis.

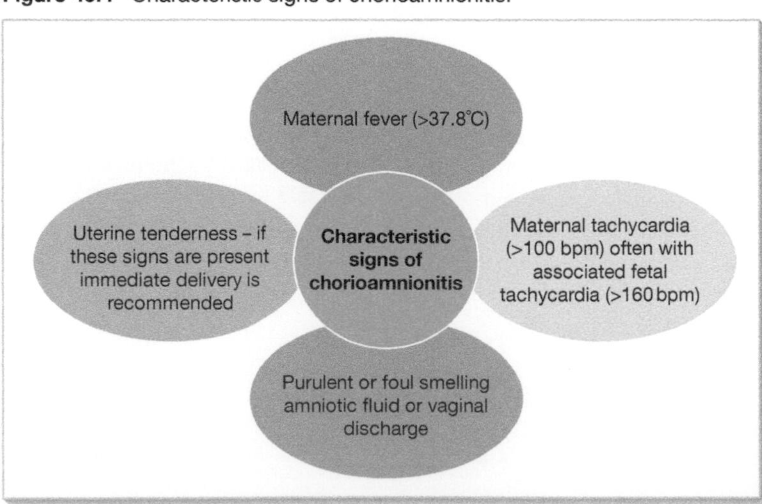

The definition of preterm labour is the commencement of painful regular contractions before 37 completed weeks of pregnancy associated with cervical shortening and dilatation. Threatened preterm labour is uterine activity without the cervical changes.

Incidence and risk factors

The incidence of preterm birth is around 7% of all births; 50% occur spontaneously, 30% occur after preterm prelabour rupture of membranes (PPROM) and 20% are iatrogenic for maternal or fetal indications. Many have no cause (idiopathic). However, there are a range of maternal or fetal contributing factors (Figure 49.1).

Risks of preterm labour and birth

Babies born before 34 weeks are most at risk of morbidity and mortality due to their prematurity. Neonatal morbidity and mortality may occur as a result of intraventricular haemorrhage, respiratory distress syndrome, systemic infections and necrotising entrocolitis; all of which are reduced with antenatal administration of corticosteroids.

The prognosis for preterm infants is dependent upon their birth weight as well as gestational age (Figure 49.2) and the condition of the neonate during labour, birth and the availability of neonatal intensive care for the immediate postnatal period (Figure 49.3).

Management of preterm labour

Any suspected preterm complication (painful regular contractions or preterm rupture of membranes, with or without contractions or vaginal blood loss) should be referred to an obstetrician, as it is outside the scope of normal midwifery practice. However, the midwife will be carrying out the initial care and observations and communicating with the woman and her family.

A full maternal history should be taken with a current assessment of the pregnancy. Precise dating of the gestation is required (confirmed by early ultrasound). If the woman has rhesus negative blood, follow local guidelines.

Maternal observations (temperature, pulse, respiratory rate and blood pressure) and abdominal palpation (remembering there is likely to be a higher incidence of breech presentation at earlier gestations) are undertaken and recorded. Ask about vaginal discharge to exclude PPROM, vaginal bleeding or infective discharge and obtain a urine sample to exclude urinary tract infection (UTI). These factors, UTI, antepartum haemorrhage (APH) and PPROM need to be excluded and treated differentially.

Monitor the contractions – their length, strength and duration – and maternal pain. Assessment of fetal wellbeing includes symphisus fundal height (SFH) measurement and auscultation of the fetal heart; usually continuous cardiotocography (CTG) is indicated on admission. Interpreting fetal CTG patterns prior to 34 weeks is more difficult.

The obstetrician will perform a speculum examination initially and a further one in 2–3 hours with cervical changes confirming a diagnosis of preterm labour. An ultrasound scan may be indicated to assess fetal size, presentation, fetal breathing movements and liquor volume to help decide on the management plan (steroids; consider tocolysis, mode and place of birth). Corticosteroids are prescribed and administered, with maternal consent, for threatened and suspected preterm labour. Even a short interval between the administration of the drug and birth has advantages for the neonate. The optimal time of birth is between 24 hours and 1 week after the administration of steroids. The optimal mode of birth is vaginal, unless contraindicated by fetal presentation, placenta praevia or other condition.

Tocolysis (relaxation of the uterine muscle) is considered and tocolytics (drugs to suppress labour) can be administered to delay the birth or transfer the woman to a hospital with intensive neonatal care facilities, depending on the gestation of the pregnancy. Some labours are too advanced to consider tocolytics, or if the woman is showing signs of infection or abruption prompt delivery is required. If the gestational age is greater than 34 weeks these drugs are not considered.

Nifedipine or atosiban are the two main drugs used to delay labour; both have side effects including nausea, vomiting, headache, cardiac palpitations and hypertension, which need to be monitored and the treatment stopped if severe.

Magnesium sulphate has a neuroprotective mechanism for the fetus and is prescribed to reduce the incidence of cerebral palsy in gestations of between 24 and 30 weeks.

Once in labour care should include continuous CTG to assess fetal wellbeing (the preterm fetus has fewer reserves in labour and is more likely to become hypoxic). Delayed cord clamping is preferred if immediate resuscitation is not required. A paediatrician should be present; as should resuscitation equipment and a plastic bag for gestations of less than 30 weeks, to create a microenvironment and prevent excessive heat loss by evaporation. Swabs from the baby are taken to exclude infection and cord bloods to assess metabolic condition. Transfer to a neonatal unit is dependent upon gestation age, weight and condition.

Management of preterm prelabour rupture of membranes

PPROM is a significant indicator of preterm birth, occurring in 2:100 births. The risks for the fetus are as for preterm labour but both the mother and fetus are at increased risk of infection or chorioamnionitis (Figure 49.4). Women with PPROM require 4-hourly observations including for contractions and fetal CTG to assess their wellbeing for 48 hours. Most women with PPROM will labour spontaneously within 1 week.

Administration of corticosteroid and prophylactic antibiotics is required if the gestational age is below 34 weeks, to mature the fetal lungs and prevent chorioamnionitis. Tocolysis is not indicated for PPROM alone, however if labour is suspected see earlier.

Optimal delivery time for woman with PPROM is usually between 34 and 37 weeks, providing a balance between enabling the fetus to mature and be in optimal condition and decreasing the risk of chorioamnionitis. Where preterm labour is excluded and women are asymptomatic, expectant management may occur with the woman at home, with daily temperature assessment and vigilance, if preferred.

50 Eclampsia

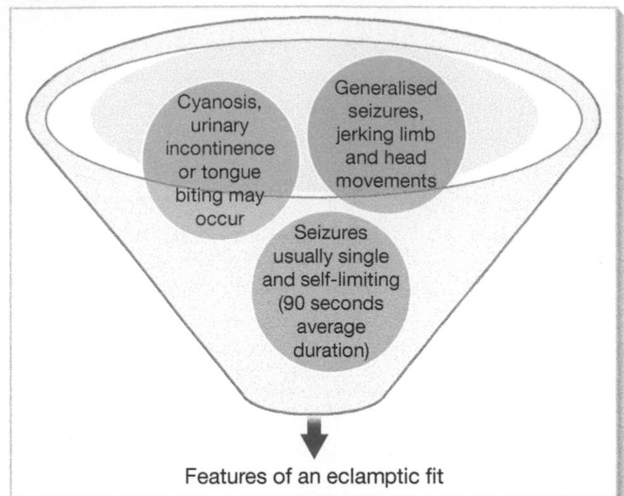

Figure 50.1 Features of an eclamptic fit.

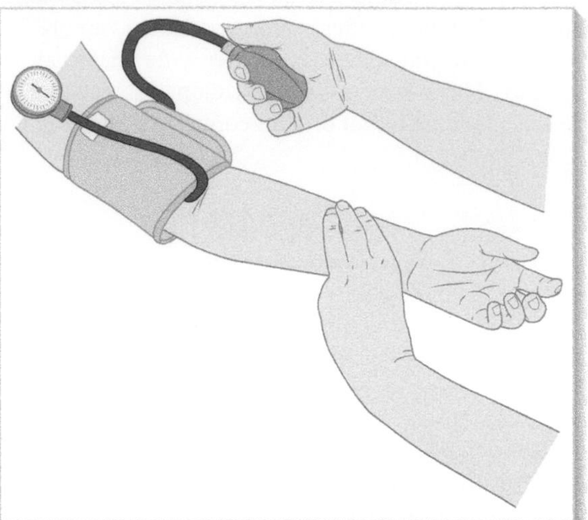

Figure 50.2 Blood pressure monitoring.

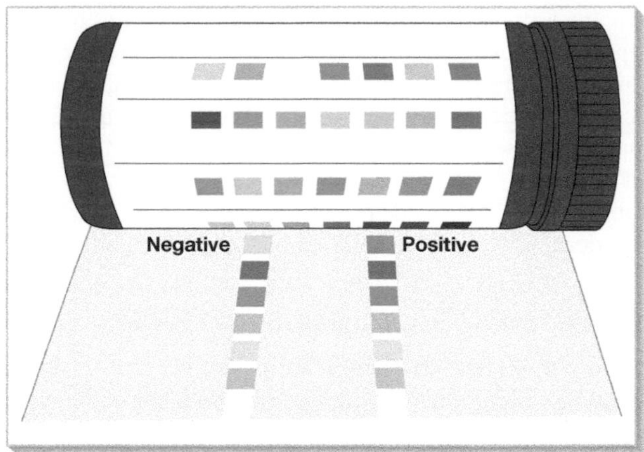

Figure 50.3 Testing for proteinuria.

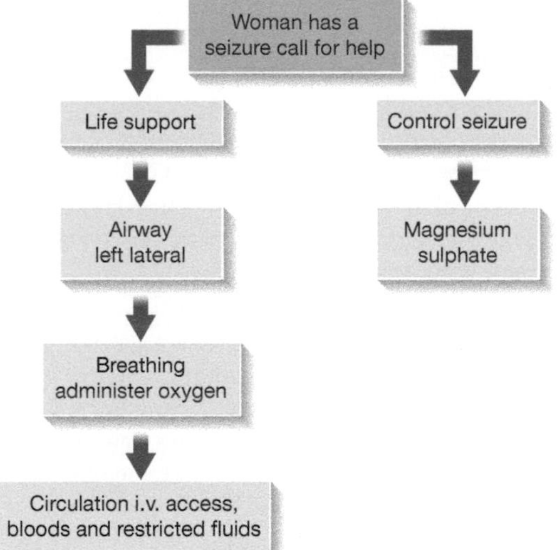

Figure 50.4 Management of eclampsia.

Table 50.1 Management of pregnancy with pre-eclampsia.

Degree of hypertension	Mild hypertension (140/90 to 149/99 mmHg)	Moderate hypertension (150/100 to 159/109 mmHg)	Severe hypertension (160/110 mmHg or higher)
Admit to hospital	Yes	Yes	Yes
Treat	No	With oral labetalol as first-line treatment to keep: diastolic blood pressure between 80 and 100 mmHg systolic blood pressure less than 150 mmHg	With oral labetalol as first-line treatment to keep: diastolic blood pressure between 80 and 100 mmHg systolic blood pressure less than 150 mmHg
Measure blood pressure	At least 4 times a day	At least 4 times a day	More than 4 times a day, depending on clinical circumstances
Test for proteinuria	Do not repeat quantification of proteinuria	Do not repeat quantification of proteinuria	Do not repeat quantification of proteinuria
Blood tests	Monitor using the following tests twice a week: kidney function, electrolytes, full blood count, transaminase, bilirubin	Monitor using the following tests three times a week: kidney function, electrolytes, full blood count, transaminases, bilirubin	Monitor using the following tests three times a week: kidney function, electrolytes, full blood count, transaminases, bilirubin

Midwifery at a Glance, First Edition. Edited by Eleanor Forrest © 2019 John Wiley & Sons, Ltd. Published 2019 by John Wiley & Sons, Ltd.
Companion website: www.wiley.com/go/forrest/midwifery

Hypertensive disorders are a leading cause of maternal morbidity worldwide, including in the UK. Substandard care is a feature of maternal deaths. Severe hypertension with a systolic BP above 160 mmHg must be treated to prevent maternal morbidity and mortality.

Eclampsia is defined as one or more convulsions associated with pre-eclampsia (Figure 50.1). Most women who have an eclamptic fit in the UK will not have the pre-eclampsia warning signs of raised BP (Figure 50.2) and proteinuria (Figure 50.3). Most eclamptic fits occur in the postpartum period (44%), with 38% occurring in the antenatal period and 18% intrapartum.

Management of eclampsia

The management of eclampsia involves basic life support as well as seizure management (Figure 50.4). Call for multidisciplinary help, including an obstetrician, anaesthetist and senior midwife. Contact the consultant obstetrician and anaesthetist too. Note the time of seizure and time help arrives.

Life support consists of airway management, breathing and circulation. As most seizures are self-limiting often the need for resuscitation is short lived. Place the women in the left lateral position or with a lateral tilt, especially in pregnancy to prevent pressure from the gravid uterus restricting blood back to the heart via the inferior vena cava. Do not restrain the woman, but maintain her safety through the fit. Once she has finished seizing, leave her to recover in the left lateral position. Administer facial high-flow oxygen. Intravenous access is required for the life support and to administer anticonvulsants, as 5–30% of women will seize again.

Insert a large bore cannula, take bloods for full blood count (FBC), urea and electrolytes, liver function tests, clotting and group and save. Start i.v. magnesium sulphate treatment. This prevents more recurrent seizures than other drugs. However, if the woman has another seizure diazepam or thiopentone may be administered if an anaesthetist is present. Magnesiun sulphate is administered in three phases, first a loading dose, then a maintenance dose and more is administered if seizures reoccur.

Document all care and drugs given and the timing of events. Consider mode and timing of birth when the woman is stable.

Pre-eclampsia

More frequently women are admitted to hospital with signs and symptoms of pre-eclampsia. The severity of their pre-eclampsia will determine where the woman should be cared for (Table 50.1).

Severe pre-eclampsia is defined by BP above or equal to 160/110 mmHg and proteinuria *or* mild to moderate hypertension, which is defined as BP between 140/90 and 159/109 mmHg, and proteinuria with one other feature:

- Severe headache
- Blurred vision
- Severe epigastric pain or vomiting
- Papilloedema
- Signs of clonus
- Liver tenderness
- HELLP syndrome (haemolysis, elevated liver enzymes and low platelet count)
- Platelet count falling to less than 100×10^9/litre
- Abnormal liver enzymes.

Management of severe pre-eclampsia

If a woman presents with severe pre eclampsia alert medical staff as it is outside the remit of a midwife. The care and treatment will be based around three principles:

1 Stabilise BP and prevent seizures.

2 Monitor vital signs, urine output, fluid balance, blood picture, neurological status and fetal condition.

3 Plan for labour and birth, including external fetal monitoring and possibly an epidural to reduce BP, a short second stage if BP is symptomatic, use of syntocinon (*not* syntometrine or ergometrine) and post birth consider thromboprophylaxis.

The rational for these management principles is to reduce the chance of intracranial haemorrhage associated with severe systolic hypertension. Pre-eclampsia can become more severe rapidly and a threshold of systolic pressure below 150 mmHg is preferred. Pressures above 160 mmHg should be considered an emergency and treated promptly.

The usual antihypertensive drugs are nifedipine or labetalol; these can be continued in labour. Automated BP machines often underestimate the BP so a manual BP measurement with the appropriate cuff size should be taken. Consider magnesium sulphate if indicated to prevent seizures.

As the woman's condition can deteriorate rapidly, observations are taken initially every 15 minutes and calculated as a MEOWS (modified early obstetric warning system) score, then every 30 minutes if the woman's condition is stable. The fetal condition will also be monitored. Urine output is measured hourly via an indwelling catheter. Oxygen saturations are also taken hourly. Bloods are taken 12–24 hourly. If the woman is on magnesium sulphate, continuous monitoring of the oxygen saturation is required. Strict fluid balance and restricted intake (of 80 ml/h) helps prevent pulmonary oedema, balanced by the risk of renal failure if there is not enough urine production (oliguria), that is less than 100 ml in 4 hours.

Planning for birth occurs when the woman's condition is stable. The mode of birth depends on the woman's condition. If a preterm birth is considered give corticosteroids to mature the fetal lungs (Chapter 49).

Post birth

Mothers will require continuous monitoring following birth if they have had an eclamptic seizure or management of severe pre eclampsia. The timeframe depends on the severity of their condition. Most seizures occur in the postnatal period and pre-eclampsia can worsen for several days after birth. Non-steroidal drugs should be avoided as they can precipitate renal failure. Consider thromboprophylaxis as severe pre-eclampsia is a risk factor. Even though the antihypertensive drugs will be continued in the postnatal period they are safe to take while breastfeeding. The midwife will support the woman and her family in the postnatal period as the events prior to birth may have been very frightening, especially if the woman had a seizure.

The long-term sequelae are an increased risk of raised BP later in life and increased risk of pre-eclampsia in the next pregnancy.

51 Disseminating intravascular coagulopathy, shock and high dependency care

Figure 51.1 Purpura and petechiae.

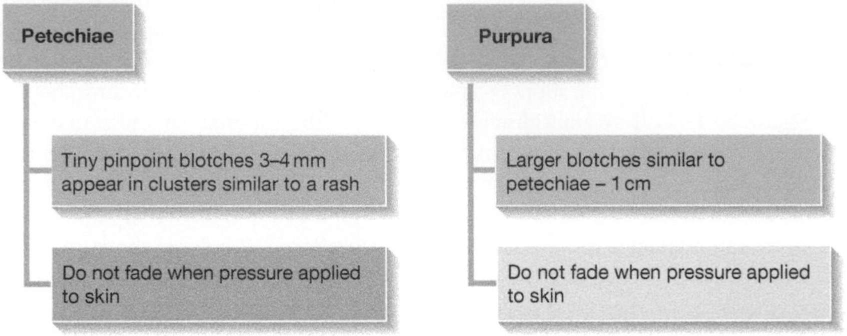

Figure 51.2 Types of shock.

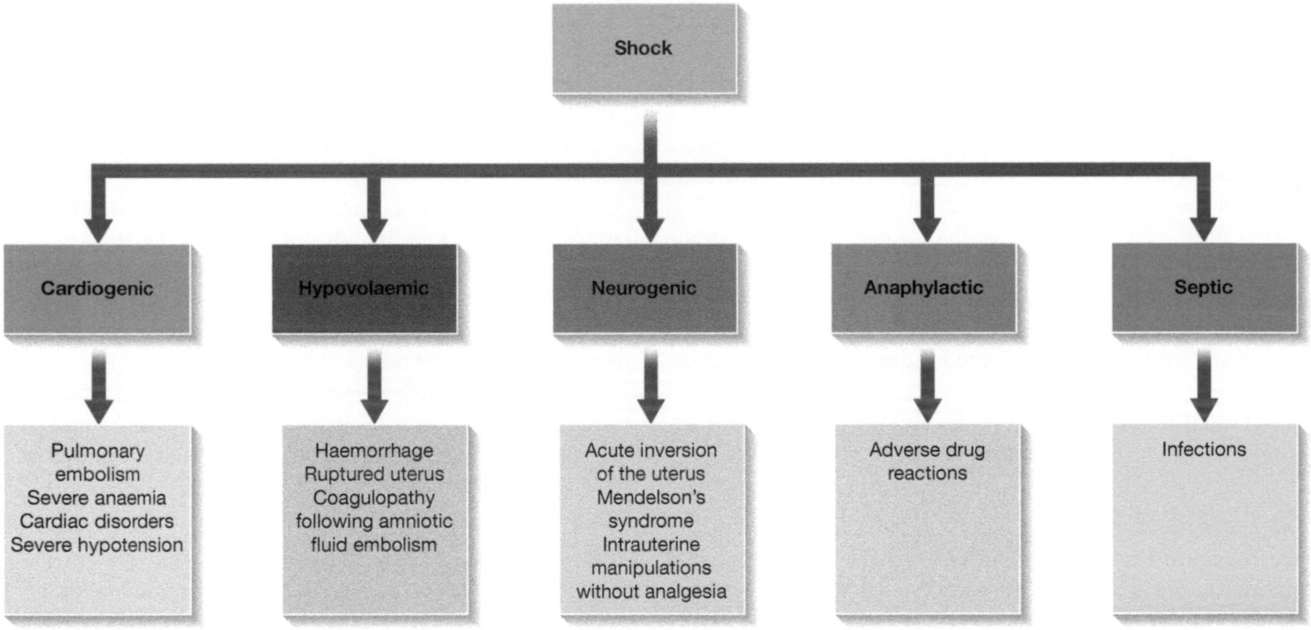

Table 51.1 Blood picture for DIC.

Reduced	Prolonged
Platelets, fibrinogen and clotting factors	Prothrombin times, as the plasma takes longer to clot, and activated partial thromboplastin time

Disseminating intravascular coagulopathy (DIC) may occur as a result of many of the preceding obstetric topics, such as abruption, sepsis, massive blood loss, severe pre-eclampsia or amniotic fluid embolism. It is a pathological process that occurs as a complication of the previously mentioned conditions and blood transfusion reactions. It affects the clotting cascade and creates small blood clots throughout the vascular system. This leads to the tissues of the body not being properly oxygenated by the blood and ultimately organ failure (ischaemia). In addition to this, as the body creates clots, it uses up all the clotting factors and severe bleeding ensues. The bleeding can be internal, within the organs or visible externally such as under the surface of the skin (Figure 51.1). For laboratory results see Table 51.1. Treatment is to fix the underlying cause of the DIC.

Signs and symptoms of DIC

One of the most common signs is purpura or petechiae, (purple spots or rashes) caused by bleeding under the skin (Figure 51.1). Any unexpected bleeding from the nose, mucosal membranes or venepuncture sites also needs reporting as well as haematuria.

Maternal observations will often demonstrate hypotension, as there is less circulating blood volume, and tachycardia as the heart rate increases to pump more blood to the organs to oxygenate them. The woman may be sweating and have cold and mottled fingers as the extremities are not perfused. When the cardiovascular system fails to perfuse the tissues adequately the condition is called shock. Untreated shock can lead to death, so the midwife must be vigilant undertaking and reporting maternal observations and understand the implications of changes.

Modified early obstetric warning system (MEOWS) scores are used to identify women who are critically ill, either with DIC, shock or other critical cases. These observation score sheets were introduced as too many midwives were failing to recognise the deteriorating condition of women who needed more urgent medical review and treatment. The respiratory rate is one of the most sensitive observations. Each hospital MEOWS will have a clear pathway for the midwife to follow should the woman's observations trigger a certain score, when often she will be exhibiting signs of shock.

Shock

There are several types of shock (Figure 51.2). These are summarised as cardiogenic, hypovolaemic, neurogenic, anaphylactic and septic.

Heart failure usually due to myocardial infarction is the main cause of cardiogenic shock. However, in childbearing this is rare and pre-existing cardiac conditions may be more common. As the cardiac output decreases, the kidneys produce a hormone so sodium and water are retained. The blood vessels constrict to help maintain the blood pressure. The body still needs nutrients and oxygen, so when the demand outweighs the heart's capacity to provide this, metabolism inside the cells fails and shock is evident.

Hypovolaemic shock is the most common type of shock in midwifery/obstetrics. Shock develops when the woman has lost 15% of her intravascular volume. Initially the pulse is thready, as vasoconstriction helps keep blood supplied to the vital organs and reduces the flow to the peripheries. A sharp decline in maternal blood pressure is usually a late serious sign of shock.

Neurogenic shock occurs when the balance between the parasympathetic and sympathetic nervous system is disturbed and results in vasodilatation of the smooth blood vessels. Although the blood volume does not change, the systemic vascular resistance falls, and if the sympathetic system cannot respond, the mother will become bradycardic and have a very low blood pressure. Fainting is one way the body copes initially to this to equalise the blood pressure across the body.

Anaphylactic shock is a severe reaction to a pollen, insect or snake bite or peanut but it can also be hospital induced by administering drugs that the woman is allergic to. The circulatory system and bronchus constricts, making this shock a rapid emergency as death can occur within minutes. Adrenaline will reverse the airway constriction initially, but other treatments such as volume expanders and steroids may be used to reduce the other effects.

Septic shock is complex; an infection usually invades the respiratory, gastrointestinal or genital tract. The infection develops and enters the blood system, leading to bacteraemia and shock.

High dependency care

Women who develop DIC have an underlying condition and may develop hypovolaemic shock as well. While midwives are competent and trained to care for women experiencing the obstetric emergencies mentioned earlier in this chapter, when shock or DIC is diagnosed a high dependency unit (HDU) bed is usually needed. Not only is this woman critically ill, she needs invasive monitoring of her body systems to ensure minimal organ damage occurs and she survives.

Invasive blood pressure treatment is frequently needed to maintain blood pressure and prevent further ischaemia or renal failure. Arterial or central venous blood pressure monitoring is frequently used. Ventilatory support is often required after surgery for critically ill women. The average length of stay for women is short, around 2 days, and their care, when stabilised, will be transferred back to the midwifery department for a further couple of days.

While the mother and baby may be separated, the advantages of HDU care are that all the staff, nursing, anaesthetic and theatre staff are familiar with the equipment and treatments required. The midwife will visit the unit to perform postnatal checks (Chapters 27 and 28) and the baby will be able to visit if he or she is stable.

52 Malposition and malpresentation

Figure 52.1 Occipitoposterior presentation.

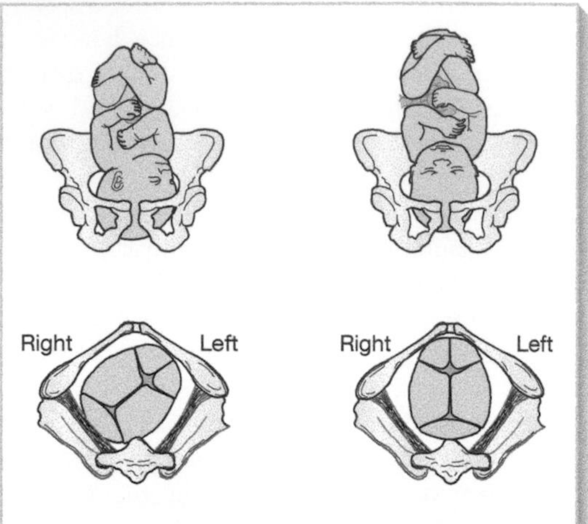

Figure 52.2 Breech positions.

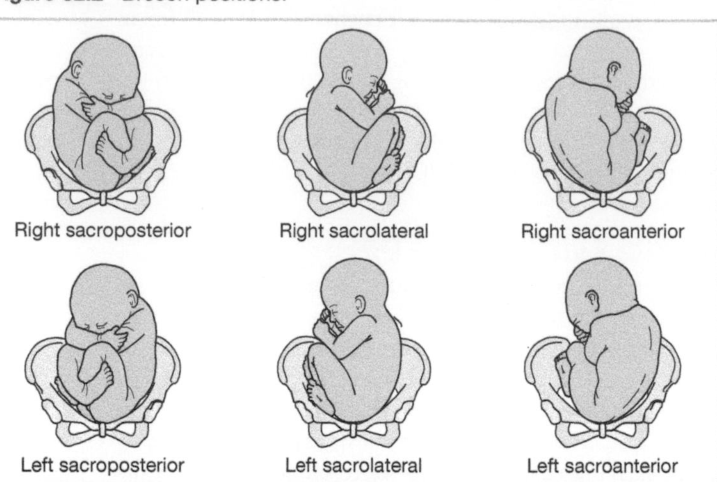

Figure 52.3 Breech presentation.

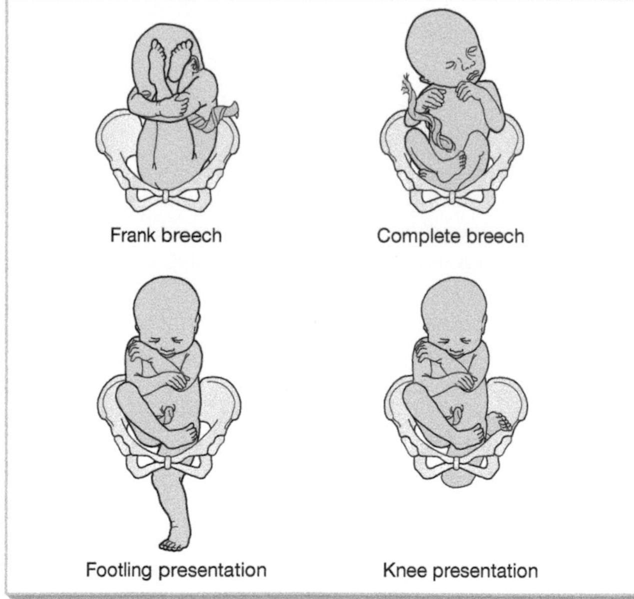

Figure 52.4 Shoulder presentation.

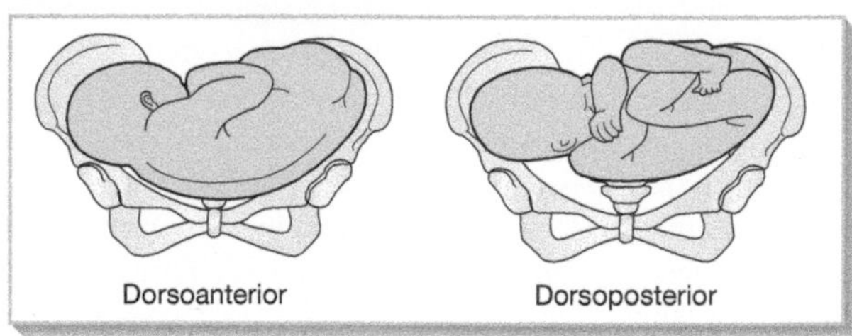

Figure 52.5 Brow presentation.

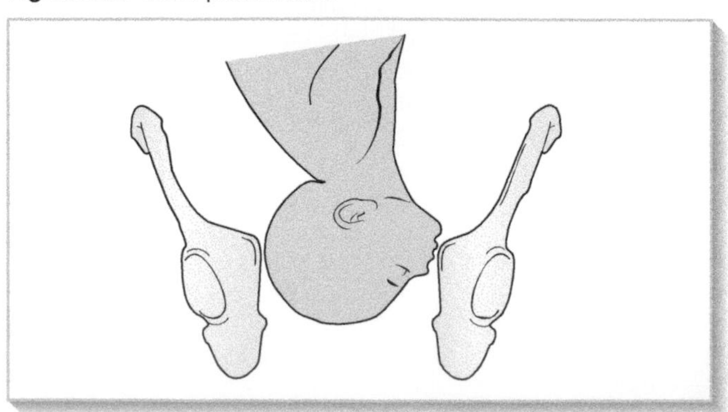

Figure 52.6 Face presentation.

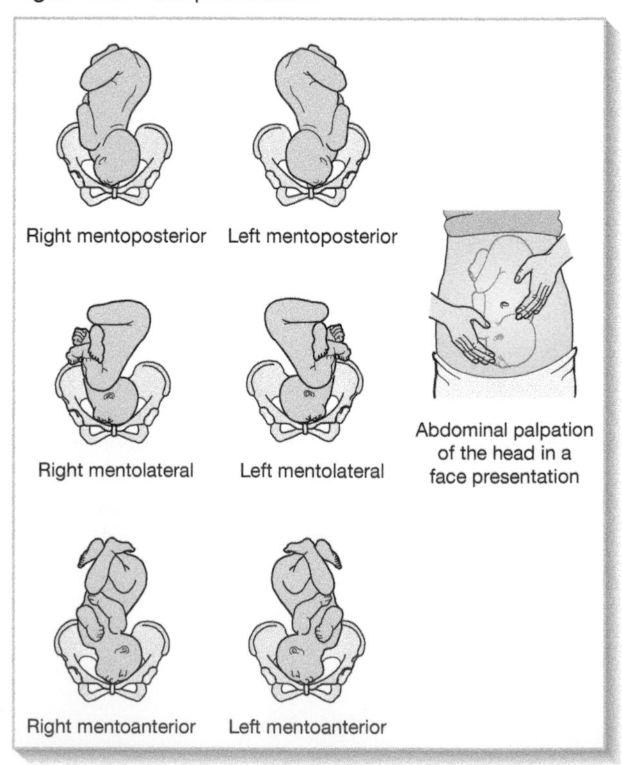

Malposition is a position other than an occipitoanterior (OA) position. Malpresentations are fetal presenting parts other than vertex.

Malposition

Malpositions include occipitoposterior (OP) (Figure 52.1) and occipitotransverse positions of the fetal head in relation to the maternal pelvis and asynclitism. Factors that increase the likelihood of malposition are:

- Pendulous abdomen – in multiparous women
- Anthropoid pelvic brim – favours OP/OA positions
- Android pelvic brim
- A flat sacrum – favours transverse position
- Placenta on the anterior uterine wall
- Asynclitism.

Occipitoposterior position

The OP labour and birth is not remarkably different from that of an OA one. When the fetal head is well down into the pelvis and a persistent OP position, the possibilities for vaginal birth are:

- Spontaneous birth in the OP position
- Forceps delivery in the OP position
- Manual rotation to the OA position and delivery
- Forceps rotation to the OA position and delivery.

Spontaneous birth

If the pelvic outlet is a good size and the vaginal outlet and perineum are somewhat relaxed from previous vaginal births, spontaneous birth often occurs. As the OP position places more strain on the perineum, the head is pushed against the perineum with more force than in the OA position. The second stage of labour may be prolonged. An episiotomy may be needed. Alternative assisted deliveries are forceps delivery in the OP position, manual rotation and forceps rotation.

Malpresentation

Malpresentations consist of breech, shoulder, brow or face presentations.

Breech presentation

Breech presentations (Figures 52.2 and 52.3) may be classified into:

- Frank – hips flexed and legs extended over the anterior body surface
- Complete – hips and legs flexed
- Footling – foot presenting
- Knee – knee presenting.

Diagnosis will usually occur during pregnancy through the palpation of the head in the apex of the uterus, however sometimes it may not occur until labour has commenced via vaginal examination. If diagnosed early in pregnancy, external cephalic version (ECV) can be performed.

External cephalic version

Conversion of breech to vertex presentation is undertaken to lower the liklihood of breech presentations in labour. Version is usually attempted about the 36th week and is performed where there are emergency caesarean section facilities. Tocolytic agents are used to aid in relaxation, the fetal heart rate is continuously monitored and the procedure is performed with ultrasound guidance. The success rate of ECV varies greatly; however when performed after 36 weeks, the gain in vertex presentations at delivery is about 30%. If the breech is to be birthed vaginally, specific mechanisms for assisting with a breech birth are required.

Shoulder presentation

Shoulder presentation is when the fetus lies with its long axis transverse to the long axis of the mother's body and with the shoulder (scapula) presenting at the pelvis (Figure 52.4). The denominator can be in one of the following positions: left scapuloanterior, right scapuloanterior, right scapuloposterior and left scapuloposterior.

Scapuloanterior is the most common because the concavity of the front of the fetus tends to fit with the convexity of the maternal spines. This is usually diagnosed during pregnancy – on inspection when the abdomen is broader from side to side and on palpation. ECV can be done in late pregnancy or even early in labour if the membranes are intact; vaginal delivery may then be feasible. During labour, if not noted on palpation, vaginal examination will reveal a high presenting part, bulging membranes or premature rupture of membranes with prolapsed arm or cord. An emergency caesarean section needs to be performed.

Brow presentation

Brow presentation results from extension of the fetal neck so that the sinciput lies below the occiput (Figure 52.5). The fetal head therefore presents with its largest mentovertical diameter (13 cm) to the maternal pelvis. There is the possibility that it will spontaneously convert to either a vertex or face presentation by flexion or further extension with advancing labour, especially if the fetus is small.

Diagnosis can be made on abdominal examination if a lot of the fetal head is palpable, however engagement of the fetal head can occur. Definitive diagnosis is usually made at vaginal examination when the anterior fontanelle, the orbital ridges and the nose are felt. Usually diagnosis occurs late in labour because feeling such landmarks can be difficult in early labour and also because extension to a brow presentation can occur during labour due to further extension of a deflexed vertex as it descends.

Face presentation

Face presentation can occur in a normal fetus (Figure 52.6). However, structural anomalies that cause hyperextension of the neck, such as anencephaly or neck tumours, are associated with face presentation. The fetal head will present with a small submento-bregmatic diameter. The chin is the reference point (denominator) in describing the position of the head in relation to the maternal pelvis. The majority of face presentations are mentoanterior in the maternal pelvis. In these cases a spontaneous vaginal birth can occur with the fetal head being born by flexion of the neck. In those with persistent mentoposterior faces, vaginal birth is impossible. Diagnosis can be on abdominal examination if a sharp angulation is felt between the occiput and the back. However, vaginal examination is the usual means of diagnosis by feeling landmarks such as the mandible.

53 Postpartum haemorrhage

Box 53.1 Antenatal risk factors.

- Previous retained placenta or PPH
- Praevia, percreta/accreta
- Previous lower uterine segment caesarean section with above
- Antepartum haemorrhage from abruption
- Overdistention of pregnant uterus
- Pre-eclampsia
- BMI >35
- Increased maternal age
- Uterine abnormalities, e.g. fibroids
- Grand multiparity
- Low haemaglobin (reduce anaemia in pregnancy to reduce risk)

Box 53.2 Intrapartum risk factors.

- Induction of labour
- Prolonged 1st, 2nd or 3rd stages of labour (+ 'non-active' management of 3rd stage)
- Oxytocin use in labour
- Retained placenta
- Precipitate labour
- Operative vaginal birth
- LSCS particularly 2nd stage
- Placental abruption
- Pyrexia in labour

Box 53.3 Management.

- Call for help
- Lie flat (administer oxygen)
- Rub up uterus (bimanual compression?)
- i.v. access 2x large bore cannulae
- Take blood (full blood count, group, cross-match, coagulation screen)
- Replace fluid (2 litres Hartmans/saline first)
- Measure observations (temperature, pressure, respiration, blood pressure, oxygen saturations)

Box 53.4 Professional issues.

Consideration must be given to:

- Documentation
- Incident form completed as per unit policy
- Debriefing for the woman and partner
- Reflecting on own experience
- Ensuring all staff are up to date: PPH policy and completion of mandatory training

Figure 53.1 Bimanual compression.

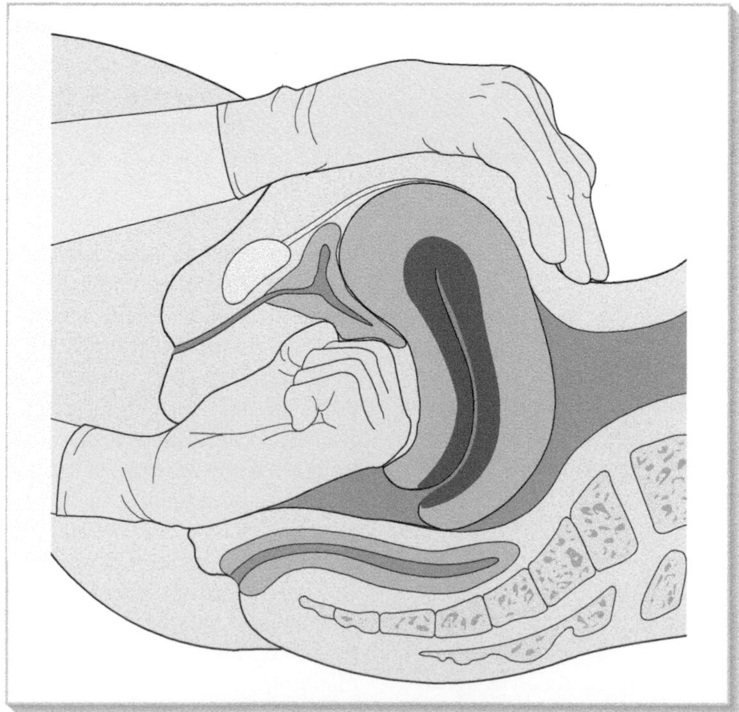

Midwifery at a Glance, First Edition. Edited by Eleanor Forrest © 2019 John Wiley & Sons, Ltd. Published 2019 by John Wiley & Sons, Ltd.
Companion website: www.wiley.com/go/forrest/midwifery

A postpartum haemorrhage (PPH) is an obstetric emergency that a midwife will face following complex and straightforward births. It is stressful for the woman, family and the midwife and can have devastating effects. It is one of the causes of maternal mortality.

Definitions

A PPH is defined as bleeding from the genital tract occurring any time from the birth of the baby to the end of the puerperium. It can be primary or secondary.

- **Primary PPH** – blood loss of 500 ml or more within the first 24 hours after delivery. This can be minor (500–1000 ml) or major (> 1000 ml); the latter can be divided to moderate (1000–2000 ml) or severe (> 2000 ml)).
- **Secondary PPH** – blood loss of 500 ml or more after 24 hours postpartum.

Blood, like any fluid, is difficult to measure with accuracy when soaked into bedding and spilled on a floor. Most healthy women can cope with a 500 ml loss, but any blood loss, however small, that affects a woman adversely should constitute a PPH. Therefore clinical appearance of shock helps establish if the woman is coping with the blood loss.

Risk factors

- Pre-labour (Box 53.1)
- Intrapartum (Box 53.2).

Causes

The causes of PPH are attributed to tone, tissue, trauma or thrombin (known as the 4 'T's).

Tone

Tone of the uterus and poor contracting of the uterus is the most common cause of PPH. If the uterus is not contracted this could be because the bladder is full and is displacing the uterus in the pelvic cavity and therefore preventing it from contracting fully. In this case the midwife should ensure that the bladder is emptied by inserting an indwelling catheter. If the uterus is not well contracted the midwife should rub up a contraction and give first line management drugs.

Tissue

Tissue could be the reason for the PPH when the placenta or membranes have been left in the uterus after expulsion has occurred. This will prevent the uterus from contracting effectively. The midwife should ensure that the placenta is examined carefully to confirm completeness and hence no retained products. If on examination the placenta is incomplete, the medical team and woman need to be notified and the woman should be prepped for exploration and evacuation under anaesthetic.

Trauma

The perineum and vaginal wall should be examined for any tears and the genital tract observed for any signs of trauma which the bleeding could be attributed to. If there is a perineal tear this should be repaired. However, if a cervical or vaginal tear is suspected then the medical team need to be notified and the woman should be transferred to theatre.

Thrombin

PPH can be caused due to blood clotting irregularities either known or as a result of the excessive bleeding. In such cases the medical team and especially a haematologist need to be contacted immediately

Signs

- Visible bleeding
- Maternal collapse.

More subtle signs include:

- Pallor
- Rising pulse rate
- Falling blood pressure
- Altered level of consciousness, restless, drowsy
- Enlarged uterus, distended and lacking tone.

Management

Management of a PPH should follow a very structured process (Box 53.3). This involves getting help immediately, lying the woman flat and administering oxygen. This should be followed by rubbing up a uterine contraction, gaining intravenous access and obtaining blood for testing and grouping, replacing fluid loss and, if necessary, undertaking bimanual compression (Figure 53.1) and measuring observations.

Fluid replacement and the use of blood and blood products should be strictly monitored and the amount given should be dictated by the lead clinician (consultant anaesthetist or consultant obstetrician) aided by the results of full blood count and clotting screen under the guidance of a haematologist and/or consultant in transfusion medicine.

A urometer should be used to measure urinary output, as a reduced output of < 30 ml could indicate hypovolaemic shock.

Drug management

The first drugs given are: syntometrine (if BP not raised); syntocinon 10 IU; or ergometrine 500 μg i.m. or slow i.v. This would be followed by: syntocinon infusion 40 units via pump over 4 hours; carboprost 250 μg i.m. every 15 minutes up to eight times; and misoprostol 800 μg per rectum.

Later management

- B-lynch suture (braces the uterus)
- Packing (tamponade)
- Radiology
- Hysterectomy.

Additional midwifery care

- Reassure woman
- Communicate with woman/family
- Communicate with team
- Keep woman warm
- Professional issues (Box 53.4).

54 Multiple pregnancy

Figure 54.1 Monozygotic twin pregnancies.

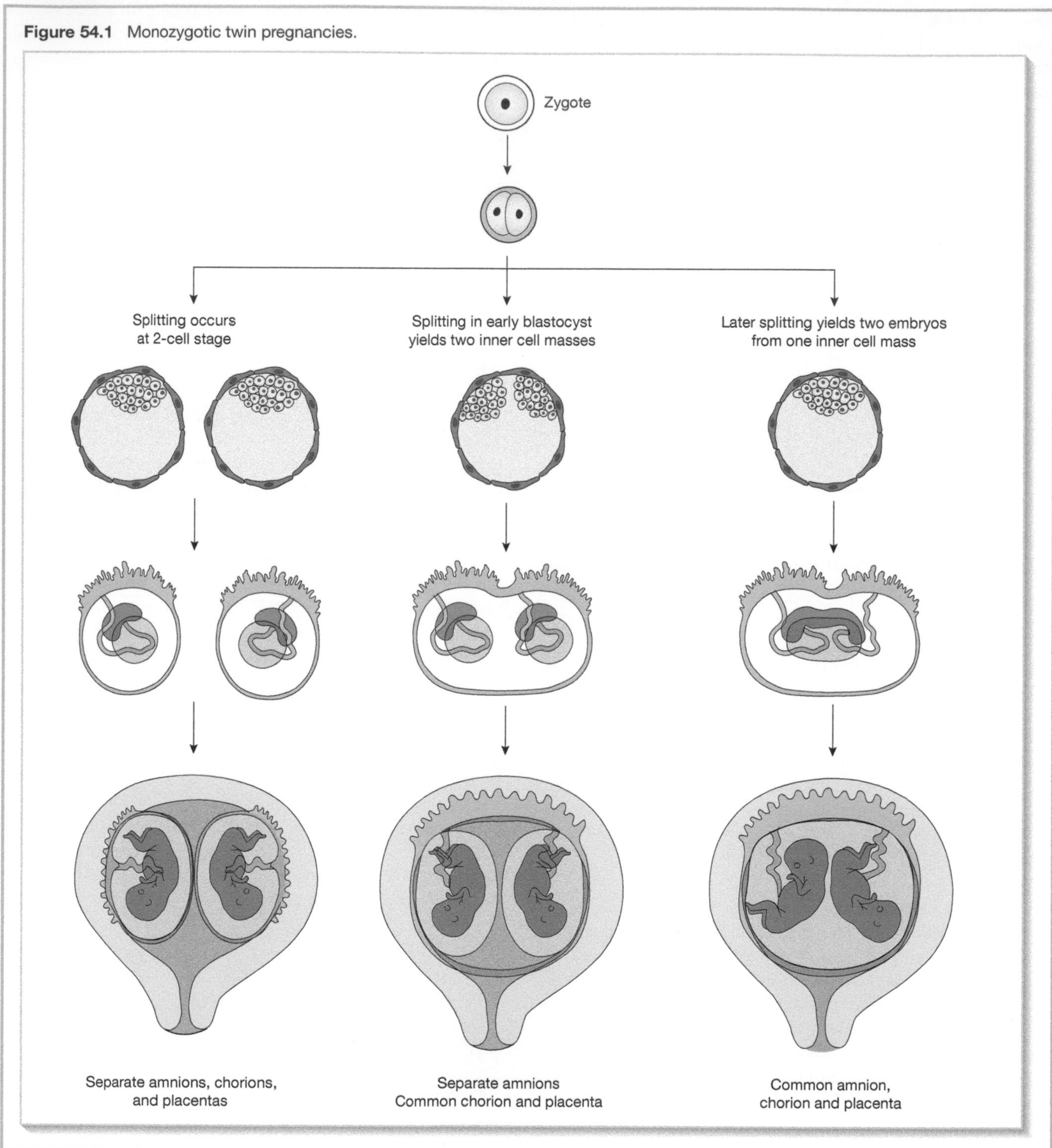

Midwifery at a Glance, First Edition. Edited by Eleanor Forrest © 2019 John Wiley & Sons, Ltd. Published 2019 by John Wiley & Sons, Ltd.
Companion website: www.wiley.com/go/forrest/midwifery

Incidence and variation of type

A multiple pregnancy refers to the situation where more than one fetus develops in utero. In the majority of cases this will be a twin pregnancy. The naturally occurring incidence of twin pregnancy is generally reported as being 1:100 pregnancies although the incidence of twinning within different populations varies, with low incidences reported in Asia and the highest incidence in sub-Saharan Africa. The incidence of twin pregnancies within Europe lies between these extremes but varies between different countries. As the incidence of monozygotic pregnancy occurs at a constant rate of 4:1000 pregnancies across all populations, variations in incidence between populations are attributed to dizygotic twinning.

Various factors have been traditionally viewed as being influential in the incidence of spontaneously occurring twinning such as increasing maternal age and familial tendency. Recent discontinuation of the combined oral contraceptive is associated with a higher incidence of twin pregnancies. More recently, a marked increase in the incidence of multiple pregnancies has been associated with the use of fertility treatments. The increasing use of early scanning in pregnancy has demonstrated that the incidence of twin conception is probably far greater than the incidence of twins born; suggesting that early demise of a twin is a fairly common occurrence (vanishing twin syndrome).

Twin pregnancies fall broadly into two main types: dizygotic and monozygotic. Two-thirds of all twin pregnancies will be dizygotic. This form of twinning is also known as non-identical or binovular and results from the fertilisation of two separate ova by two different sperm. The resulting fetuses are totally independent of each other in terms of genetic material and are no more similar that other siblings. Consequently dizygotic twins each have their own placenta, chorion and amnion (dichorionic-diamniotic), and may be of the same or different sex.

In contrast monozygotic twins, also known as uniovular or identical, result from the fertilisation of one ovum (Figure 54.1). This fertilised ovum then divides at an early stage into two separate pregnancies derived from the same genetic material, resulting in identical twins of the same sex. The timing of the division of the fertilised ovum into two separate pregnancies is crucial in determining the extent to which the twins will share their placenta and membranes. The earlier the division, the more independent the two twins will be from each other and the greater the chance of two healthy babies resulting. Division of the zygote into two separate pregnancies will result in both twins having their own placenta, chorion and amnion. Later division of the dividing cells results in variations of shared physiology. Slightly later division, at the blastocyst stage, is likely to result in a shared placenta and chorion but individual amniotic sacs (monochorionic-diamniotic), whereas even later division may result in the twins sharing a chorion, amnion and placenta (monochorionic-monoamniotic). Very late division of the embryonic disc may result in co-joined twins. This occurs in 1% of monochorionic-monozygotic twinning.

Complications of pregnancy

The incidence of complications of pregnancy increases proportionately to the number of fetuses present. From the maternal perspective the incidence of minor disorders such as nausea, morning sickness and heartburn are amplified, whilst complications such as pre-eclampsia and antepartum haemorrhage are increased. The incidence of maternal mortality associated with multiple pregnancies is 2.5 times greater than that associated with singleton pregnancies.

Risk to the fetuses is also greatly increased. Early pregnancy loss is common and demise of one twin after the first trimester can lead to the release of thromboplastin which may have a serious impact on the development of the remaining twin and has the potential to initiate disseminated intravascular coagulation in the mother. The rate of congenital malformations is increased in twin pregnancies with the incidence of major abnormalities being significantly higher in monozygotic twins. Monoamniotic twins are particularly at increased risk of complications as a result of their shared circulation, which can lead to twin–twin transfusion, and shared space, which often results in fetal loss from cord entanglement. Extreme situations such as fetal acardia, in which one twin has no heart and the circulation for both twins is maintained by the remaining twin, results in severe compromise of the donor twin. Such situations require highly specialised intervention but may still result in a poor outcome. Even in fairly uncomplicated twin pregnancies discordant growth between the fetuses may occur. In addition, the onset of labour may be preterm and the presentation of the fetuses may make vaginal delivery more challenging. The stillbirth rate associated with multiple pregnancies is considerably higher than that of singleton pregnancies and the likelihood of preterm delivery, growth restriction and increased risk of developmental abnormalities increases the need for specialist neonatal care.

Management

Given the potential for complications, the antenatal management of multiple pregnancies needs to be tailored to meet the challenges presented by each case. This is to a large extent driven by the chorionicity of the pregnancy which should be determined at an early stage by ultrasound. Thereafter care from a multidisciplinary team including a specialist obstetrician, midwife and sonographer with expertise in the management of multiple pregnancies will be required to ensure an appropriate care plan is developed. This plan should include referral to a perinatal mental health professional, specialist physiotherapist, dietician and infant feeding specialist. Care should be evidence based and should be co-ordinated to minimise the number of visits required and should be organised as closely to the mother's home as possible. It is important that parents are involved in the decision-making process throughout the pregnancy and are empowered to make informed choices around issues such as screening for Down's syndrome, the use of targeted corticosteroids and the timing and mode of delivery. The midwife should also direct parents to other agencies that may provide additional support such as the Twin and Multiple Birth Association and local twin groups.

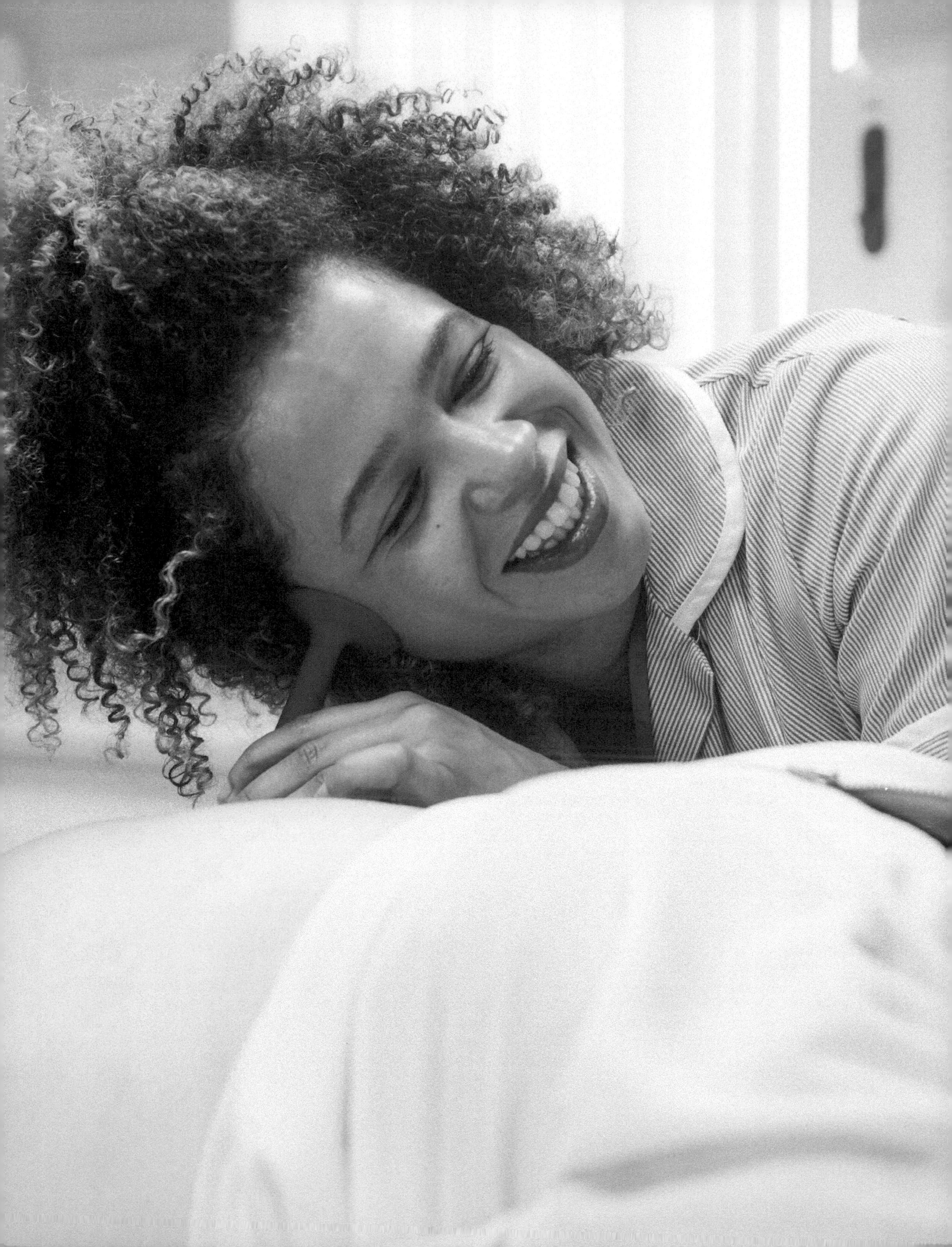

Fetus and baby

Chapters

55 Intrauterine growth restriction

Box 55.1 Fetal causes.

- Genetic disorders
- Infection
- Multiple gestation
- Trisomy: 21 (Down's syndrome, 18 (Edward's syndrome), 13 (Patau syndrome)
- Turner's syndrome (sex linked)
- Single gene disorders: Russell
- Silver syndrome
- Infections: toxoplasmosis, rubella, cytomegalovirus, herpes, syphilis

Box 55.2 Maternal causes.

- Chronic hypertension
- Pregnancy-induced hypertension
- Cyanotic heart disease
- Diabetes
- Haemoglobinopathies
- Autoimmune diseases (systemic lupus erythematosus, antiphospholipid syndrome)
- Protein/calorie malnutrition
- Substance abuse
- Uterine malformation
- Thrombophlebitis
- Prolonged high altitude exposure
- Maternal age
- Ethnicity
- Placental/umbilical cord:
  - Twin to twin transfusion
  - Placental abnormalities
  - Chronic abruption
  - Placenta praevia
  - Abnormal cord insertion
  - Cord anomalies

Box 55.3 Morbidity from IUGR.

- Hypoxia
- Meconium aspiration
- Necrotising enterocolitis
- Thrombocytopenia
- Temperature instability
- Insulin instability
- Renal failure
- Cerebral palsy 4–6 times more likely

Box 55.4 Long term effects.

- Obesity
- Hypertension
- Respiratory
- Hypercholesterolemia
- Cardiovascular disease
- Type II diabetes
- Impaired mental health/cognitive function

Midwifery at a Glance, First Edition. Edited by Eleanor Forrest © 2019 John Wiley & Sons, Ltd. Published 2019 by John Wiley & Sons, Ltd.
Companion website: www.wiley.com/go/forrest/midwifery

Intrauterine growth restriction (IUGR) is defined as when a fetus's size or weight is equal to or less than the 10th percentile for weight of all fetuses of that gestational age, when plotted on a recognised growth chart. Other terminology is often used synonymously for IUGR, such as small for gestational age (SGA), small for dates (SFD) and fetal growth restriction (FGR). There are also different types of IUGR. Symmetrical is where the head and abdomen are equally small and is thought to happen early in the pregnancy. It is associated with infections or congenital anomalies (Box 55.1). Another type is asymmetrical, where the head is larger than the abdomen and occurs later in the pregnancy. For example in a non-growth restricted infant the brain weighs three times the liver; in asymmetrical IUGR it can weigh 5–6 times the liver. In 40% of these cases the cause is unknown but it is thought to be mainly due to placental insufficiency (maternal/placenta/umbilical cord causes (Box 55.2).

Pathophysiology

The gas exchange and nutrient delivery to the fetus is not sufficient to allow it to thrive in utero. Depending on the cause this can be due to reduced oxygen-carrying capacity (congenital heart disease, haemoglobinopathies), a dysfunctional oxygen delivery system (secondary to maternal vascular disease) or placenta damage (thrombophlebitis). Blood flow that is redistributed to develop vital organs is known as the brain-sparing effect. This leads to increased relative blood flow to the brain, heart, adrenals and placenta and decreased relative blood flow to the bone marrow, lungs, gastrointestinal tract and kidneys.

Neonatal outcome

Mortality statistics in 2012 (ONS) stated that infant mortality rates for very low birth weight babies (< 1500 g) and low birth weight babies (< 2500 g) were 173.0 and 35.2 deaths per 1000 live births, respectively. This is higher than the rate of 1.3 deaths per 1000 live births among babies of normal birth weight (> 2500 g). These statistics do not differentiate between IUGR and prematurity.

Morbidity from IUGR involves many areas of the body (Box 55.3). Long-term hypoxia due to placental dysfunction may result in polycythaemia and thrombocytopenia. Polycythaemia from the hypoxia-induced synthesis of erythropoietin results in high red cell mass and possible placental to fetal transfusion at birth. Although hypoxia is thought to be the reason for the thrombocytopenia, the actual mechanism for this is not known.

Meconium aspiration may occur during perinatal asphyxia. SGA fetuses, especially those who are post mature, may pass meconium into the amniotic sac and begin deep gasping movements. The consequent aspiration is likely to result in meconium aspiration syndrome, which is most severe in growth-restricted or post-mature babies, because the meconium is contained in a smaller volume of amniotic fluid. If meconium aspiration syndrome occurs this is often accompanied by persistent pulmonary hypertension. As the disease process evolves, babies can develop secondary surfactant deficiency related to surfactant inhibition by meconium or, in the case of pulmonary haemorrhage, by blood. Pulmonary hypertension is right-to-left shunting at the level(s) of the ductus arteriosus and the foramen ovale, requiring higher oxygen levels and positive pressure ventilation. This can result overall in damage to the lung tissue and chronic lung problems.

The abnormalities of the fetal mesenteric circulation from the circulatory redistribution and hypoxia may result in hypoxic ischaemic injury of the bowel and contribute to necrotising enterocolitis.

Temperature instability is not fully understood in IUGR babies and is not necessarily due to brown fat deposits, which are not always reduced. It is possibly due to hypoxia and hypoglycaemia which interfere in heat production.

Metabolic problems with glucose and fatty acid metabolism lead to hypoglycaemia due to poor glycogen stores and diminished glucose product. Alternatively, insulin instability can also occur due to low insulin secretion and low plasma insulin concentration and can lead to hyperglycaemia.

Renal failure or reduced renal function are a possibility due to alteration of fetal physiology (fetal programming) in utero. Adaptive outcomes observed in response to placental insufficiency include reduced nephron number and marked increases in blood pressure. This is possibly due to hypoxia increasing renal sympathetic nerve activity alterations in the renin–angiotensin system.

Long-term health effects

Many of the long-term effects of IUGR are still being explored and the theories are not fully developed. There are many areas of long-term health problems that have been found to be more prevalent in adults who were born with IUGR (Box 55.4). Obesity is thought to occur due to deficient leptin neuronal signals, which favours weight gain, in conjunction with body fat distribution, adipocyte maturation and changed glucose insulin metabolism.

Type 2 diabetes, due to increased insulin sensitivity and accelerated growth following birth, is thought to lead to glucose intolerance later in life.

Hypertension, as a result of an insult during kidney development, leads to 'programming' of the kidneys. Studies suggest that this results in an abnormal outcome in the complex mechanisms associated with blood pressure regulation.

Respiratory problems are due to the chronic restriction of nutrients and oxygen in late pregnancy. This can cause abnormalities in the airways and lungs such as enlarged alveoli with thicker septal walls and membranes. The impaired lung function seen at birth may persist or progress with age and cause lung problems and quicken lung ageing. Cardiovascular disease is thought to be due to changes in gene expression patterns of the cardiovascular and renal system and metabolic issues, already discussed in relation to obesity and diabetes.

Osteoporosis is another outcome of the abnormal leptin signalling on bone growth.

Cognitive function impairment, including learning difficulties and behavioural problems, has also been found in children who were born with IUGR.

Intrauterine growth restriction monitoring

Table 56.1 Biophysical testing scores.

Parameter	Normal (2 points)	Abnormal (0 points)
NST/Reactive FHR	At least two accelerations in 20 minutes	Less than two accelerations to satisfy the test in 20 minutes
US: Fetal breathing movements	At least one episode of >30 or >20 seconds in 30 minutes	None or less than 30 or 20 seconds
US: Fetal activity/gross body movements	At least three or two movements of the torso or limbs	Less than three or two movements
US: Fetal muscle tone	At least one episodes of active bending and straightening of the limb or trunk	No movements or movements slow and incomplete
US: Qualitative amniotic fluid volume/index	At least one vertical pocket >2 cm or more in the vertical axis	Largest vertical pocket ≤2 cm

Figure 56.1 Deterioration of fetal cardiovascular system.

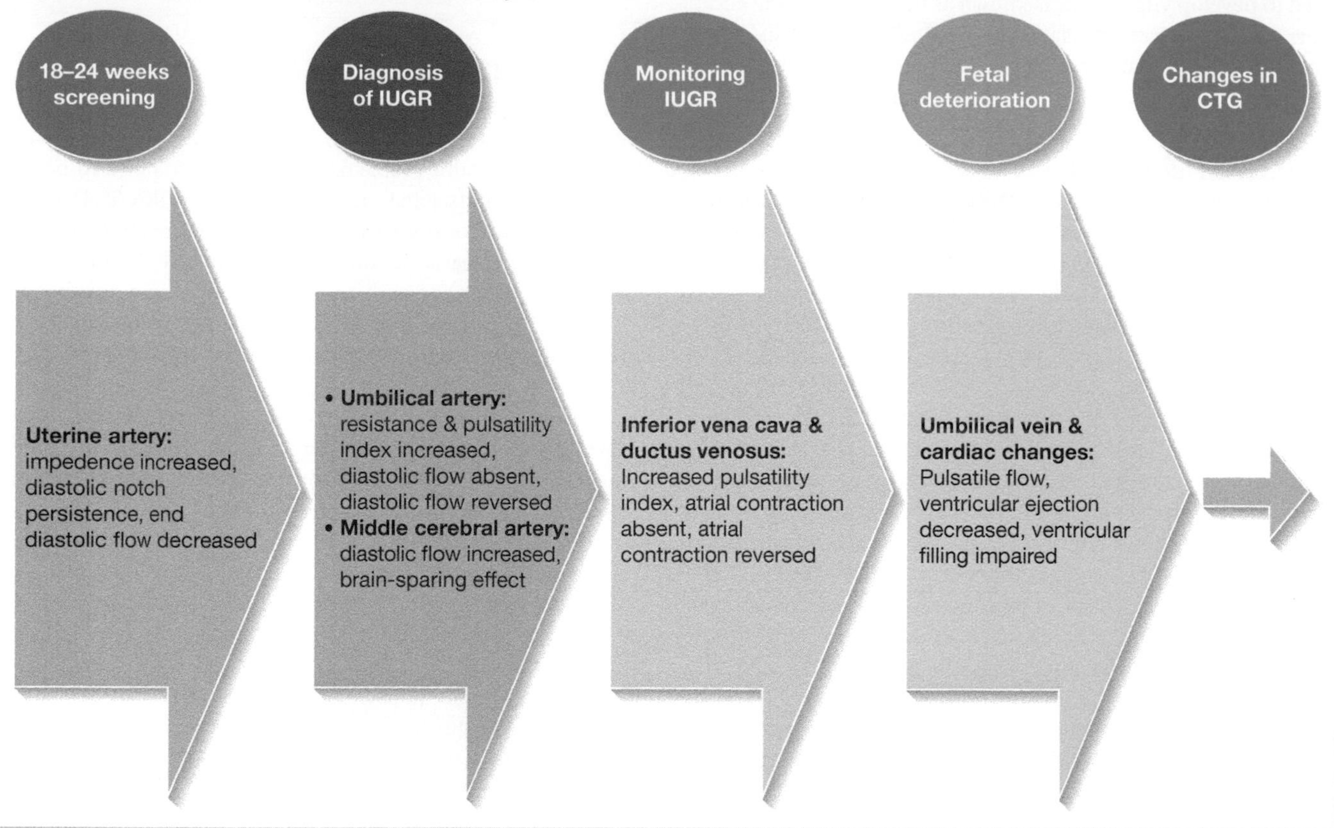

Midwifery at a Glance, First Edition. Edited by Eleanor Forrest © 2019 John Wiley & Sons Ltd. Published 2019 by John Wiley & Sons, Ltd.
Companion website: www.wiley.com/go/forrest/midwifery

Monitoring growth antenatally can be done by several means. However, currently there is no robust evidence to inform best practice for fetal surveillance regimens, when caring for women with pregnancies affected by impaired fetal growth. Ultrasound by serial measurements of the fetus's abdominal circumference is one method of surveillance. The Perinatal Institute and Royal College of Obstetricians and Gynaecologists (RCOG, 2008) recommend that a fetal growth scan should be offered if the first fundal height measurement is below the 10th centile on the customised chart or serial measurements have shown a slowing of growth. The results of the ultrasound biometry, expressed as estimated fetal weight (EFW), should be plotted on the customised growth chart to assess relative size for gestation (or growth if a previous EFW has been plotted)

Symphysis–fundal height measurements

The use of fundal height is controversial because some research concludes that its use is debatable, however it is still commonly used. The National Institute for Health and Care Excellence (NICE, 2008a) recommend that it should be measured and recorded at each antenatal appointment from 24 weeks. Other recommendations are that the fundal height be measured at each antenatal visit from 26 weeks' gestation, plotted on customised growth charts and adjusted for maternal height, weight in early pregnancy, parity and ethnic origin.

Non-stress and contraction stress tests

Neither should be used until the fetus is a viable age. Both tests are not currently commonly used on their own. The non-stress test (NST) is the monitoring of the fetal heart for periods of not less than 10 minutes and not more than 90 minutes under specific conditions, ensuring possible influences are controlled such as time of day, maternal activity, medication, dietary status and observation techniques. These are especially important if serial testing is used for management. In the contraction stress test (CST) the process of monitoring is similar, but oxytocin is administered to induce contractions for 20–30 minutes once satisfactory uterine activity is established (three moderate contractions in 10 minutes). The observer will look for acceleration and deceleration of the fetal heart during and after the contractions.

Biophysical profiles

Biophysical profiling (BPP) involves five elements: four ultrasound (US) assessments (fetal movement, fetal tone, fetal breathing and amniotic fluid index (AFI)) and one NST in the form of cardiotocography (CTG) to evaluate fetal heart rate (FHR) and response to fetal movement (Table 56.1), with scores from 0 to 10. If there is a score of <2 induce labour; <4, induce labour if gestational age >32 weeks or repeat the test on the same day if <32 weeks, then delivery if score <6. If the score is 6, induce labour if >36 weeks and if the cervix is favourable and normal AFI or repeat the test in 24 hours if <36 weeks and cervix is unfavourable; then deliver if score is <6, and follow-up if >6. If the score is 8 induce labour only in the presence of oligohydramnios.

Amniotic fluid volume

This can be measured in two ways by ultrasound. The AFI is an estimate of the amniotic fluid volume in a fetus. It is measured by adding the values of individual amniotic pocket depths in centimetres for each of the four quadrants and is part of the fetal biophysical profile. The normal range for amniotic fluid volumes varies with gestational age. As a rule an AFI of <8 implies oligohydramnios, and an AFI of >25 implies polyhydramnios. The maximum pool or the maximal vertical pocket (MVP) depth is considered a reliable method for assessing amniotic fluid volume on US. It is performed by assessing a maximal depth of amniotic fluid. The usual accepted values are <2 cm: indicative of oligohydramnios; 2–8 cm: normal but should be taken in the context of subjective volume; >8 cm: indicative of polyhydramnios, although some centres use a cut off of 10 cm. Controversially, neither approach is well supported by research but both have been compared and the maximum pool has been considered the better choice.

Umbilical arterial blood flow

Umbilical arterial blood flow (absence or reversal of end diastolic flow) or middle cerebral artery blood flow change as gestation advances. Diastolic flow gradually increases in intrauterine growth restriction (IUGR) with a large increase in end diastolic flow due to brain sparing or the ductus venosus causing abnormal blood flow due to hypoxia conditions. An EFW below the 10th centile on the customised chart, or slow EFW growth, is an indication for assessment of umbilical artery Doppler flow (Figure 56.1).

Timing of birth

Decisions about the optimal timing of birth of the fetus require consideration of the severity of growth restriction and its impact on fetal wellbeing balanced against the gestation. There is general consensus that the fetus needs to be born when the risk of death or significant morbidity from continuing intrauterine life is greater than the risk of prematurity. The decision-making process has been informed by the findings of the Growth Restriction Intervention Trial (GRIT) which concluded that, in general, in gestations of less than 31 weeks, birth is best delayed if there is any uncertainty about the severity of such an intervention. The GRIT study did not provide evidence that early birth to avoid severe hypoxia and acidosis reduces any adverse outcome. Before 36–37 weeks, birth should be deferred if end diastolic flow is present on umbilical artery Doppler and other surveillance findings are normal. Before 34 weeks, if diastolic flow disappears or reverses then the pregnant women needs to be admitted for close surveillance and steroids given. If other surveillance results (BPP, venous Doppler) are abnormal, then birth is needed. If more than 34 weeks, even if other results are normal, birth is considered a good option. Beyond 36–37 weeks, if IUGR is certain, end diastolic flow is present and AFI is normal, birth may be deferred until the Bishop's score is adequate for induction. If the AFI is reduced, delivery should be expedited. However, if growth is static between two scans taken 2 weeks apart in a fetus of more than 32 weeks, birth may be appropriate (once steroids have been administered).

Intrapartum

If induction takes place continuous CTG monitoring is required. The NICE 2008b guideline on induction of labour indicated that if fetal growth restriction was identified between 24 and 36 weeks of gestation, there was insufficient evidence to determine whether immediate or delayed birth was beneficial. The recommendation was made that if there was severe IUGR with confirmed fetal compromise, induction of labour was not recommended.

57 Fetal circulation

Figure 57.1 The adult heart structure.

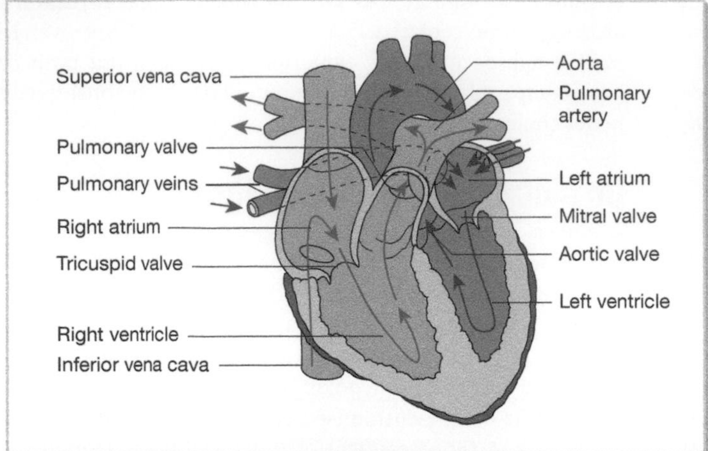

Figure 57.3 Blood flow into the aorta.

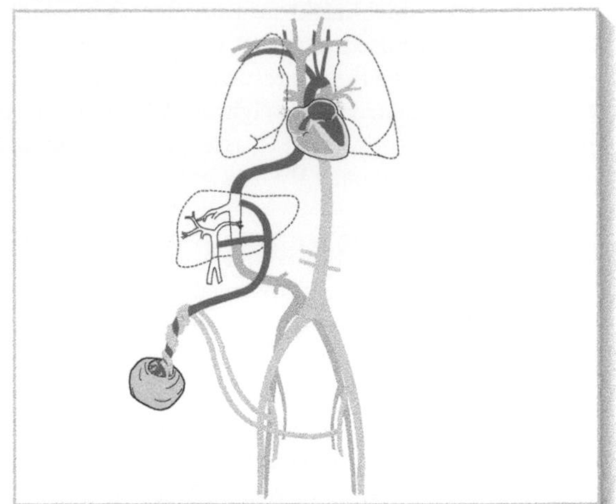

Figure 57.2 The fetal heart structure.

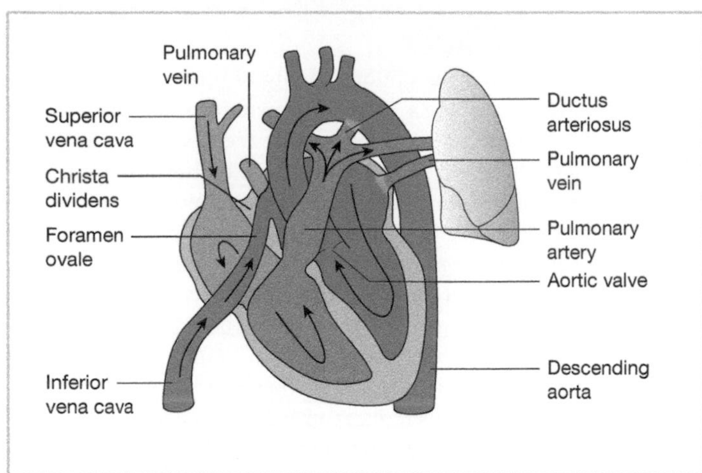

Figure 57.4 Route of the mixed blood.

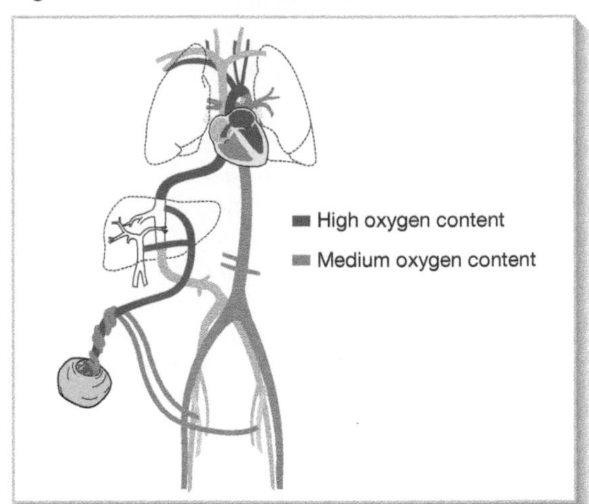

Figure 57.5 Full fetal circulation.

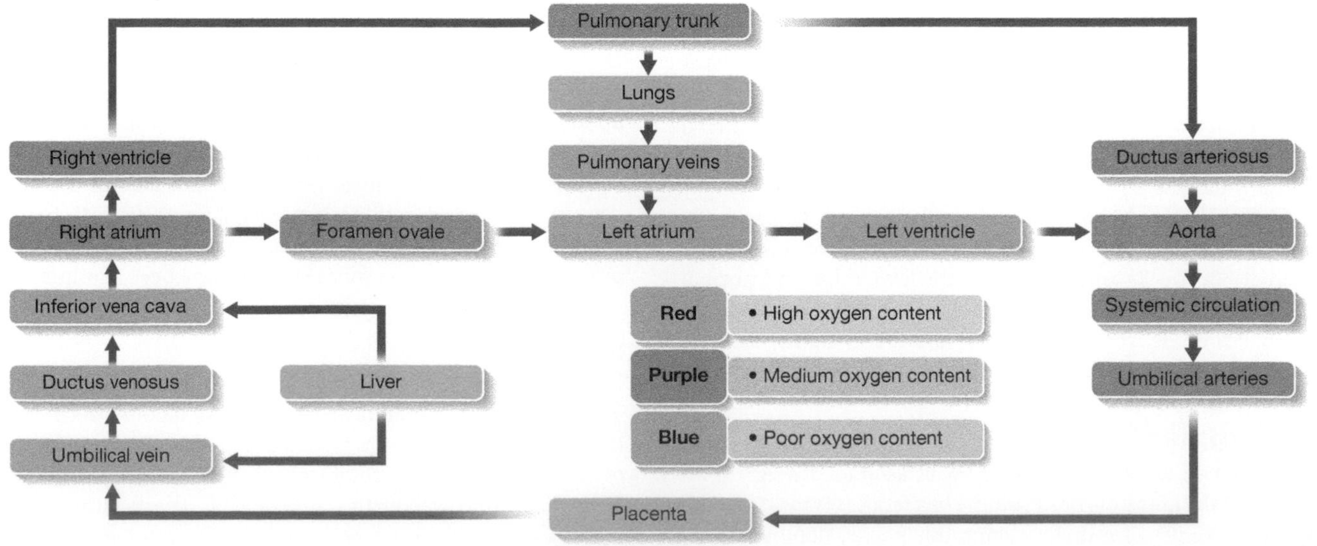

There are major differences in the structure of the fetal heart and the circulation of fetal blood. This is due to the fact that the majority of the circulating blood does not pass through the fetal lungs to be oxygenated but needs the maternal blood supply to do this. The umbilical vein and arteries from the placenta are used to exchange gases within the fetus which would normally occur through the lungs by breathing. Oxygenated blood is supplied from the mother via the umbilical vein and the umbilical arteries return deoxygenated blood to the mother for excretion.

Differences in the fetal and adult heart structure

There are several structures that exist in the heart and in the circulatory system that will change and in most cases disappear in early infancy. Some differences in the heart structures are shown in Figures 57.1 and 57.2, whilst the following differences are not depicted.

One other difference in structure is the ductus venosus which shunts most of the left umbilical vein blood flow directly to the inferior vena cava and allows most of the oxygenated blood from the placenta to bypass the liver. After it closes, the remnant is known as the ligamentum venosum.

The foramen ovale is an opening in the septum between the two atria of the heart which allows the majority of the oxygenated blood from the placenta to bypass the pulmonary artery and therefore the lungs and go into the left atrium. The closure of the foramen ovale is initially a functional change but later is an anatomical closure from proliferation of endothelial and fibrous tissues. In the adult this is called the fossa ovalis.

The ductus arteriosus is an opening between the pulmonary artery and aorta which allows most of the blood from the right ventricle to bypass the fetus's fluid-filled non-functioning lungs. The ductus arteriosus constricts at birth, but there is often a small shunt of blood from the aorta to the left pulmonary artery for a few days in a healthy, full-term infant. In the adult this is called the ligamentum arteriosum.

The two umbilical arteries supply deoxygenated blood from the fetus to the placenta in the umbilical cord. The umbilical arteries surround the urinary bladder and then carry all the deoxygenated blood out of the fetus through the umbilical cord. In the adult the umbilical artery is a branch of the anterior division of the internal iliac artery (patent part). The non-patent obliterated part of the artery is the medial umbilical ligament. The umbilical artery is found in the pelvis, and gives rise to the superior vesical arteries. In males, it also gives rise to the artery to the ductus deferens.

The umbilical vein carries oxygen and nutrient-rich blood derived from the fetal–maternal blood exchange at the chorionic villi.

Blood flow

Figure 57.3 shows the route of the oxygenated blood which comes to the fetus from the placenta via the umbilical vein. Some of the blood goes into the liver and the remainder goes via the ductus venosus into the inferior vena cava and enters the right atrium of the heart. Once in the right atrium some of the blood goes down into the right ventricle and the rest passes across the foramen ovale to the left atrium.

Blood in the right ventricle is pumped into the pulmonary vein to the lungs via the pulmonary veins. Some of the blood will go across the ductus arteriosus to the descending aorta and mix with the oxygenated blood from the aorta.

The blood that has gone into the left atrium and then to the left ventricle across the foramen ovale is pumped up into the aorta. From the aorta some of the blood then goes up into the brain and the rest into the descending aorta, which mixes with the blood that has entered via the ductus arteriosus (Figure 57.3).

The blood in the descending aorta then travels down to oxygenate the gut, kidneys and legs. The blood finally goes back into the placenta via the umbilical arteries.

The oxygenated blood from the placenta mixes with deoxygenated blood from the legs and the lower body which goes into the liver and back out into the inferior vena cava. This combines with the deoxygenated blood from the head and neck and goes via the superior vena cava and enters the right atrium before travelling down into the right ventricle.

Some deoxygenated blood will also come back from the lungs into the left ventricle from the pulmonary veins. The route of the mixed blood is shown in Figure 57.4.

Figure 57.5 shows the full fetal circulation with the different types of blood being represented by the three colours: red for oxygenated, purple for mixed and blue for deoxygenated blood. The blood circulation of the fetus is not well oxygenated in to this system. As a result, the fetus has higher haemoglobin levels and a different type of haemoglobin which has a higher affinity to oxygen and better access to oxygen from the blood than that of the adult.

58 Changes at birth

Box 58.1 Heat loss.

Babies lose heat through:
- Conduction (contact with objects)
- Evaporation (wetness)
- Convection (draughts)
- Radiation (not direct contact, e.g. windows)

Box 58.3 Action of peptide hormones.

- Enteroglucagon: growth of intestinal mucosa
- Gastrin: growth of gastric mucosa and exocrine pancreas
- Motilin and neurotensin: gut activity

Box 58.2 Brown adipose tissue deposit.

- Around the nape of the neck
- Under the clavicle
- In the axillae
- Around the kidneys
- Adrenal glands
- Large vessels in the neck
- Mediastinum

Box 58.4 Content of meconium.

- Fatty acids
- Amniotic fluid
- Vernix caseosa
- Epithelial cells
- Lanugo
- Bile
- Other intestinal secretions

Figure 58.1 Heat production from BAT.

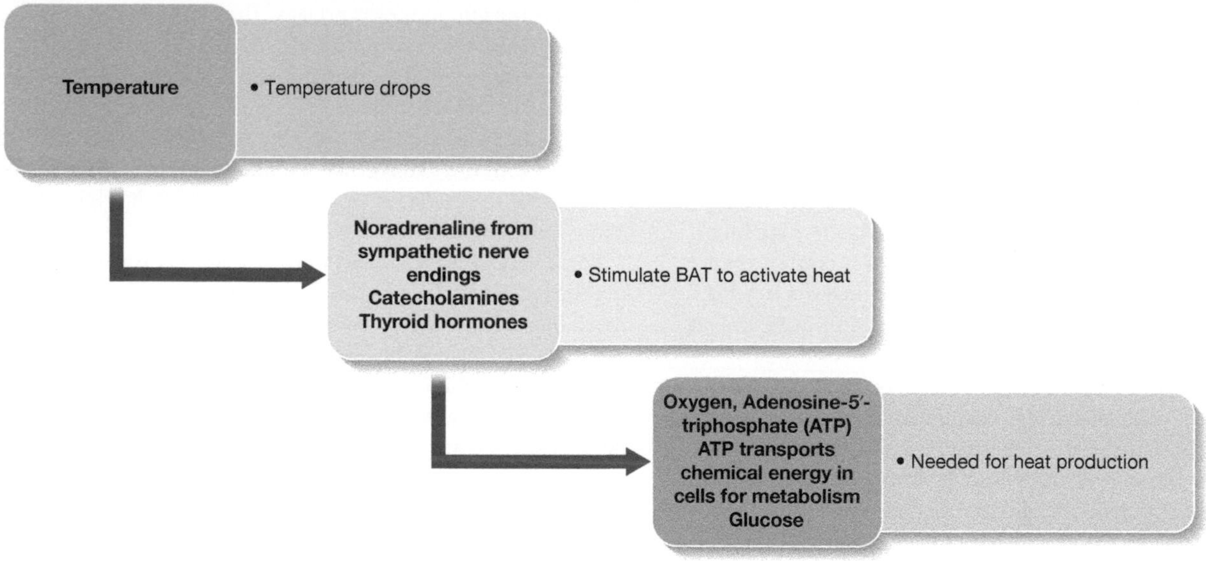

Figure 58.2 Causes of gastric reflux.

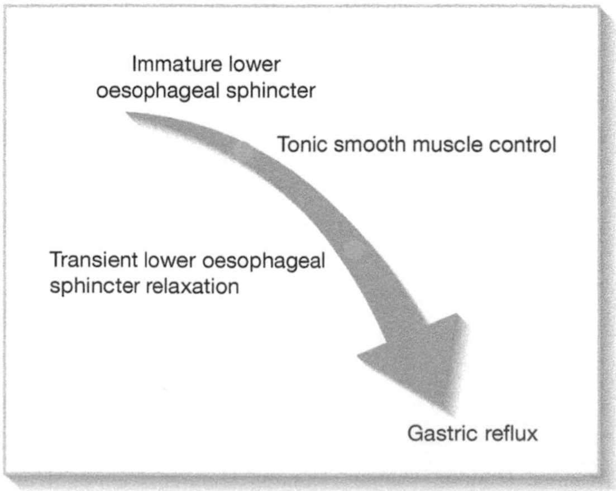

Figure 58.3 Sucking.

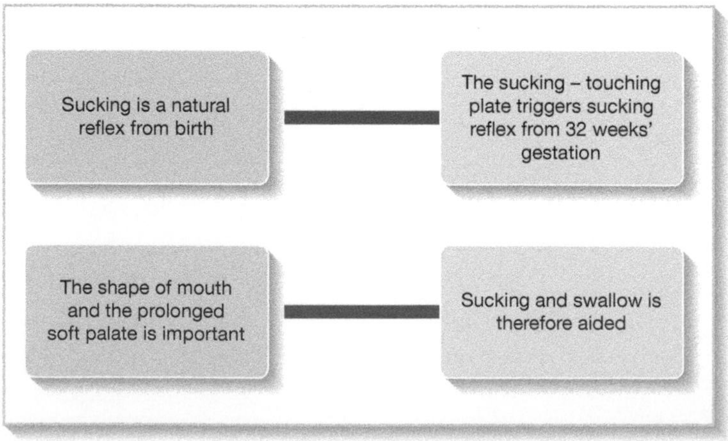

Midwifery at a Glance, First Edition. Edited by Eleanor Forrest © 2019 John Wiley & Sons, Ltd. Published 2019 by John Wiley & Sons, Ltd.
Companion website: www.wiley.com/go/forrest/midwifery

There are many different physiological changes that occur within the baby at birth. These changes refer to the adaptations that the newborn's body undergoes to adapt to life outside the uterus.

Heart and pulmonary system

In utero, oxygen and carbon dioxide flow through the placenta to the fetus. At birth the baby's lungs are not inflated and are filled with amniotic fluid. The baby's first breath is taken due to: response to mild asphyxia and acidosis, cord clamping, the medullary chemoreceptors increasing ventilatory drive, changes in temperature and tactile stimulation. Usually the first breath occurs within 6 seconds and is normal in 15 minutes. Following the first breath and the expansion of the lungs there is a decrease in the pressure (pulmonary vascular resistance) in the lungs; therefore more blood flows into the lungs from the pulmonary artery where it is oxygenated. More blood then flows back to the left atrium, increasing the pressure in that chamber causing the foramen ovale to close – this is also due to a decrease in venous return from the contractility pressure in the right atrium which falls. The high oxygen content of the blood in the aorta causes the ductus arteriosus to close.

In utero, the lungs are filled with fluid and the alveoli are collapsed. With the first breath the diaphragm contracts and fluid is forced into the alveoli and disperses surfactant. This lines the alveoli and keeps them from collapsing each time they exhale; it is then reabsorbed into the pulmonary lymphatic vessels. Thoracic compression during vaginal birth gets rid of fluid from the upper airways. Normal breathing is irregular with some shallow breathing.

Thermoregulation

Thermoregulation is not fully developed at birth and maintaining the baby's temperature is important. Babies only have half the amount of internal subcutaneous fat compared with adults but have a large surface area through which heat can be lost (Box 58.1). Initially, normal term babies have limited response to temperature changes; by 24–48 hours they can produce heat in response to a cold environment. Newborns do not shiver but generate heat through increasing their metabolic rate using muscular activity and non-shivering thermogenesis (NST); this is the metabolism of brown adipose tissue (BAT). BAT comprises 2–7% of the baby's body weight and is deposited in the fetus from 26 weeks' gestation. BAT is found in several areas of the body; it is not renewable once used (Box 58.2). When the temperature drops, noradrenaline is released with other catecholamines and thyroid hormones, stimulating BAT activation and heat production (Figure 58.1). Skin-to-skin contact is a good way of reducing heat loss.

Hepatic system

The newborn liver is immature; this can give rise to hyperbilirubinaemia from poor excretion of bilirubin (Chapter 63). Unconjugated bilirubin is insoluble and is transported by plasma albumin to the liver to be metabolised to be conjugated and excreted in bile and through the intestines. Glucose regulation occurs when lipids and glycogen are stored in skeletal muscle and liver. Glucose levels fall after birth and are irregular due to extra usage and slow breakdown of stored glycogen and fat and immature thyroid hormone production.

Gastrointestinal system

Postnatal maturation of the gut is stimulated by the initiation of feeding, the composition of the milk and hormonal regulation. Early feeding stimulates the increase of peptide hormone concentration in the plasma (Box 58.3). Milk in the newborn stomach stimulates the epithelial lining to mature by promoting rapid cell turnover and producing amylase, trypsin and pancreatic lipase. The newborn relies on additional means for digesting protein, carbohydrates and fats by the use of enzymes in saliva and the intestines in addition to that in breast milk. Colostrum is non-irritating to the gut and enhances the passage of meconium.

Reflux is due to several causes (Figure 58.2). Sucking is a natural reflex from birth (Figure 58.3). Meconium is the first stool passed within 12–48 hours. It is formed in utero from intestinal debris (Box 58.4). After meconium, the next stool is a changing stool; when feeding is established this stool should be soft and yellowish. The gut is sterile and breast milk helps colonise the gut with vitamin K-producing bacteria. The newborn has a low storage of vitamin K and requires supplementation.

Renal system

At birth the kidneys are immature, especially the renal cortex. Glomerular filtration rate and ability to concentrate urine is low. A newborn needs to urinate within 24 hours – between 20 and 30 ml per day rising to 100–1200 ml by the end of the first week. The newborn will lose water and sodium equivalent to 5–10% of their birth weight in 4–5 days. Due to the immature kidneys there is a chance of a possible imbalance of solids such as urea and sodium chloride, especially if they become dehydrated. Imbalance is less likely if demand fed. The elimination of drugs such as antibiotics is decreased meaning that the half-life is increased. Kidney function matures by 1–2 years.

Excretory system

The full term infant's skin is well developed, opaque with few visible veins and has limited pigmentation due to low melanin production. Its function is as a temperature regulator, a barrier to infection and a sensory organ. The newborn will have some vernix caseosa, a moisturiser which is a thick, white, creamy substance found in varying amounts usually in the creases such as the neck axilla and groin. Lanugo is present at birth. Vernix is an in utero barrier to amniotic fluid, prevents loss of water and electrolytes, insulates the skin and reduces friction at birth. Drying of the skin is keratinisation, which is a normal maturation process and enhances its role as infection barrier.

Nervous system

After the first 24 hours the grasp and moro reflexes are used to assess reflexability. The newborn has limited visual acuity, with focus at 20 cm, and can usually hear sounds which are noticed by turning towards the sound or being startled.

59 Fetal skull

Figure 59.1 Regions of the fetal skull.

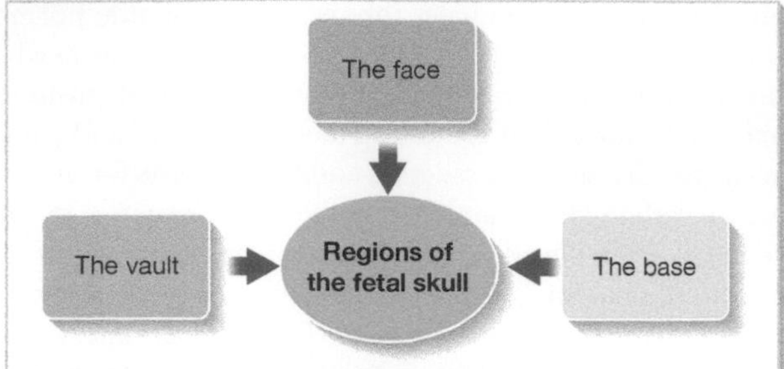

Figure 59.3 Landmarks of the fetal skull.

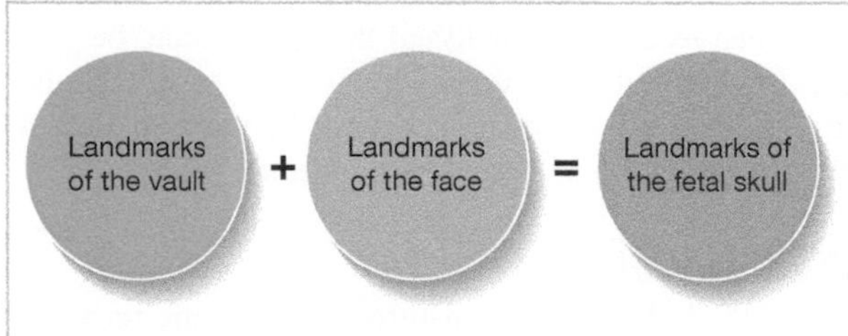

Figure 59.5 The (a) longitudinal and (b) transverse diameters of the fetal skull.

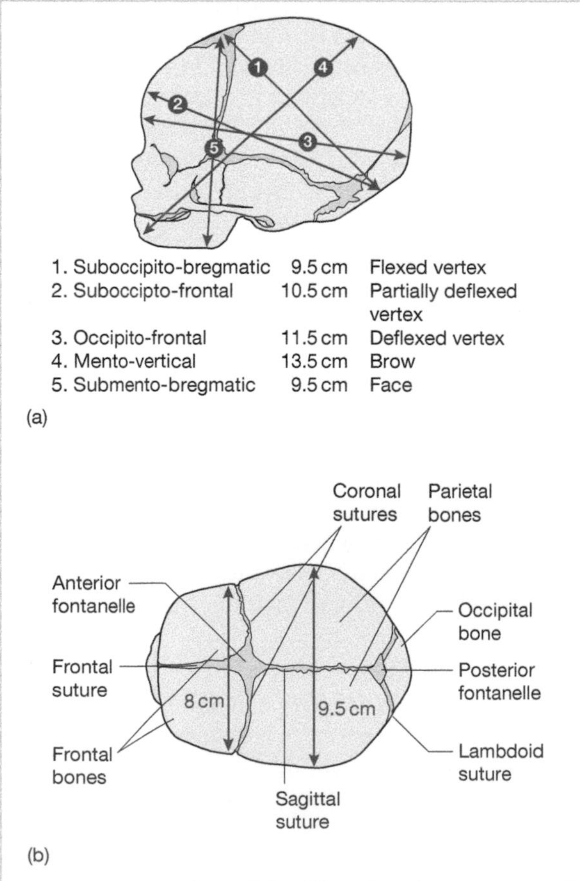

Figure 59.2 Bones and sutures of the fetal skull (lateral view).

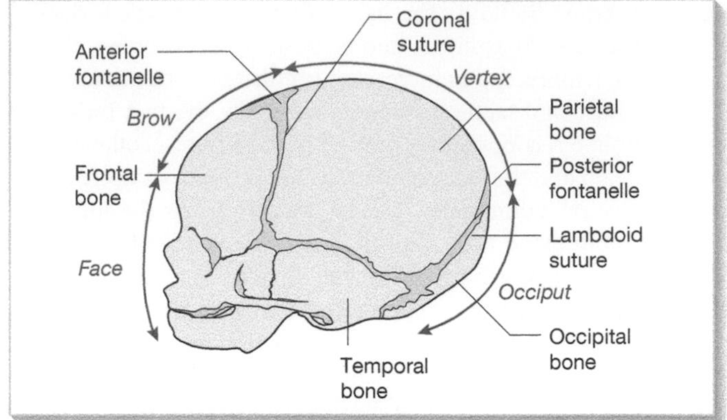

Figure 59.4 Areas of the fetal skull.

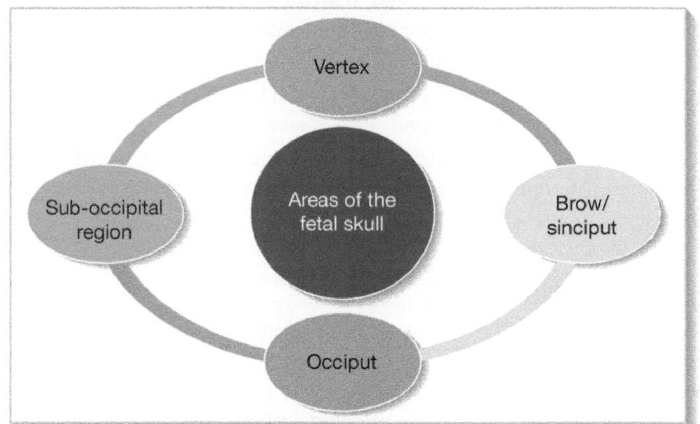

Table 59.1 Diameters of the fetal skull.

Diameter	Landmarks measured between	Measurement
Biparietal	Between the parietal eminences	9.5 cm
Bitemporal	Between the widest points on the coronal suture	8.2 cm
Suboccipito-bregmatic	Directly under the occipital protuberance to the centre of the bregma	9.5 cm
Suboccipito-frontal	Directly under the occipital protuberance to the centre of the sinciput	10.5 cm
Occipito-frontal	From the occipital protuberance to the glabella	11.5 cm
Submento-bregmatic	From the junction of the chin with the neck to the centre of the bregma	9.5 cm
Submento-vertical	From the junction of the chin with the neck to the highest point on the vertex	11.5 cm
Mento-vertical	From the tip of the chin to the highest point on the vertex	13.5 cm

The fetal head is the largest and least compressible part of the fetus and the part of the fetus that is likely to present the most challenges in terms of delivery regardless of whether the presentation is cephalic or breech. The fetal head is subject to considerable pressure during the process of birth and the potential for damage to the head and brain should not be underestimated. As the majority of fetuses are cephalic presentations, a good knowledge of the bones, sutures and fontanelles of the fetal skull will enable the midwife to:

- Determine the level of the head in relation to the maternal pelvis and thus estimate the degree of descent
- Determine the position of the head in relation to the maternal pelvis and thus monitor the rotation of the head during labour
- Determine the degree of flexion of the head and the reduction in engaging diameters as the head descends and rotates.

Regions of the fetal skull

The fetal skull is divided into three regions: the vault, the face and the base (Figure 59.1).

The vault

The vault is the most important part of the fetal skull from a midwife's perspective as it contains the brain and is usually the part of the skull that will be felt during internal examinations to assess progress in labour. Knowledge of the landmarks of the vault, and an ability to identify these by touch, is essential if the midwife is to determine the level, position and rotation of the fetal skull. Most bones develop from cartilage but the individual bones that comprise the vault of the skull develop from a membrane that covers the brain in early fetal life. The gradual ossification of this membrane leads to the development of the individual bones that form the vault of the skull. By term, this process is incomplete and membranous gaps, known as sutures, exist between the bones (Figure 59.2). Where sutures meet a widened area of membrane is found. This is known as a fontanelle.

The bones of the vault are:

- The frontal bone, which is divided into two halves
- Two parietal bones
- Two temporal bones
- The occiput.

The sutures are:

- The frontal suture – located between the two halves of the frontal bone
- The sagittal suture – located between the parietal bones
- The coronal suture – located between the frontal and parietal bones
- The lambdoidal suture – located between the occiput and the parietal bones.

The fontanelles are:

- The anterior fontanelle or bregma – located at the junction of the coronal, frontal and sagittal sutures. This fontanelle is diamond shaped and measures 2.5 × 1.25 cm
- The posterior fontanelle or lambda – located at the junction of the lambdoidal and sagittal sutures. This fontanelle is triangular.

The sutures and fontanelles allow a degree of overlap to occur between the bones during labour. This is known as moulding and is an important adaptation that allows the shape of the fetal skull to alter slightly as it descends through the pelvis. Although the shape of the skull may change, the volume of the skull does not as this would cause compression of the brain.

The face

The area from the root of the nose to the junction of the chin and neck is the face (Figure 59.2).

The base

The base is an internal fusion of bones that surrounds the medulla.

Landmarks of the fetal skull

Digital palpation of the landmarks of the vault and face are useful in determining position, descent and rotation during labour (Figure 59.3). The landmarks of the vault are:

- The lambda
- The bregma
- The parietal eminences – a raised area in the middle of each parietal bone where ossification started
- The occipital protuberance – the raised area in the centre of the occiput where ossification started.

The landmarks of the face are:

- The glabella – the bridge of the nose
- The mentum or chin.

Areas of the fetal skull

The landmarks are used to describe different areas of the fetal skull (Figure 59.4):

- The vertex – the area enclosed by the anterior and posterior fontanelles and the two parietal eminences. This is the part of the skull that will present in the majority of cephalic presentations
- The brow or sinciput – the area between the coronal suture and the ridge above the eyes
- The occiput
- The suboccipital region – the area below the occipital protuberance.

Diameters of the fetal skull

The landmarks are also used to describe various measurements of the fetal skull. These are known as diameters (Figure 59.5). The diameters that negotiate the maternal pelvis will vary depending on how the fetal head is positioned within the pelvis. For example, when the fetal head is positioned with the occiput to the front of the pelvis, the fetal chin will be on the chest, the head well flexed and the diameters of the skull small and favourable for a normal birth. If the head is positioned with the occiput to the back of the maternal pelvis, then the head is likely to be less well flexed and larger diameters will present. This may result in a longer labour often accompanied by backache. See Table 59.1 for a summary of the variations of diameters in relation to different positions, presentations and mouldings.

Immediate care of the newborn

Figure 60.1 Instinctive newborn behaviour.

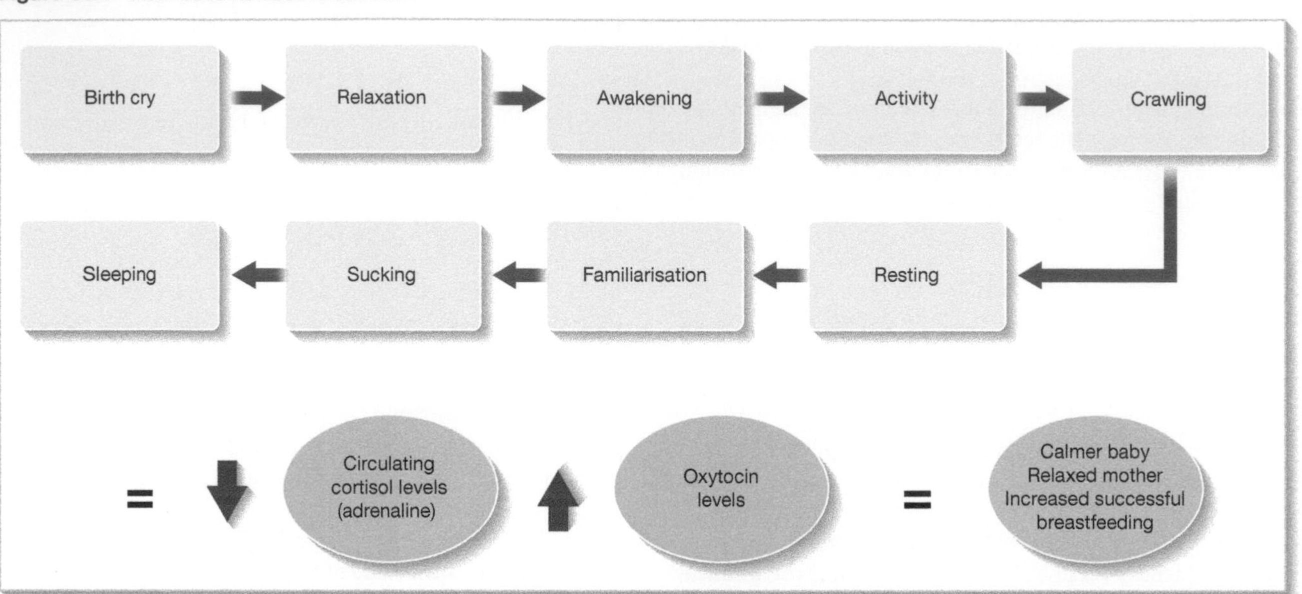

Figure 60.2 Neonatal heat loss.

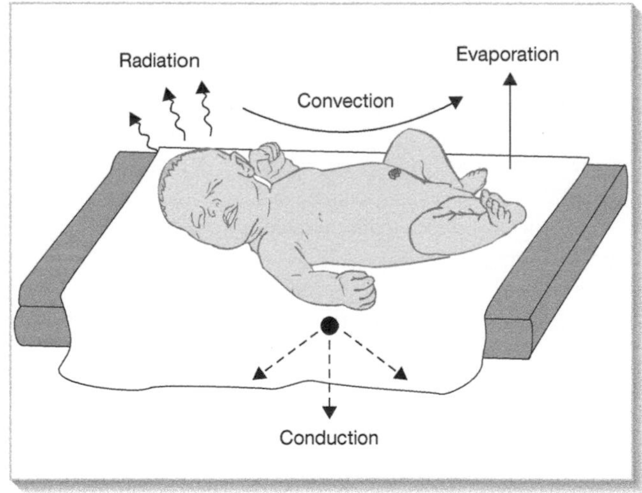

Table 60.1 Apgar score.

Acronym	Score of 0	Score of 1	Score of 2
A Appearance	Pale or blue	Pink body, blue extremities	Body and extremities pink, no cyanosis
P Pulse	Absent	<100 Slow	>100 Fast
G Grimace	No response from stimulation or reflex	Grimace present	Crying and/or coughing
A Activity	Limp, no muscle tone	Little flexion of the extremities	Active baby
R Respiration	No respiratory effort	Irregular and slow	Good effort, crying

Box 60.1 Skin-to-skin contact.

- Regulates breathing
- Regulates heart rate
- Temperature
- Stimulates digestion/feeding in the baby
- Improves protection from infection
- Facilitates bonding and attachment
- Enables breastfeeding

It is essential that newborn babies are seen as individuals and treated as such, they have entered a new environment following birth that may cause them fear, stress and discomfort. It is therefore important that the care given in the first hours following birth promotes the physiological and psychological wellbeing of the baby.

Instinctive newborn behaviour

It has been identified that newborn babies go through nine distinctive behavioural changes following birth: birth cry → relaxation → awakening → activity → crawling → resting → familiarisation → suckling → sleeping (Figure 60.1). Midwives should delay any unnecessary separation of the baby from his or her mother to facilitate this process. By allowing this time it will reduce the circulating cortisol levels (adrenaline) and increase the levels of oxytocin in the mother. Both will be more relaxed, importantly reducing fear and anxiety in the baby. Breastfeeding will then be established in a calm and beneficial way (Chapter 34 and 83).

Skin-to-skin contact

Skin-to-skin contact relaxes both baby and mother: it regulates breathing, heart rate and temperature, and stimulates digestion and feeding in the baby (Box 60.1). Furthermore, it connects the baby's skin with the mother's friendly bacteria enabling protection against infection. It is beneficial for both parents to provide this bonding and comfort intervention and infants show improved attachment behaviours if they receive this comfort. Moreover, babies who receive immediate uninterrupted skin-to-skin contact are more likely to be breastfed successfully for longer periods. Routine care that interferes with skin-to-skin contact should be minimised and hospital practice, for example weighing, should not take priority. Midwives should consider encouraging the woman's partner to provide skin-to-skin contact as it will be of benefit to the baby should separation from the mother happen, for example having to go to theatre for a procedure post-delivery.

Thermoregulation

The temperature of the birthing environment should be > 25°C. All doors and window should be closed; fans turned off and if possible warm towels available. Initially the baby should be dried with a warm towel whilst the receiving skin-to-skin comfort from the mother; dry warm blankets can then be placed over to cover the baby. The baby's temperature should be recorded and bathing delayed until temperature is maintained.

Thermoregulation is important in the newborn as a hypothermic baby will have a decreased suck ability, which can lead to impaired feeding. This impaired feeding will lead to a decrease in heat production as a result of reduced energy intake. As the body temperature decreases further, the baby becomes lethargic, hypotonic, the effort to cry becomes weaker and overall the baby becomes less active. Respiration starts to slow and becomes shallow and the heart rate decreases. The on-going care of thermal management of the well term baby will involve daily temperature recording by midwifery staff and attention should be paid to cot position so that it is not near an outdoor wall or doorway as heat can be lost through conduction, convection, evaporation and radiation (Figure 60.2). The baby should be clothed and wrapped depending on the environmental conditions.

Vitamin K

Vitamin K helps blood to clot so that should an injury occur the body is able to stop the bleeding. Babies are born with a much lower level of vitamin K than adults; however it is usually sufficient to stop any bleeding should this occur. Formula milk contains significantly more vitamin K than breast milk, however this should not deter women from breastfeeding as the benefits overall need to be taken into consideration.

Occasionally, a small number of babies do not have enough vitamin K to help blood clot and prevent internal bleeding; this is known as vitamin K deficiency bleeding (VKDB). This is a very rare but serious disease of the newborn and is most common in the first 13 weeks of life. Prophylactic vitamin K is recommended for all newborn babies at birth via 1 mg intramuscular injection or following an oral vitamin K regimen. The oral regimen is not suitable for high risk (such as forceps delivery), premature or sick infants. This may also be an unsuitable route for babies whose mothers are on certain drugs at time of birth such as warfarin. All interventions with the baby at birth should be discussed with the parents and consent sought.

Initial examination of the newborn

In 1952 a scoring system was developed by anaesthesiologist Virginia Apgar which defines the appearance of the newborn. The assessment tool is called Apgar (Table 60.1), after the doctor who devised it, and takes into account five key elements:

- Respiration, crying
- Reflexes, irritability
- Pulse, heart rate
- Skin colour of body and extremities
- Muscle tone.

Each element gets a score of 0 to 2; the higher the score, the better condition the baby appears to be in. A baby born with a score of 8–10 is in good condition, a score of 4–7 would require careful observation, and for a score < 4 immediate resuscitation measures are required.

The midwife in attendance for the birth should carry out an initial examination of the newborn including temperature and weight. This is a top to toe look at the baby, checking for any abnormalities or birth injuries – all of which will be discussed with the parents and documented.

61 Normal neonate and care needs

Figure 61.1 Neonatal needs to develop and grow.

Neonatal needs

- On-going physical & emotional support
- Sleep, stimulation, exercise & rest appropriate to age
- A safe, supportive & nurturing environment
- Nutritional requirements to be met

Figure 61.2 Infant massage. Source: YogaBellies, Reproduced with permission.

Infant massage is suitable from birth in the well, term baby. Research has shown improved mother – infant interaction, it helps postnatal depression, improved sleep and relaxation, reduced stress hormones, reduced crying and possible improved psychological outcomes and weight gain. Using gentle massage strokes can help alleviate colic, wind and constipation as well as teething and cold symptoms

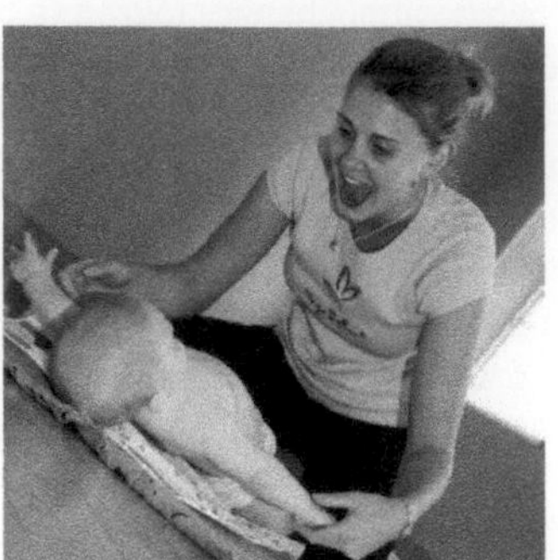

Box 61.1 Crying baby.

- Offer comfort; a baby should be given a cuddle
- Respond to a crying baby; she may just be looking for reassurance
- Check for wet or soiled nappies & ensure no clothing garment may be causing discomfort
- Offer a feed as a baby will almost always cry if she is hungry
- Overstimulation: dim the lights & quieten down background noise – consider that she may just want to be left alone
- Unwell cry? Assess baby's wellbeing and encourage the parents to trust their instinct
- Offer parents support & reassurance as it is more beneficial if they remain calm when handling the baby

Box 61.2 Benefits of breastfeeding.

Breastfed babies are at a lesser risk of:

- Respiratory, ear, urinary tract and gastrointestinal infections
- Eczema and wheezing
- Insulin-dependent diabetes mellitus
- Sudden infant death syndrome
- Childhood leukaemia
- Necrotising enterocolitis
- Sudden unexpected death in infancy (SUDI)

Breastfeeding mothers are at a lower risk of:

- Rheumatoid arthritis
- Breast cancer
- Ovarian cancer

Box 61.3 Reducing the risks of SUDI.

- Minimise or stop cigarette smoke both maternal (whilst baby is in utero) & passive smoking postnatally
- Baby to sleep supine (on their backs) and feet to bottom of cot/pram
- For the first 6 months of life baby to sleep in their own cot in their parents' room
- Do not bed share especially if one of the parents has consumed alcohol, drugs that make them drowsy, illegal drugs, if they are over tired or if either of them smoke
- The room temperature should be around 18°C. Care should be taken to not allow the baby to get too warm or cold

A newborn baby is limited both physically and psychologically and is solely reliant on its parents to provide care to secure on-going survival and development (Figure 61.1).

Sleep

Newborn babies are asleep more than they are awake; babies under the age of 6 months need on average 14 hours of sleep in a 24-hour period. Sleep patterns vary from baby to baby; some sleep for long periods whilst others have short naps; some settle to sleep through the night fairly quickly whilst others take longer. Established circadian rhythms are not present in neonates (this occurs around 12 weeks of age) therefore their sleep phases will be distributed throughout the night and day and they generally sleep for short periods of time due the frequency of feeding. When babies are asleep they develop their learning and memory skills, are of better mood when awake and have improved immune systems.

Crying baby

Humans are biologically programmed to respond to the sound of the crying baby. Crying is the most effective and powerful way a baby can summon attention. Babies cry when they are bored, lonely, hungry and tired and they sometimes just like to know people are around them and want a cuddle (Box 61.1). Prompt response to a crying baby in the first year of their life may facilitate more advanced communication skills and outgoing behaviour in the child as they have established a sense of security. They also cry less, learn to self-sooth and, should the baby need comfort, it will settle more quickly once the care giver provides it. An attachment to the care giver will be created by the age of 1 year.

Infant feeding

Breastfeeding

Breast milk is best for baby (Box 61.2). Breast milk contains a unique formula for brain growth such as omega 3 fatty acids, cholesterol and amino acids, along with immune properties that cannot be matched with any substitutes. From around 16 weeks' gestation colostrum is produced which lasts until mature milk comes in around day 10–14 postnatal. Colostrum has a yellow/orange, thick, sticky appearance and has a lesser calorie content than mature milk. Colostrum has, however, a higher concentration of protective properties such as immunoglobulins and growth factors (Chapters 34 and 62).

Formula feeding

When discussing formula milk it should always be reiterated that breast milk is the optimal means of infant feeding for the first 6 months of their life. Whilst around 80% of mothers' breastfeed at birth, this falls to 70% at 1 week with a further drop to about 35% at 6 months. This decline in breastfeeding rates means that many parents use formula feeding as a source of nutrition for their babies. In order to formula feed safely it is important that parents receive correct information and have support regarding their choice to formula feed. Should parents receive little or wrong information regarding the preparation, reconstitution, storage and delivery of feeds, dehydration, malnutrition, infection and hypernatraemia of the baby could result.

The main formula brands are made of modified cow's milk. Whey-based formulas, also known as first stage formulas, are considered to have a protein profile closer to breast milk than cow's milk. Casein-based formulas, also known as second stage 'hungry baby' formulas, have a composition closer to cows' milk. They are not recommended and there is little evidence to support the use of 'hungry baby' formula (Chapters 34 and 62).

Colic and wind

A baby who is well fed and appears healthy may at times suffer from excessive and frequent crying (colic). A colicky baby has sporadic muscles spasms of the gastrointestinal or genitourinary tracts; around one in five babies suffer from this condition. It generally starts at around 3 weeks old and lasts until around 3 months and is almost certainly gone by 6 months. Babies display restlessness, pulling up of legs and crying as though in pain. Although it appears distressing, there is no evidence to show that babies suffer any long-term health effects and will continue to feed and grow as normal.

Almost all babies experience wind and this is not to be confused with colic. Infant massage has shown to be effective to reduce both (Figure 61.2). Midwives should encourage parents to be aware of feeding practices, particularly if they are giving a feed through a bottle as air bubbles can get into the teat and be ingested.

Sudden unexpected death in infancy (SUDI)

There are approximately 300 babies who die suddenly in the UK each year (SUDI). However, despite the alarming statistic, the risk of a baby dying is low; 90%, of deaths occur during the first 6 months of a baby's life, with the likelihood peaking between 2 and 4 months of age. SUDI is more common in baby boys (60:40), and babies with a low birth weight or born prematurely are at greater risk. There is no complete understanding of what causes SUDI although research has shown factors that, if introduced, can reduce the risk of it occurring (Box 61.3).

Spotting signs of an ill baby

The following can be indicators of an unwell baby and should always be treated as serious and medical attention sought:

- High pitched continuous cry or weak cry
- Reduced activity or increased floppiness, lack of responsiveness, listlessness
- Not taking any fluids for more than 8 hours
- Temperature of 38°C for a baby less than 3 months old
- Fit, convulsions or seizures
- Pale complexion, ashen, mottled or turning blue
- Repeated vomiting
- Bulging fontanelle.

Observe babies breathing; these signs indicate that they are working hard to breathe and medical attention should be sought:

- Difficult, fast, grunting breaths or evidence of nasal flaring or sucking in their stomach under the rib cage.

Observe babies skin for rashes, in particular:

- Purple, red rash that does not disappear when observed through a glass.

62 Infant nutrition

Table 62.1 Supplements in pregnancy.

Supplement	Dosage	Duration
Folic acid	400 μg/day	3 months prior to conception to 12 weeks pregnancy
Folic acid (where there is a family history of neural tube defect, maternal diabetes, maternal epilepsy, maternal coeliac disease or maternal BMI >30)	5 μg/day	Throughout pregnancy
Vitamin D	10 μg/day	For the duration of pregnancy until the cessation of breastfeeding

Box 62.1 Cleaning and sterilising feeding equipment.

- Wash hands before cleaning and sterilising feeding equipment
- Wash all equipment in hot soapy water
- Scrub inside and outside of bottles and teats with brush to remove any remaining feed
- After washing feeding equipment, rinse it thoroughly under the tap
- If using a commercial steriliser, follow manufacturer's instructions
- If sterilising bottles by boiling: fill a large pan with water to allow complete submersion of all feeding equipment and make sure there are no air bubbles; put lid on and boil for at least 10 minutes, making sure the pan always has water. Keep the pan covered until equipment is needed
- Wash hands and surface near the steriliser before removing equipment
- To prevent contamination of bottle and teat: assemble with the teat and lid in place if the bottles are not to be used immediately

Box 62.2 Additional guidance for preparing feeds.

Note: each bottle should be made up fresh for each feed; do not store made-up formula milk as it may increase the chances of a baby becoming ill

- Wash and dry hands
- Clean surfaces where feed is to be prepared
- Boil water in a kettle
- Note: allow the boiled water to cool to no less than 70°C. This means in practice using water that has been left covered, for less than 30 minutes after boiling
- Add water to the bottle first before powdered infant formula
- Only use the required amount of boiled water in the sterilised bottle
- Add the exact amount of formula as per manufacturer's instructions
- Assemble bottle and shake well to mix the contents
- Cool quickly to feeding temperature by holding under a running tap, or placing in a container of cold water
- Check the temperature by shaking a few drops onto the inside of your wrist – it should feel lukewarm, not hot
- Discard any feed that has not been used within 2 hours

Box 62.3 Developmental readiness for weaning.

- Ability to hold their head unsupported for complementary foods
- Sit with minimal support
- Have no tongue thrust
- Form a food bolus and move food from the front to the back of their mouth
- Pick food up and put in their mouth
- Have interest in food when others are eating

Breastfeeding

Immunisation is preventative medicine par excellence. If a new vaccine became available that could prevent one million or more child deaths a year, and that was moreover cheap, safe, administered orally with no cold chain, it would become an immediate public health imperative. Breastfeeding could do all of this and more, but requires its own 'warm chain' of support – that is skilled care for mothers to build their confidence and show them what to do and protection from harmful practices. If this warm chain has been lost from the culture, or is faulty, then it must be made good by health services (Dobbing et al., 1994).

Preconceptual nutrition

Women of child-bearing age should pay special attention to ensuring they are in optimal nutritional health prior to embarking on a pregnancy. Evidence suggests that there is a critical window of fetal development that occurs in the earliest days of pregnancy, before a woman even knows she is pregnant. Any deficiency of the mother's nutritional state can impair fetal brain growth and function, lead to the baby being born small for gestational age and have long-term consequences for health outcomes. For 3 months prior to conception until the 12th week of pregnancy women are advised to supplement their diet with folic acid 400 µg daily to reduce the risk of neural tube defects.

Nutrition in pregnancy

During pregnancy there is an increased demand for several key nutrients such as vitamin D, folate, iron and calcium. Once pregnancy is confirmed, women are advised to take a further supplement of 10 µg of vitamin D daily (Table 62.1). This supplement of vitamin D should continue until the cessation of breastfeeding. Vitamin D is required as it cannot be sourced from food alone. Provided the mother had adequate iron and calcium stores prior to the pregnancy and eats foods rich in these nutrients, the increased demand for iron, folate and calcium can be derived from the diet. Women are advised to eat foods rich in folate and folic acid to increase their nutrient intake to 300 µg per day for the duration of their pregnancy.

Pregnant women should avoid eating pate, certain types of cheese, raw or partially cooked eggs, raw shellfish and raw and uncooked meat. Pregnant women are advised to limit their caffeine intake to less than 200 µg daily, which is equivalent to two mugs of instant coffee, two mugs of tea or five cans of cola; avoid alcohol completely.

World Health Organisation guidance

The WHO recommends exclusive breastfeeding for the first 6 months of infant life. Breastfeeding should continue, with the introduction of appropriate solid foods, for up to 2 years of age and beyond.

Breast milk is more than a source of nutrition to a growing infant: it contains a wide range of bioactive substances including transfer factors such as lactoferrin, which support the development of the brain, digestive and immune systems, enzymes, hormones, immunoglobulins, leucocytes and anti-inflammatory molecules. None of these bioactive substances can be replicated; therefore, none are present in infant formula. Breastfeeding supports the development of a responsive, symbiotic relationship between mother and child and hence also assists attachment.

Infant formula feeding

Despite evidence demonstrating that breastfeeding is the healthiest choice for mothers and infants, many women will choose to formula feed their infant; healthcare professionals need to actively support this choice. Infant formula is produced from the modification of cow's milk and as a consequence contains none of the active and protective properties of breast milk described previously.

Reconstitution of powdered infant formula

Powdered infant formula is not a sterile product and can provide a medium for the growth of harmful bacteria. Parents choosing to formula feed their infants require information and support to reconstitute powdered infant formula in ways that reduce the inherent risks to their infant (Boxes 62.1 and 62.2).

Types of infant formula

There are two main types of infant formula which can be used as a substitute for breast milk.

1 **Whey-based infant formula** – this should be used throughout the first year of life. There is no medical or nutritional reason to change either type or brand of infant formula.

2 **Casein-based infant formula** – this is less modified than whey-based formula and is less suitable for use as a breast milk substitute.

Follow-on milk is also available and is promoted for use for infants between 6 and 12 months of age. There is no advantage to be found for infants in relation to follow-on milk and it should not be recommended to parents. Infants should continue on a whey-based formula until 12 months of age and full fat cow's milk should be gradually introduced into the infant diet.

Weaning

Weaning is the gradual introduction of food alongside breast milk or infant formula. For the first 6 months exclusive breast milk or infant formula provides adequate nutrition for most infants. After 6 months infants are no longer able to obtain all the nutrients they require such as iron, from milk alone. At about 6 months old most infants' renal and gastrointestinal systems are mature enough to digest and absorb nutrients from non-milk food so can start weaning. Infants are developmentally ready at around 6 months, as indicated in Box 62.3.

Suitable first weaning foods include soft foods which the infant themselves can pick up and mashed family foods (no added salt or sugar). Early weaning is associated with an increased likelihood of obesity in later life and developing respiratory and gastrointestinal illness compared with those given complementary foods at a later stage. Weaning before 4 months is associated with a risk of eczema, and with type 1 diabetes if foods containing gluten are introduced before 3 months.

Neonatal jaundice

Box 63.1 Factors associated with physiological jaundice.

- Haemoglobin level is higher than required
- Red blood cells have shorter life
- Hepatic immaturity
  - Reduced glucuronyl transferase activity
  - Reduced active uptake of urobilinogen
  - Reduced intracellular transport system
  - Reduced active secretion of conjugated bilirubin
  - Large enterohepatic circulation of bilirubin to add to the load of urobilinogen in the hepatocyte

Box 63.2 Other contributing factors to physiological jaundice.

- Drugs-antibiotics (penicillin)
- Bruises
- Caput
- Cephalhaematoma
- Hypoxia/asphyxia
- Hypoglycaemia
- Hypothermia

Table 63.1 Appearance of jaundice.

Timing	Cause
From birth to 24 hours	Sepsis, TORCH, haemolytic disease
48–72 hours	Physiological, polycythemia, bruising
72 hours to 1 week	Sepsis, TORCH, cytomegalovirus (CMV)
After 1 week	Breast milk, hypothryroidism, atresia, G6PD
Persisting 1 month	Cholestasis (total parenteral nutrition), hepatitis, CMV

Table 63.2 Kramers rules.

Blanch the skin in each of the five zones and observe the colour of the blanched skin (will be yellow if jaundiced). This indicates what the serum bilirubin (SB) level could be. The zones indicate the progression of jaundice levels as they increase

Score	Area	SB levels
1	Face	4–6 md/dl
2	Chest, upper abdomen	8–10 mg/dl
3	Lower abdomen, thighs	12–14 mg/dl
4	Arms, lower legs	15–18 mg/dl
5	Palms, soles	15–20 mg/dl

Neonatal jaundice is the medical term for jaundice in babies. This condition, which affects newborn babies, is common and normally does not cause harm. It is defined by a yellow discoloration of the skin, sclera and mucous membrane due to an increase in the serum bilirubin level. This becomes clinically evident when serum bilirubin reaches about 80–100 μmol/l.

Physiology of bilirubin metabolism

Bilirubin is formed from the breakdown of haemoglobin. There are two types of bilirubin: unconjugated and conjugated. When bilirubin is first formed it is unconjugated and fat soluble. It cannot be excreted in bile or urine and travels in the plasma, bound to albumin. It enters the liver cells with the aid of Y and Z carrier proteins and becomes conjugated with glucoronic acid. The reaction is catalysed by an enzyme called glucuronyl transferase. Hypoxia or hypothermia may compromise bilirubin conjugation.

Conjugated bilirubin is water soluble and is excreted through the biliary tree into the gut. Conjugated bilirubin is further catabolised by intestinal flora into urobilinogen and stercobilin. It forms a major component of bile in faeces; this gives the characteristic orange colour to faeces. A small amount is also passed in the urine.

Causes of hyperbilirubinaemia

There are many causes of unconjugated hyperbilirubinaemia; the most common being physiological. Other causes are: breast milk, excessive bruising, polycythaemia due to delayed cord clamping or twin-to-twin transfusion, haemolytic disease from rhesus or ABO incompatibility, glucose 6 phosphate dehydrogenase (G6PD) and congenital hypothyroidism.

There are also many reasons for conjugated hyperbilirubinaemia such as sepsis, hepatitis, TORCH (toxoplasmosis, other agents, rubella, cytomegalovirus and herpes simplex), cystic fibrosis and biliary atresia. The timing of the appearance of jaundice is associated with the cause (Table 63.1).

Aetiology of physiological jaundice

In a newborn the haemoglobin level is usually 18–19 g/dl and in adults it is 11–14 g/dl. There is an increased red blood cell (RBC) count in infants; haemoglobin is a constituent of RBC and is broken into: globin, a protein that is conserved and utilised, and haem, which cannot be used and is degraded and excreted. Bilirubin is a product of this degradation and it causes yellow staining of the tissues. The high haemoglobin level and the shorter life of the RBCs in the newborn, combined with a decreased hepatic blood flow, immature liver and an immature breakdown system for bilirubin, causes jaundice. Due to the gastrointestinal tract lacking bacteria to breakdown waste, this therefore increases reuptake of bilirubin (Box 63.1).

Physiological jaundice is jaundice occurring in the immediate newborn without signs of illness. It will usually peak at 2–4 days and rises slowly to a bilirubin blood level of less than 100 μmol/l. It will generally disappear by 1 week and does not normally present before 24 hours of birth. Physiological jaundice responds well to single phototherapy, if used. The incidence of this type of jaundice is 80% in preterm infants, and 30–50% in term infants in the first week of life, and only 10% will require phototherapy. Other factors that can contribute to physiological jaundice are shown in Box 63.2.

Investigations

There are different tests for jaundice and tests that are required once jaundice is detected. Initially it is important to check the naked baby in bright and preferably natural light, examing the sclera, gums and blanched skin in all skin tones. Kramer's rules, which are a simple way to assess the degree of jaundice, can be applied to this process (Table 63.2). However, this is a guide only and serum bilirubin levels should always be obtained.

In some health settings a jaundice meter or icterometer is used to assess jaundice level. If used these need strict criteria as to when they are used and at what levels further action is required to be taken. Serum bilirubin levels are the most common method of assessing jaundice levels. The importance of the level depends on the baby's gestation and hours after birth and if the bilirubin is unconjugated (indirect) or conjugated (direct). Therefore, the level needs to be plotted on a specific chart. Other important factors for investigation are: clinical history of mother and family, history of labour, bruising, cephalohaematoma, birth trauma, blood group and rhesus factor, haemoglobin, reticulocyte count (raised levels in cases of haemolysis), feeding pattern, infection, G6PD and drug use.

Care of baby

Increase the frequency of breastfeeding and offer regular artificial feeding to maintain nutrition and hydration. Maintain a neutral thermal environment, prevent hypoglycaemia and hypoxia and avoid constipation. If physiological jaundice requires phototherapy (if level is >340 μmol/l), then single phototherapy or biliblanket should be used and the baby should only be out of the light for short feeding times. When using phototherapy:

- Place the baby in a supine position where possible
- Provide eye protection and routine eye care
- Use 'blue light' phototherapy
- Ensure treatment is applied to the maximum area of skin; monitor temperature and hydration; weigh daily; assess nappies
- Support parents and carers, and encourage interaction with the baby
- regular measurements of serum bilirubin.

Kernicterus

Kernicterus is the yellow staining of the basal ganglia of infants, influenced by serum bilirubin levels greater than 340 mmol/l in term babies and rapidly rising bilirubin levels of greater than 8.5 μmol/l per hour.

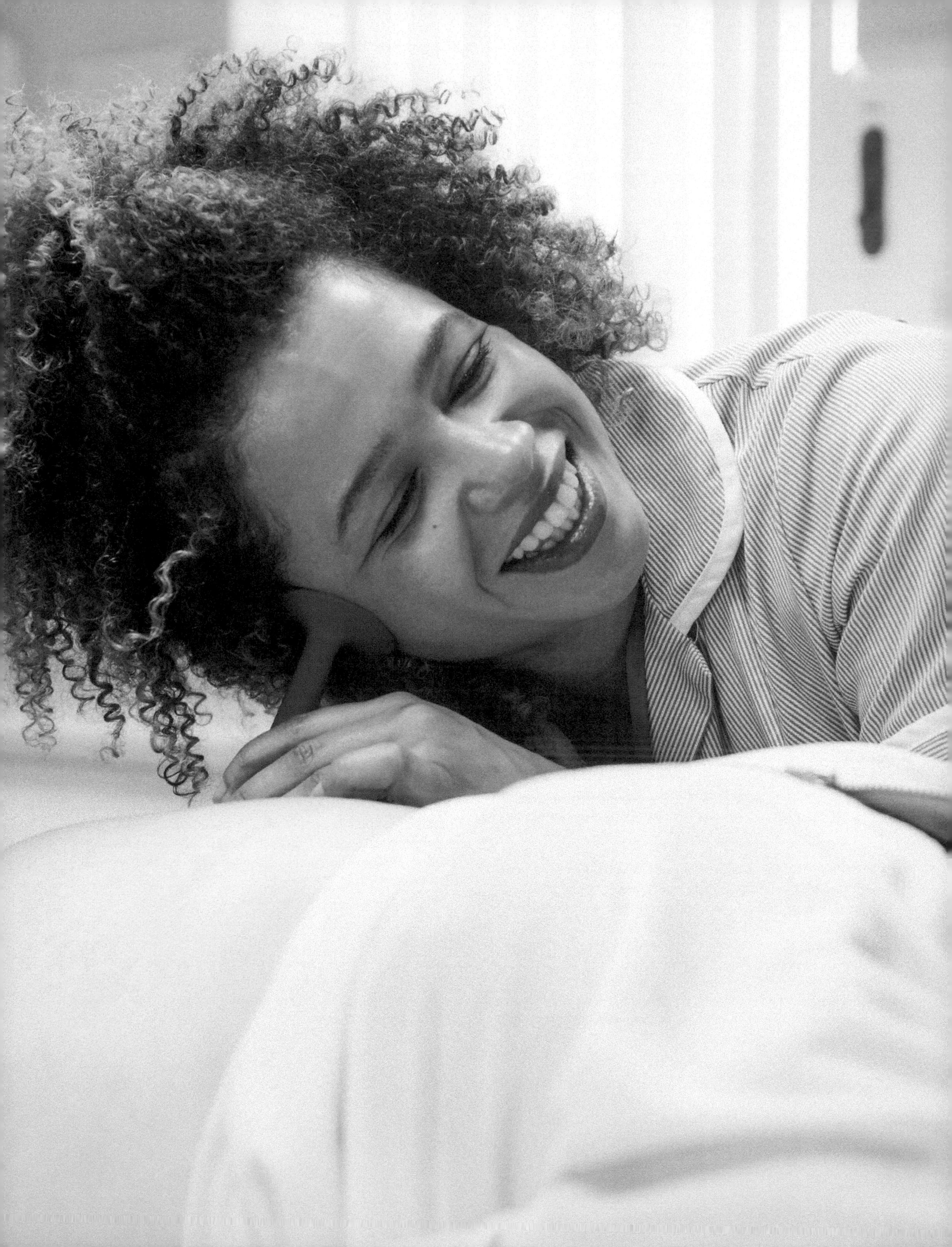

Psychological dimensions

Chapters

64 Becoming a parent

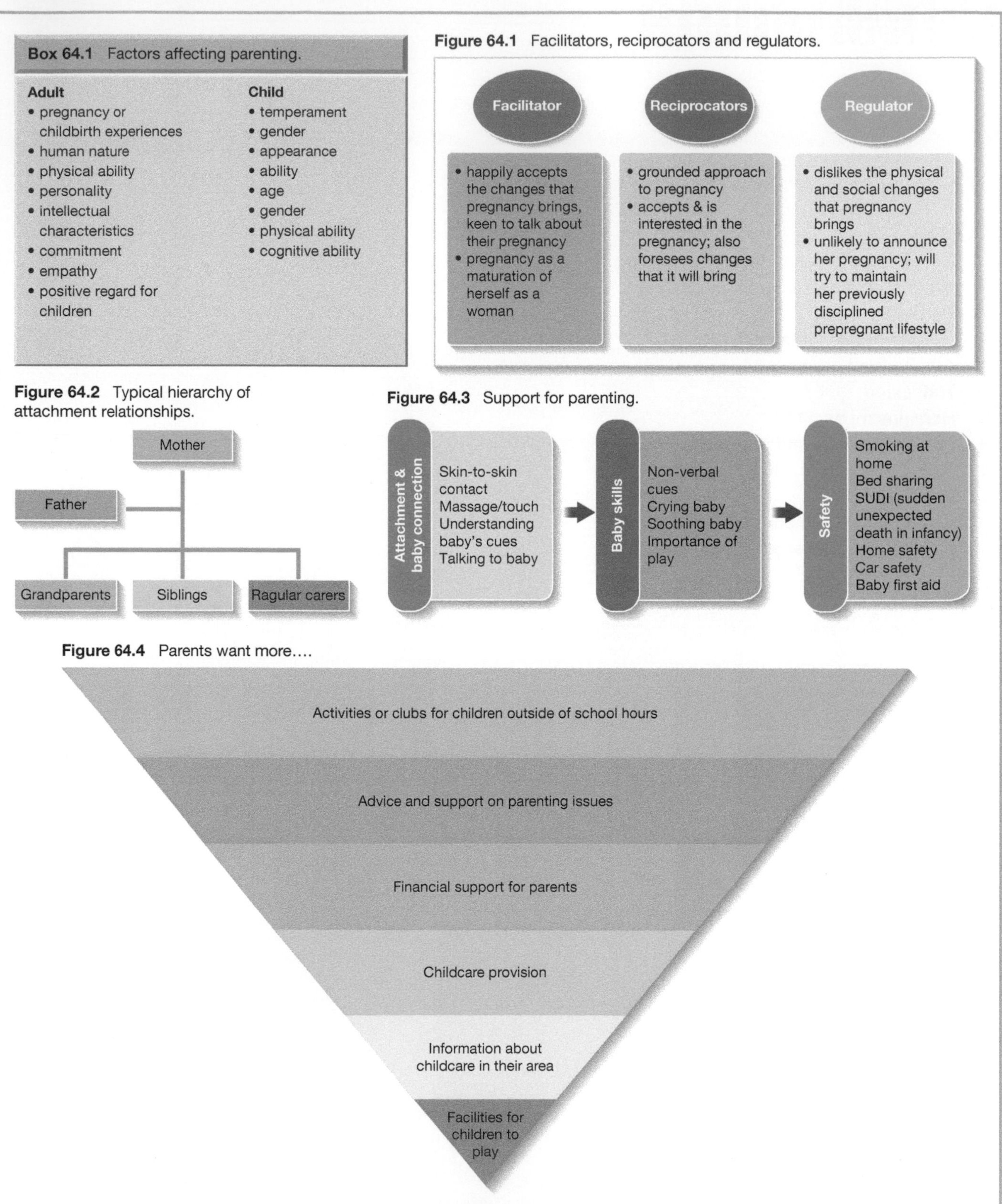

Figure 64.1 Facilitators, reciprocators and regulators.

Figure 64.2 Typical hierarchy of attachment relationships.

Figure 64.3 Support for parenting.

Figure 64.4 Parents want more....

Worldwide, millions of people become parents every day, so it is an extremely common occurrence and one which is generally accepted as being an event within the cycle of life. Parenting brings a range of emotions, experiences and challenges; many of which can be difficult but also rewarding. Each individual's experience of their upbringing and being parented is different and this can influence how the practice of parenting is passed on. Parenting is about nurturing, caring and protecting the child, showing love and kindness. The act of parenting is a responsible job that focuses on the development of the child. Although parents will have their own needs, parenting involves placing the child at the centre of care.

Although traditionally and across cultures the mother's role is at the forefront of parenting, fathers have an important role too and many children are parented by both. Parenting is not unique to biological parents, however, as children can also be parented by significant others in their lives. Families, regardless of their make-up, are the basis of society and influence our future. Although parents mostly do a great job in bringing up children, it can sometimes be a difficult process resulting in difficulties and dysfunction for children. Parenting can also be affected by the children, for example temperament, gender, appearance or ability. Additionally, pregnancy or childbirth experiences can influence perceptions of the child and affect parenting (Box 64.1).

Becoming a parent

The concept of becoming a parent normally begins for the individual at the beginning of pregnancy or even earlier, when the pregnancy is being planned. It is not until the baby has arrived that being a parent becomes a reality for most people. Although having a set of rules to follow might make this process easier for some people, becoming a parent involves adaptation and is a personal learning process about developing relationships.

It has been suggested that women fall broadly into three groups – facilitators, reciprocators and regulators (Figure 64.1) – and that this can influence how they adapt to pregnancy and develop an identity as a mother. In reality women do not fit neatly into these groups and by 24 weeks' gestation most women will develop an increasing attachment with their fetus.

Many mothers voice aspirations for their fetus as the pregnancy continues based on apparent characteristics of fetal behaviour: for example, lively fetus if experiencing a lot of fetal movement, will be a night owl if experiencing a lot of night movement. Many mothers hold, stroke and talk to their growing 'bump'. The developing relationship with the fetus makes the mother appear more focused on herself and the fetus than others around her. These psychological adaptations may be the start of the bonding process and initiate some initial preparations towards becoming a mother.

Bonding and attachment

The relationship from the parent to the child is often called bonding, and from the child to the parent, attachment. However, the term attachment also relates to the quality of the relationship and can be used for both as they need to be synchronous to be effective.

Attachment focuses on the relationship and not the person and is the term used to describe the very early relationship formed between an infant and carer. The physical and emotional development of the child is dependent on a secure attachment relationship. In fact it is said to be the single most important factor influencing a child's development. An infant's early experiences of attachment can affect later expectations and capacity to make further relationships. Therefore, secure parenting at this early stage to ensure good attachment is extremely important to an infant's future wellbeing. For example, when an infant's needs are responded to positively, attachment occurs.

Depending on who provides the most consistent care for the infant, a hierarchy of attachment will develop (Figure 64.2). If a child has a consistent, small number of regular carers, secure attachments are likely to occur, allowing the child to develop to their full potential to learn and be able to regulate their own behaviour. Inconsistencies, too many carers or negative experiences with carers can result in the formation of insecure relationships. Good parenting is important to help prevent this. However, many people struggle as parents and require additional support.

Support for parenting

Generally, parents depend on health professionals, such as midwives, health visitors and GPs for advice when the baby and child are young. However, parenting advice can be provided initially by midwives throughout the antenatal period. Each contact with women provides an opportunity for discussion, such as how she is feeling about the baby, about becoming a mother and how she perceives this might change her routine and life. Antenatal classes can also provide information on parenting skills and safety, for example, and allow women to meet other future parents to share ideas and express their feelings. In the postnatal period, the midwife can support women and families to focus on the infant's cues to encourage early bonding and attachment and provide positive encouragers when appropriate responses are made. Early skin-to-skin contact, touch and communication are also some approaches the midwife can encourage to help forge early attachment and parenting skills (Figure 64.3).

Health visitors have a key role in the early years to ensure that the child's and family's needs are identified, early intervention is implemented and referral made to specialist services. However, approximately 30% of parents with a child less than 2 years of age use the internet for advice and support. When providing support, it is important to know what parents want and what is available locally. Often parents want play facilities, clubs, parenting advice, financial support and childcare provision (Figure 64.4).

65 Maternal mental health

Figure 65.1 Whooley questions: During the past month…

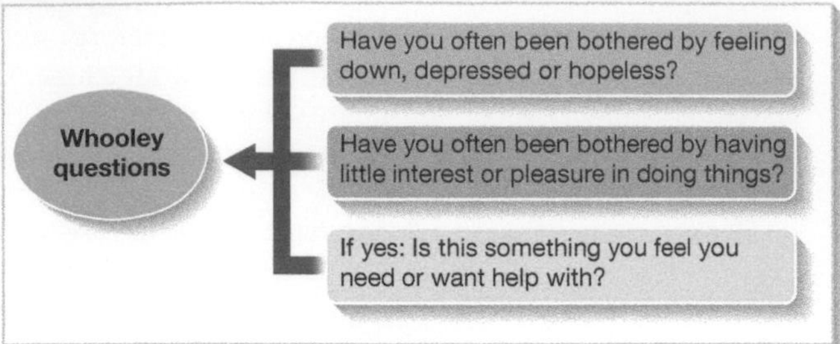

Figure 65.2 The baby blues'.

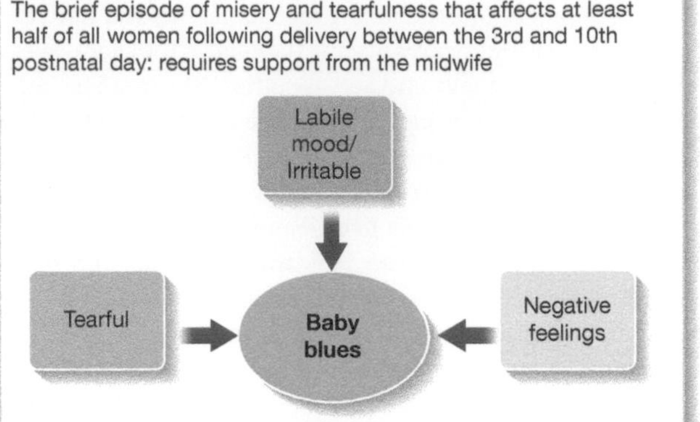

Figure 65.3 Postnatal depression.

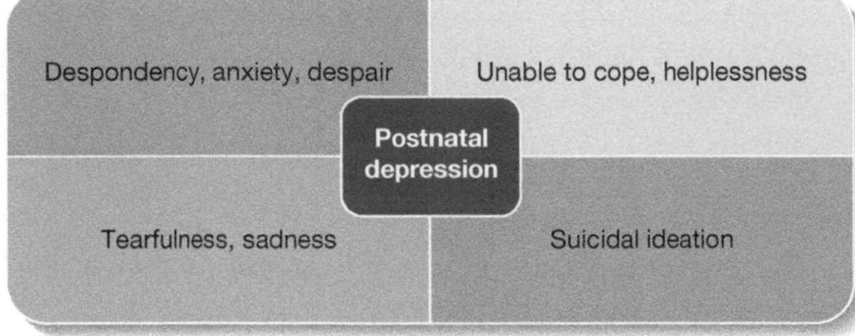

Figure 65.4 Postpartum/puerperal psychosis.

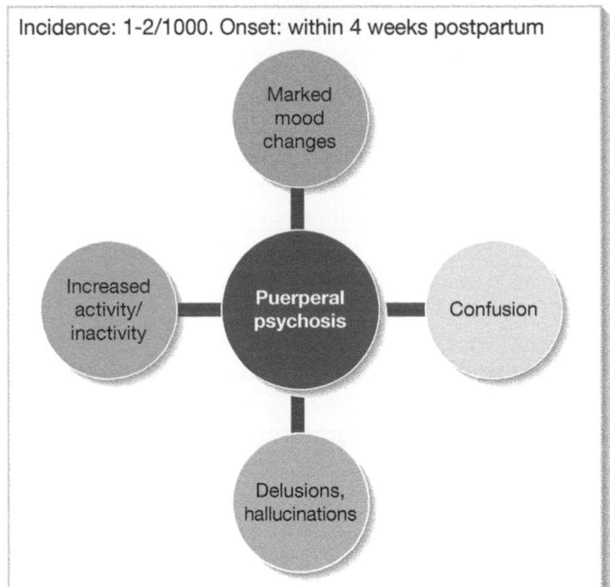

Figure 65.5 Features of post-traumatic stress disorder (PTSD).

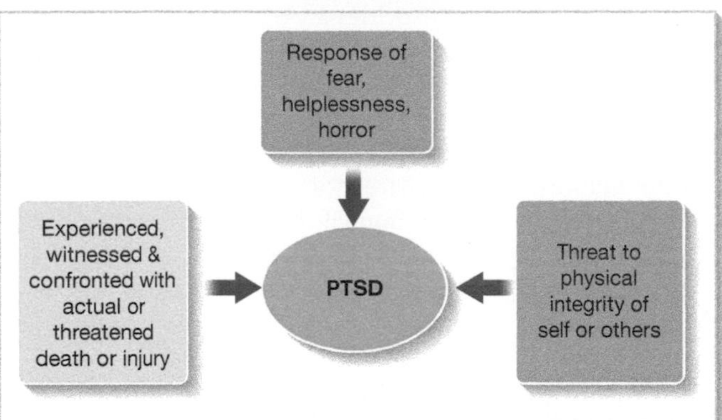

Box 65.1 Midwifery role in perinatal mental health (PMH).

- Development of improved services through development of integrated care pathways (ICPs) and care networks
- Organisation of professionals' planning meetings and liaison meetings with psychiatry and obstetrics
- Development of care plans
- Providing continuing professional development (CPD) training
- One to one and group support

Box 65.2 Hormone changes.

- Oestrogen rises to 50 times normal level by last 3 months of pregnancy
- Oestrogen falls back to normal level in the 3 days following the baby's birth
- Progesterone rises to 10 times the normal level in pregnancy
- Progesterone falls back to normal level in the week following the baby's birth
- Cortisol rises 2–3 times normal level in pregnancy
- Cortisol levels slowly decrease after birth
- Prolactin goes up to 7 times its normal level in pregnancy
- Prolactin falls back to normal level in the 3 months following birth

Box 65.3 Myths of motherhood.

- Pregnancy or becoming a mother is always wanted or needed
- Being a mother is natural
- A mother should be beautiful & radiant whilst being a good cook & housekeeper
- Good mothers always have time to play with their children
- Good mothers have the wisdom to guide and discipline their children
- A mother is supposed to have infinite feelings for her baby

The mental health of women in the perinatal period is a public health issue that midwives have a responsibility to address as childbearing has a relationship with mood disorders. To ensure that women's on-going mental health needs are met, the midwife will have to liaise with other health professionals. Due to the complexity of mental health problems, a multiprofessional approach to care is required which may include midwifery, perinatal mental health midwife (Box 65.1), obstetric, psychiatric, social services, health visitors, GP, clinical psychologists, community mental health services and voluntary services. Services for women should be ascertained and accessed according to individual need. Many women present to maternity services with pre-existing mental health problems, whilst others develop mental health problems during pregnancy or the postnatal period. Childbearing is known to be a risk factor for maternal mental ill health. For example, during the period 2003–2005, the most common cause of indirect deaths and the largest cause of maternal death overall in the UK was psychiatric illness.

Men can also be affected by mental illness, such as depression as a result of becoming a father due to the added anxiety and stress this may cause, especially if his partner has developed a mental health problem at this time.

A detailed plan for psychiatric management for late pregnancy and early postnatal should be made for women at high risk of postnatal mental illness. This should be agreed with the woman and subsequently shared with the mulitdisciplinary team.

Perinatal mood disorders

Antenatal and postnatal period

There are many misconceptions that pregnancy is always wanted, or a happy time for women. Pregnancy and becoming a mother are life changing events which women have to adjust to but can cause anxiety. There are many hormonal changes in pregnancy (Box 65.2) that women have to adjust to and the effect of these are often combined with financial stresses, lack of social support and anxiety. There are many myths of motherhood that can perpetuate women's anxiety about their ability to be a good mother which often begin during pregnancy (Box 65.3). Weight gain is required and considered normal in pregnancy, but many women, and in particular those with an eating disorder, often struggle with this and require specialist support. Women can also have fears about the birth and in extreme situations may even suffer from tokophobia, a pathological fear of pregnancy which can lead to avoidance of childbirth. Depression and anxiety can be onset by pregnancy, or exist prepregnancy.

Screening for mental ill health is important (Figure 65.1) and the midwife must ensure that a robust history, which ascertains a woman's past and current mental health, and her family's mental health, is obtained (Chapter 15). Of significance is a personal or family history of bipolar affective disorder, schizophrenia or severe depressive disorder; these can indicate that a woman is at greater risk of developing mental illness in pregnancy or the postnatal period and requires referral to a specialist perinatal mental health team for assessment.

The postnatal period is a time of major change and physical, social and emotional adjustment for new mothers, partners and their families.

Postpartum 'baby blues'

This is a transient, self-limiting condition that occurs usually around the third but can be up until the 10th postnatal day (Figure 65.2). It affects about 70% of women. As such it is considered a normal reaction, usually associated with hormonal changes. However, persistent or severe feelings might indicate the onset of postnatal depression.

Postnatal depression

Postnatal depression (PND) is a non-psychotic depressive illness affecting between 10% and 20% of women within the first postpartum year and can vary in severity; it is the most common perinatal mood disorder (Figure 65.3). Symptoms often occur within the first 4 weeks but can appear up to the end of the first postnatal year. If diagnosed and treated early, this condition usually resolves within 6 months, but can last much longer if not detected early. Women often feel guilty and inadequate about having negative feelings towards motherhood or their baby and often do not admit to being depressed. Midwives therefore have a duty to screen for risk during pregnancy and the postnatal period. The causes are often multifactorial – physical and psychosocial, but current or previous history of depression increases the risk for women. Detrimental effects on infant cognitive, emotional, social and behavioural development have been associated with untreated postnatal depression. Fewer positive and more negative responses are given to infants by mothers with depression.

Postpartum (puerperal) psychosis

This is a severe affective psychotic mood disorder of acute onset, linked to the postnatal period (Figure 65.4). It is accompanied by features such as loss of contact with reality and abnormal behaviour. Although relatively rare, this severe mental illness requires urgent psychiatric attention. Risk factors are personal or close family history of bipolar affective disorder or previous psychotic episode. Treatment is normally with antipsychotic, mood stabiliser drugs and admission to a specialist mother and baby unit if possible.

Post-traumatic stress disorder (PTSD)

In relation to the perinatal period, PTSD can be caused by pain associated with childbirth, fear and feeling out of control. It can also be linked to previous traumatic experiences of childbirth or gynaecological examinations or sexual abuse. Although not well researched, midwives should be aware of how this can affect the mental health and wellbeing of childbearing women and adopt an appropriately sensitive approach to care. PTSD can occur with exposure to a traumatic event with two key elements: (i) experienced, witnessed and confronted with actual or threatened death or injury; and (ii) threat to physical integrity of self or others and the response involved fear, helplessness and horror.

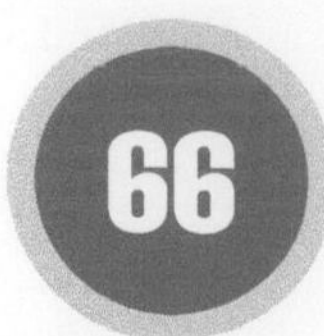

66 Bereavement care

Figure 66.1 Kübler-Ross grief stages.

GRIEF STAGES
Loss
Denial, shock and isolation
Don't cry
Avoid mention of loss
Return to normal life quickly
Sense of shock continues
Non believing
Anger
Unresolved anger
Easily roused to anger
Bargaining
Continuing lack of acceptance
Trying to change outcome
Depression
Depression worsens
Appetite affected
Disturbed sleep
Lack of energy
Suicidal thoughts
Acceptance

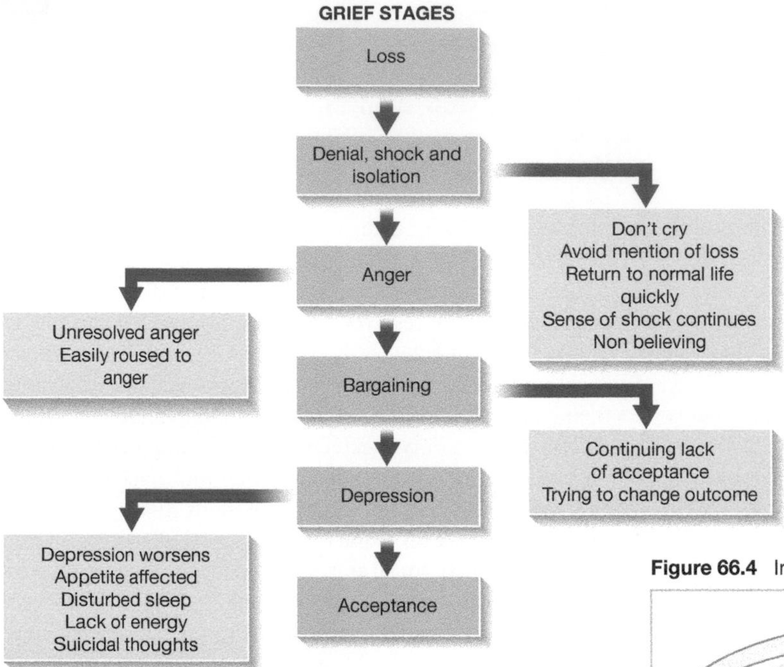

Figure 66.2 Examples of grief stage emotions.

Shock: 'This can't be happening'
Denial: 'The midwives don't know what they are talking about'
Anger: At self, relative or midwife/obstetrician
Bargaining: 'If only I had listened and not continued to cycle – I won't do it again'
Depression: Tired, withdrawn, apathetic
Acceptance: Coming to terms with loss; learning to live with it

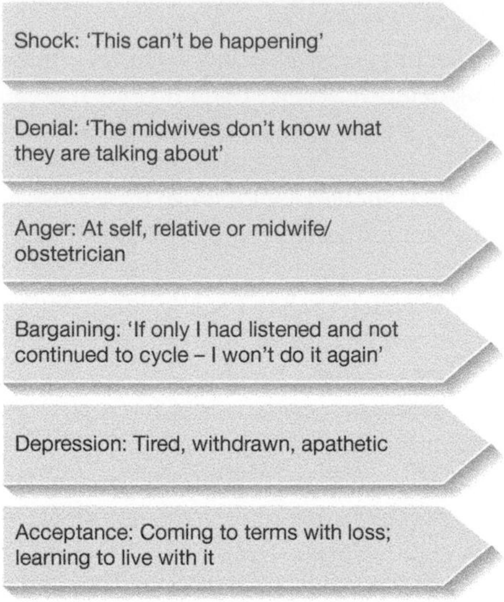

Figure 66.3 Disenfranchised grief.

When a relationship is not recognised
When a death/loss is difficult to publicly accept
Disenfranchised grief
When a loss is not recognised
When a grieving person is not recognised

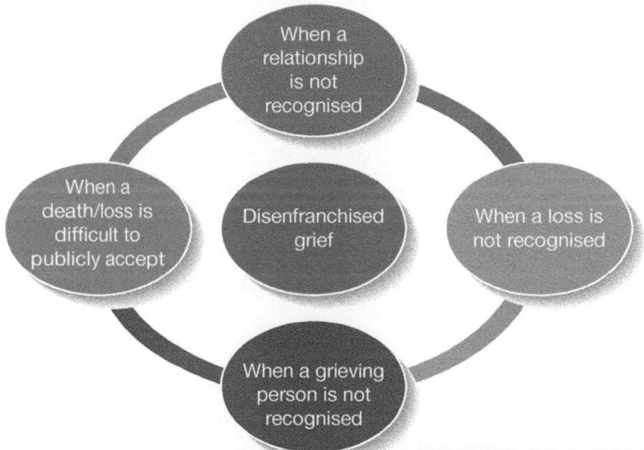

Figure 66.4 Initial reactions to bad news.

1. Shock
2. Protest
3. Disorganisation
Reorganisation

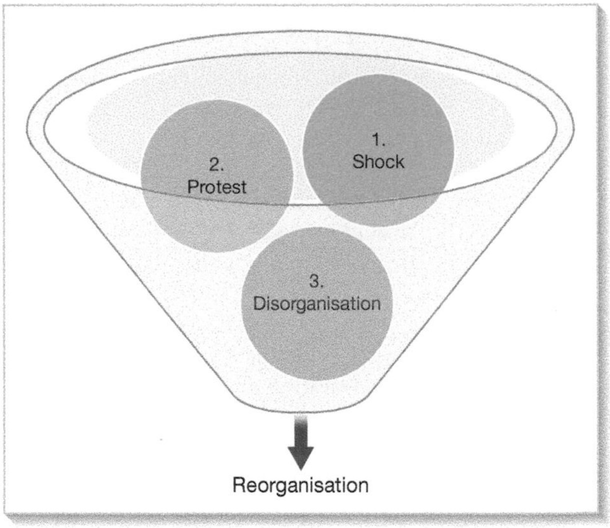

Figure 66.5 Encourage memories with hand and foot prints.

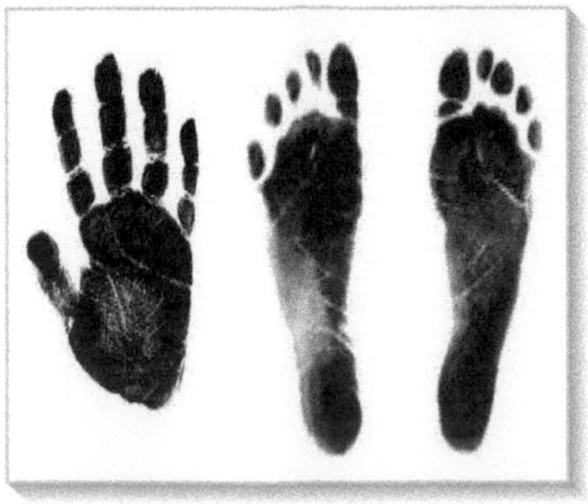

Box 66.1 Areas that incur bereavement.

- Infertility
- Ectopic pregnancy
- Miscarriage
- Stillbirth
- Termination of pregnancy
- Perinatal and neonatal death
- Sudden infant death syndrome
- Death of another child
- Child fostered or adopted
- Loss of relationship
- History of abuse
- Loss of identity
- Loss of trust
- Loss of expectations, such as normal childbirth

Box 66.2 Some support services.

Samaritans:
https://www.samaritans.org/
Bliss:
https://www.bliss.org.uk/
Sands:
https://www.sands.org.uk
Miscarriage Association:
https://www.miscarriageassociation.org.uk/
Cruse Bereavement Care:
https://www.cruse.org.uk/
Bereavement Counselling Service:
http://bcsplymouth.co.uk/

Midwifery at a Glance, First Edition. Edited by Eleanor Forrest © 2019 John Wiley & Sons, Ltd. Published 2019 by John Wiley & Sons, Ltd.
Companion website: www.wiley.com/go/forrest/midwifery

Midwives and maternity care professionals have responsibility for delivering holistic, evidence-based bereavement care to childbearing women. It is important to recognise the physical, psychological and social components of bereavement, loss and grief to be equipped with appropriate skills to deal with related adversity. Although used interchangeably, the term bereavement refers to the state of loss, and grief to the reaction to the loss of someone or something important. In maternity care settings, this loss of someone important could be a miscarriage or stillbirth (Box 66.1), and the loss of potential motherhood and associated social identity could be identified as being the loss of something important to the woman and her family. Bereavement in the perinatal period generally originates from two main areas: actual loss of a baby and loss of idealisation through events such as traumatic birth or an ill baby, for example. Women who have experienced such losses in the childbearing period will go through a period of bereavement in which there will be associated grief and personal adjustment to the loss.

Grief

Grief is a multifaceted response to the loss of someone or something to which there is a bond. Grieving for the death of a baby or child is considered one of the most difficult. Childbearing women need support to adapt and recover from this loss and midwives have an important role to play in this. Being aware of different cultural and religious approaches to grieving will allow the midwife to provide support to meet the individual needs of parents and their wider extended family.

There are many models of grieving, but the well-known stages described by Kübler-Ross from the late 1960s is often applied to many different situations when an understanding of grief is required (Figure 66.1). It is appropriate for use within maternity care to help midwives and other professionals identify and understand the grieving process that a childbearing woman who has suffered bereavement may experience (Figure 66.2). This model demonstrates how grieving occurs in stages, although is not always linear, as parents' emotions often move back and forwards before final acceptance occurs. Although grief is a normal response to loss, there may be individual differences in the timing and responses and, for some, adjusting to the loss may be problematic. A loss in pregnancy, for example, is a form of disenfranchised grief (Figure 66.3), whereby society often makes it difficult to recognise the loss, such as in miscarriage or termination of pregnancy, or if the pregnancy was the result of sexual abuse or rape; women can often feel isolated in their grief. In situations where grief is denied or the woman's response has become maladaptive, women may not cry, may avoid talking about their loss, or continue to feel anger long after this would usually be over; they may also display symptoms of depression or anxiety (Figure 66.1). Maintaining mental health for childbearing women is an important role of the midwife (Chapter 65) and being aware of risk factors such as bereavement is something that midwives must be alert to.

Breaking bad news

It is inevitable within maternity care that bad news will have to be given to women and their families. It may be the midwife who will be that professional or who will be providing support thereafter. It is imperative that providers of such care have good communication skills and understand the importance of a sensitive and individual approach. It is the professional's duty to ensure balance between causing distress and giving essential information, providing support and making appropriate referrals. An empathic cycle of listening should be employed with the woman at the centre and the professional demonstrating that the woman has been heard and understood, that the professional knows about appropriate interventions and observes the woman's responses. The words used are key – these convey honesty from the outset. To prevent unnecessary anguish, information should be given in small amounts, with statements that will indicate the serious nature of the situation employed, for example, 'I am very sorry to have to tell you' or 'it's not good news, I'm afraid'. Following the bad news, there are a range of expected initial reactions such as shock. Then, a disorganisation of emotions occurs when despair and confusion can be felt before reality starts to be understood and reorganisation of emotions takes place (Figure 66.4).

Encouraging memories

Gathering meaningful memories of their baby may help parents in the grieving process. It enables them to formulate their baby's social identity and forge concrete memories of the time they had together. Bereavement protocols within maternity units should all have guidelines for staff and parents, facilities for professional photographs to be taken and memory boxes to be created for parents using such items as a lock of the baby's hair, hand and footprints and baby's identity bracelet. These treasured items can be looked at time and again as parents come to terms with their loss (Figure 66.5).

On-going support

On-going support for women and families that have suffered bereavement is vitally important to help them deal with their loss and ultimately recover. Midwives can support women, but ideally a bereavement care midwife should be employed in each hospital to provide tailor-made care. The bereavement care midwife will have knowledge of necessary follow-up and referral appointments that may be required: genetic counselling, prepregnancy counselling, contraception advice, obstetric consultation liaison, multidisciplinary notification, and postmortem and undertaker advice. Information about local support agencies can be given (Box 66.2) and although these might not initially be suitable for all women, they may in time be of use.

It is also important to consider the needs of a colleague who has just returned to work following a childbearing bereavement.

67

Gender-based violence

Figure 67.1 Some health consequences of gender-based violence.

Health consequences of GBV include, but are not limited to:
Physical injury
Chronic pain
Gynaecological problems
Sexually transmitted infections
Obstetric complications
Anxiety & depression
Self-harm/suicide attempts
Alcohol/drug misuse
Post-traumatic stress

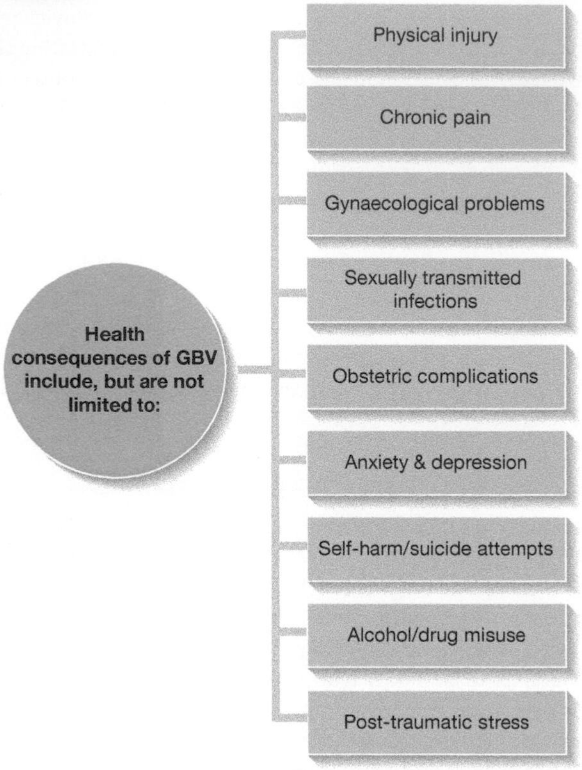

Figure 67.2 What women want from health professionals.

Women who have experienced, or are experiencing abuse do not expect health professionals to 'fix it' or to be experts in dealing with GBV. What they want is:
To be believed
To not be judged
Time to talk and be heard
Help to access services

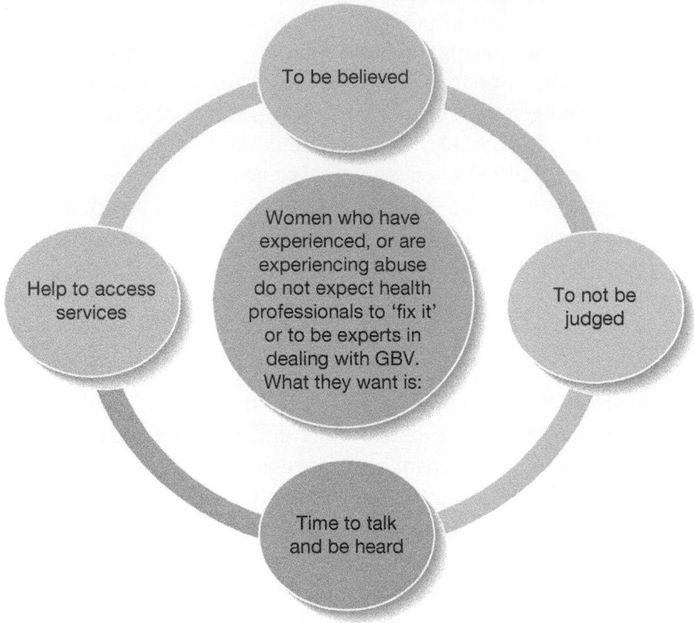

Box 67.1 What health professionals need to do.

- Ensure private, accessible, supportive environment where the woman can be seen alone
- Assess language & communication support required
- Be aware of abuse & how it can impact on health & wellbeing
- Identify & respond appropriately to disclosure
- Consider safety & risk to the woman & any children
- Provide information on support services & refer to services/agencies as required
- Safely document disclosure of abuse including actions/plan of care but never in woman's hand-held notes

Companion website: www.wiley.com/go/forrest/midwifery

Gender-based violence (GBV) is a major global public health issue that impacts on the health and wellbeing of those affected by it (Figure 67.1). Health professionals need to be aware of the crucial role they play in identifying and responding to GBV due to the impact it has on physical, psychological and sexual health. Evidence shows us that it is predominantly women and children that experience GBV and men that perpetrate such violence. This violence exists due to gender inequality between men and women where one group has been given greater power and control to the detriment of the other. This is seen in the level of fear and coercive control used by men perpetrating violence against women.

Men can be affected by GBV as some women will use violence against their male partners, although the highest risk of violence to men comes from other men. GBV can happens in same sex relationships. Evidence shows that the greatest risk to experiencing abuse is being a woman.

Disclosing abuse is never easy whether you are a woman or a man. The most important issue is the care given following disclosure, therefore health professionals need to have knowledge, understanding and be skilled in how to raise the issue and respond appropriately to support the client.

What is gender-based violence?

According to the United Nations GBV is 'violence that is directed against a woman because she is a woman, or violence that affects women disproportionately. It includes acts that inflict physical, mental or sexual harm or suffering, threats of such acts, coercion and other deprivations of liberty.'

To understand GBV the difference between sex and gender must first be understood. Sex is biological and usually people are born with male or female genitalia. Gender is socially constructed, is not biological and refers to the different social roles that define men and women. This can change through time and varies within different cultures (e.g. dressing baby girls in pink and boys in blue). GBV stems from gender inequality and by referring to it as gender-based violence this highlights the need to understand violence within the context of women's subordinate status in society and how this unequal status increases their exposure to and risk of abuse, violating many of their human rights.

GBV is a term used to cover a range of complex abusive behaviours that include the following.

Domestic abuse

This is physical, psychological, sexual and financial abuse perpetrated by partners or ex-partners. Physical abuse includes all types of assault and physical attack. Psychological abuse (emotional abuse) includes threats, intimidation, verbal and racial abuse and other controlling behaviours (e.g. isolation from family and friends). Sexual abuse includes acts that degrade and humiliate women and are perpetrated against their will, including rape. Financial abuse includes withholding or controlling money.

One in four women will be affected by domestic abuse; it is rarely a one-off incident and increases in frequency and severity over time. The woman's life is controlled by the abusive partner taking away her autonomy, slowly stripping her confidence and self-esteem. The perpetrator can micromanage her life, controlling every aspect of her daily living whether he is there or not. Threats, intimidation and isolation are often used to maintain this control.

Domestic abuse often starts or escalates in pregnancy, impacting on the health and wellbeing of the woman, fetus and any children in the family. It is important that midwives are aware of domestic abuse and are able to identify and respond to disclosure offering support, assessing the safety of the woman and children and making referral to appropriate services.

Rape and sexual assault

This can be a one-off or repeated unwanted or coerced sexual activity, including penetration, being forcibly touched in a sexual manner and sexual harassment. It is often carried out by someone known to the victim. Humiliating and degrading the victim is often an intrinsic part of ongoing sexual violence.

Childhood sexual abuse

This is exploitation of a child or young person by an adult for their own or other's sexual gratification. It involves forcing or enticing a child to take part in sexual activity whether the child is/is not aware of what is happening and can take many different forms. It can include penetrative or non-penetrative acts, involvement in or exposure to pornography, or using sexually explicit language – all impacting on the physical and emotional wellbeing of the child.

Stalking and harassment

This is unwanted, persistent, repeated behaviour which is often threatening. Repeated calls/texts, following, unwanted gifts, hanging around place of work or home and vandalism are a few of the behaviours. In most cases the stalker is known to the victim.

Harmful traditional practices

These are forms of violence that have primarily been committed against girls in certain communities and societies for so long that they are considered, or are presented by perpetrators, as being part of accepted cultural practices. They include female genital mutilation, forced marriage, dowry-related violence and female infanticide.

Commercial sexual exploitation

Such exploitation includes a range of sexual activities that harm, exploit and objectify women including prostitution, trafficking, pornography, stripping and pole and lap dancing.

Often these forms of abuse are interconnected and many women experience more than one form of abuse during their lifetime. For example, a woman may have been forced into a marriage and experienced domestic abuse within this relationship, which may also have included sexual abuse.

In order to help women living with GBV, health professionals need to understand their role and care should be woman centered (Figure 67.2 and Box 67.1). They also need to be aware of the increased risk of child abuse. When a woman is experiencing abuse, this should significantly increase suspicion that any children/young people in the family may be at risk. If there are any concerns, seek advice and follow local child protection guidelines.

68 Alcohol and drugs

Figure 68.1 Fetal alcohol syndrome features.

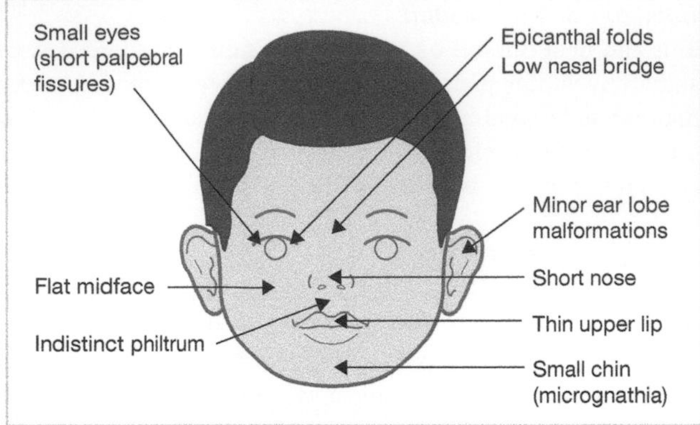

Figure 68.3 Drinking in pregnancy. Source: General Lifestyle Survey, Office for National Statistics 2011. Licensed under Open Government Licence v3.0, http://www.nationalarchives.gov.uk/doc/open-government-licence/version/3/

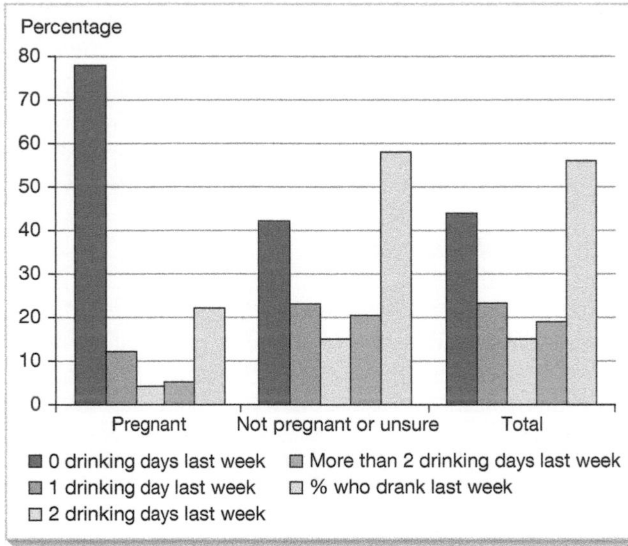

Figure 68.2 Fetal alcohol syndrome features.

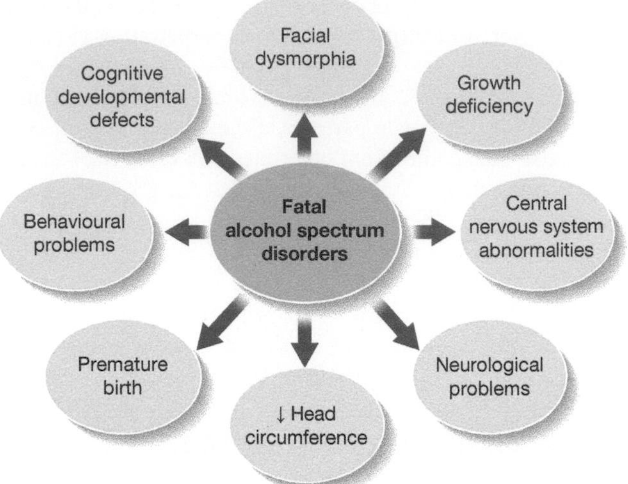

Figure 68.4 Toxins to fetus.

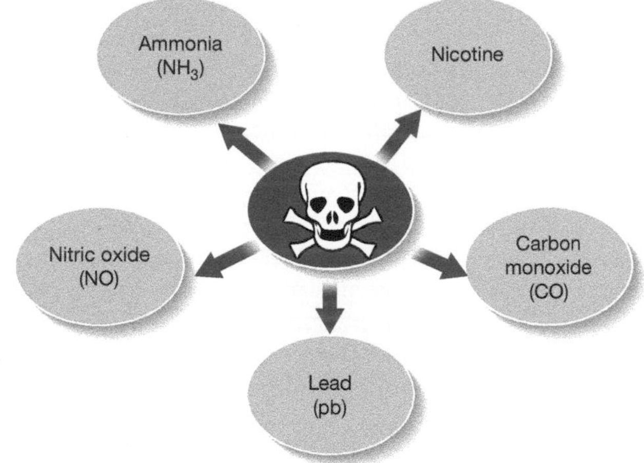

Box 68.1 Maternal heroin effects.

Drowsiness
- Respiratory depressant
- Nausea

Euphoria
- Withdrawal symptoms
- Risk of overdose

Preterm birth
- Placental abruption
- Thromboembolism

Box 68.2 Fetal and baby heroin effects.

Neurobehavioural teratogenicity
- Irritability
- Hypertonicity

Neonatal abstinence syndrome
- Tremors
- Vomiting and diarrhea
- Tachypnoea

Attention deficit hyperactivity disorder (ADHD)
- Poor feeding/excessive sucking and rooting
- Reduced learning capacities in children

Teratogenic substances such as prescribed and illegal drugs, nicotine, alcohol and infections (e.g. German measles, cytomegalovirus and irradiation) induce the formation of developmental abnormalities in a fetus. Many have public health implications, especially those that are preventable and due to the woman's lifestyle. National guidelines advocate that at the first contact with a health professional, pregnant women should be given lifestyle advice such as alcohol consumption in pregnancy, smoking cessation and the implications of recreational drug use (Chapter 15).

Alcohol consumption

Alcohol's teratogenic effects occur during the earliest weeks of embryo development. Alcohol during pregnancy can affect the embryo or fetus by causing injury to neural crest cells; the cranial neural crest cells form the facial cartilage and bone. It may cause the corpus callosum (the central tract within the brain) which unites the left and right hemispheres to develop abnormally. It also mimics the effects of stress on the maternal hypothalamic–pituitary–adrenal (HPA) axis which releases corticotrophin-releasing hormone (CRH). Cortisol secretion causes fetal growth restriction, underdevelopment and immunosuppression. If a fetus has been affected by maternal alcohol consumption the baby may have fetal alcohol syndrome, which has specific physical features (Figures 68.1 and 68.2).

Care provision

Alcohol consumption advice is controversial as it lacks robust evidence. Current advice from national guidelines is that women should avoid drinking alcohol in the first 3 months of pregnancy if possible as it may be associated with an increased risk of miscarriage. If women choose to drink alcohol during pregnancy they are advised to drink no more than 1–2 UK units once or twice a week as this enters the bloodstream and readily crosses the placenta; at this low level there is no evidence of harm to the unborn baby. Women should be informed that getting drunk or binge drinking during pregnancy (defined as more than 5 standard drinks or 7.5 UK units on a single occasion) may be harmful to the unborn baby.

The vast majority of women heed this advice, however 5% of pregnant women drink alcohol more than 2 days in the week and 9% of pregnant women consumed more than 2 units on their heaviest drinking day in that week (Figure 68.3).

Drugs

Particular legal and illicit drugs of recreation will be discussed.

Legal smoking

The 2010 Infant Feeding Survey (IFS) states that just over a quarter of mothers (26%) in England smoked at some point in the 12 months immediately before or during their pregnancy. Of the mothers who smoked before or during their pregnancy, just over half (55%) in England gave up at some point before the birth.

Smoking in pregnancy exposes the fetus to numerous toxins (Figure 68.4). Nicotine crosses the placenta quickly and is found at 15% higher concentrations in the fetus than the mother. Cigarette smoke impedes normal placental function as it reduces uterine blood flow. Nicotine is a neuroteratogen that interferes with the development of the nervous system. Smoking also deprives the fetus of oxygen which means that hypoxia-ischaemia and malnutrition results. Smoking is thought to be a cause intrauterine growth restriction (IUGR) (Chapter 55). Nicotine and nicotinic acetylcholine receptors interact when the mother smokes during early fetal life, and carbon monoxide (CO) and tobacco tar can also have direct effects on the fetal brain. Exposure to smoking during pregnancy has been found to be associated with signs of nicotine withdrawal in the early neonatal period, such as irritability, tremor and hypertonicity. Smoking has also been linked to attention deficit hyperactivity disorder (ADHD).

At first contact with the pregnant woman, healthcare professionals should discuss her smoking status and inform her of the risks to her unborn fetus and of the risks of exposure to secondhand smoke. Any concerns about smoking cessation for herself and others should then be addressed. Screening and monitoring of smoking is conducted in pregnancy through the use of tests that measure substances such as CO and serum cotinine (the primary metabolite of nicotine). In some health boards these are routinely used on women for screening, whilst in some areas screening will be carried out based on the woman's choice. Smoking cessation programmes and specialist midwives are often available to help those women who wish to stop smoking and women should be referred to this service if available.

Illicit substances

Some commonly used drugs during pregnancy are marijuana, heroin and stimulants such as cocaine/amphetamines. Drug abuse differs by city region and country and midwives need to be aware of the problem in their own area and what services exist. It is not possible to discuss each of the different drugs so the example used is heroin (diacetylmorphine) which can be sniffed, smoked and injected by the woman. This drug has an effect on the mother, as it stimulates opiate receptors, and it has the same effect on the fetus as it crosses the placenta, like many other psychoactive substances (Boxes 68.1 and 68.2).

Care provision

On first contact with a health professional all women should be asked about their illicit drug use and if necessary referred for specialist help. Known substance abusers will be referred directly to specialist care during pregnancy. They should be asked if they wish to join the rehabilitation programme available in most health boards. These programmes will usually give women methadone as a replacement for the illicit drug and they will receive a specific antenatal care regimen that may be under the care of a specialist obstetrician and/or specialist midwives. It is important that midwives are aware of the referral process and services in their own area.

69 Trafficking

Figure 69.1 Vulnerable to trafficking.

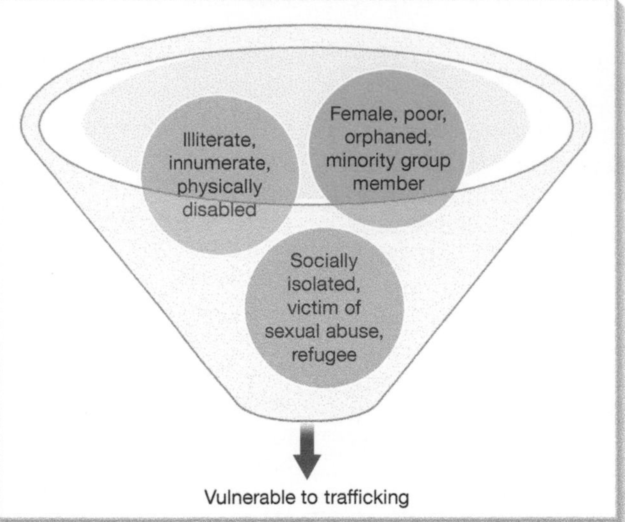

Figure 69.2 Classification.

Situational	• Documentation – absent or held by another person • Constant presence of another individual • Signs of physical abuse (scars, burns, HIV/AIDS, damage to vagina or anus) • Complication from unsafe abortion, overcrowded residence, frequent change of address or location
Story	• Individual controlled • Lack of freedom of movement • Changing employment • Forced to provide sex
Demeanour	• Fear • Depression • Evasive answering to questions

Figure 69.3 Health problems.

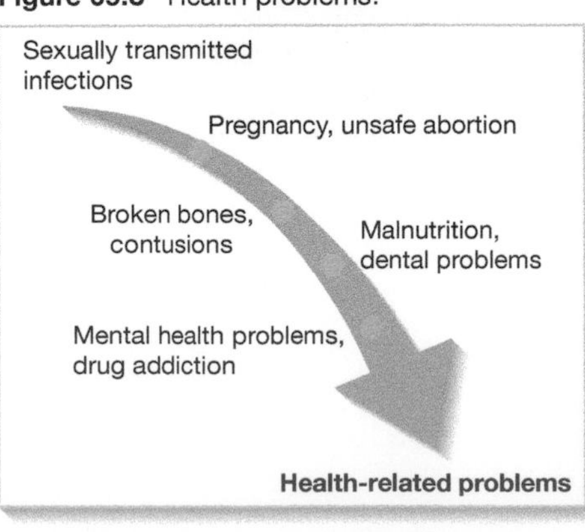

Figure 69.4 Needs care plan.

Comprehensive and coordinated care plan

Immediate needs	Ongoing needs	Long term needs
Safety services Shelter Basic needs Language services Midwifery care Medical care Legal advocacy	Physical healthcare Mental healthcare Substance abuse services Safety services Housing advocacy Language services Social services	Parental skills Life skills Job skills Long-term housing

Continued focus on safety, health, wellbeing

Midwifery at a Glance, First Edition. Edited by Eleanor Forrest © 2019 John Wiley & Sons, Ltd. Published 2019 by John Wiley & Sons, Ltd.
Companion website: www.wiley.com/go/forrest/midwifery

The number of people trafficked on a yearly basis is difficult to quantify due to the covert nature of this practice, however it is thought to be up to 1 million worldwide. Traffickers usually prey on the most vulnerable (Figure 69.1) in the poorest of countries or regions; 60–75% of trafficked people are female. It is a complex phenomenon that occurs internationally and nationally and has become a major concern worldwide.

Possible trafficking priority groups

Identification of victims is the first step in the process of helping them. Meetings with healthcare practitioners can be the window of opportunity for the start of intervention on behalf of these victims. Women coming into contact with maternity services might provide them with an opportunity to disclose their situation. Indicators that someone has been trafficked are classified in three categories: situational, story and demeanour (Figure 69.2). Victims may not want to escape because they fear reprisals against themselves or their families or they may identify with their exploiters (Stockholm syndrome) as they may believe that the traffickers care for them and look after them.

Although a difficult issue, midwives should consider trafficking if the woman is travelling with an older person who is not a partner or guardian, has material things that seem unlikely they could afford, are overfamiliar with sexual terms and practices, have tattoos that they are unwilling to discuss, or appear fearful or distrusting because of to your position. They may portray physical and emotional injuries similar to those of domestic abuse (Chapter 67). Health problems associated with trafficking are as a result of issues such as deprivation of food and sleep, stress, hazardous travelling, violence and hazardous work (Figure 69.3).

Trafficking and childbirth

It will not be easy for midwives to identify trafficked women because they either do not attend for antenatal care or present late, accompanied by their trafficker. They may not identify with being trafficked and it will only be through health issues and the midwives' knowledge that they may be identified. The midwife's role is to advise on health promotion and be proficient at providing effective midwifery care to women during the childbearing period. It is also important that they are aware of complications; both physical and social, and recognise the needs of women who require referral to other health and social care professionals. All antenatal appointments with women are opportunities for the midwife to build a trusting relationship to enable women to discuss their health, living and social issues. It allows other agencies to become involved in a less threatening way in the guise of normal antennal care.

Midwives should observe guidance about specific issues especially when a woman presents late for initial booking:

- Sexually transmitted diseases or long-term physical injuries
- Unkempt general appearance
- Poor English
- May not be registered with a GP
- Have moved frequently or unsure where they live
- Vague or inconsistent when explaining their residential situation, employment, schooling, medical history and support mechanisms
- Always accompanied by a person who appears controlling and will not let them speak for themselves
- Have old or serious untreated injuries; are vague or cannot explain how they occurred.

Trafficked women may present with sexual trauma, symptoms of psychological distress or signs of self-harm. They may appear with unspecific symptoms, poor dental hygiene and poor nutrition.

It is important that midwives gain the woman's trust and can demonstrate their commitment to providing them with midwifery care and any support they need. When discussing issues with trafficked women, use indirect phrasing of questions, for example . . . 'I was wondering if you could tell me . . . '; or, 'I would be interested to hear about . . . '. Any interaction should be on a one-to-one basis or with a professional interpreter. National guidelines indicate the need to initiate a multiagency needs assessment, including safeguarding issues, so that the woman has a co-ordinated care plan. Always respect the woman's right to confidentiality and sensitively discuss her fears in a non-judgemental manner. Tell the woman why and when information about her pregnancy may need to be shared with other agencies.

Midwives should attempt to get a trafficked woman admitted to the antenatal ward so that they can be assessed and investigated and an appropriate care pathway devised with their consent.

Vulnerable pregnant women can often have poor health and this can result in poor outcomes for the woman and the infant. It is important to risk assess their needs and to devise an appropriate care devised that is specific to that woman. This will also help to build up the trust required for the women to disclose her issues.

Health services

Women who have been trafficked need comprehensive and co-ordinated management with specific emphasis on safety, healthcare and future care. In the case of pregnancy this health situation can be used for the initial discovery and sensitive needs assessments (Figure 69.4). This should involve maternity and other health services but also language services, and social, safety, shelter and legal advocacy services. Once the woman's immediate needs are catered for, there will be on-going needs which are likely to be long term such as continuing maternity care, other physical care, dental care, mental health services, substance abuse issues, as well as social, safety, shelter and legal advocacy issues. These long-term needs may involve issues such as parenting skills, life/job skills, language skills and long-term housing.

Although the midwife is unlikely to be involved in all these issues they need to have knowledge of them so any discussion with the women can include a timeframe, and many of these processes can be commenced in a sensitive manner.

70 Homelessness

Figure 70.1 Homelessness and childbirth.

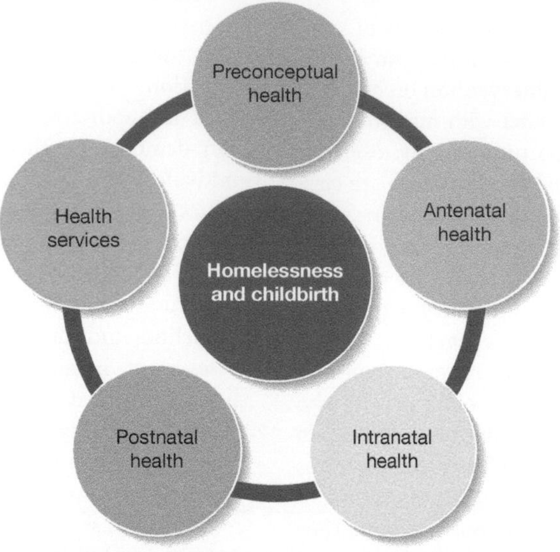

Box 70.1 Antenatal considerations.

- Ultrasound scan to confirm pregnancy and gestation
- Blood tests such as: haemoglobin, STI and HIV status
- History: obstetric and medical
- Arrange antenatal care and education
- Ascertain if social service and multiagency input required

Box 70.2 Intranatal considerations.

- Important to discuss how much they have accessed services
- Establish what and where antenatal care has been given
- Review medical/obstetric history
- Check blood test results: initiate those not done
- Discuss woman's preferences for labour and birth

Box 70.3 Postnatal considerations.

It is important to recognise that there will be a need for common assessment framework and multidisciplinary team support that includes services such as:

- Social work
- Housing
- Family support
- General practitioner service
- Midwifery input

Companion website: www.wiley.com/go/forrest/midwifery

Homelessness during the childbirth continuum is one of the many social issues in the individual woman's life that might need addressing. Therefore it is important that midwives have a clear understanding of what constitutes homelessness and how it could possibly influence the health of the woman at all stages throughout her childbearing life. Worldwide the number of people classified as homeless, especially women, are difficult to ascertain. Those countries that do collect statistics produce national figures for how many people are homeless, but each country's data are not directly comparable because they measure different variables over different time lines and many homeless people do not show up in official statistics at all.

The term homeless has many definitions, but most countries use some variation of the literal term homelessness, such as someone who does not have permanent housing. However, the stability of living arrangements also needs to be considered. Therefore the following situations are also pertinent to homelessness, where a person:

- Lives in a house that is not safe
- Is fleeing domestic violence
- Has been stopped from accessing their house by a landlord
- Lives in a house that is overcrowded and a danger to health
- Is at risk of abuse or a threat of abuse
- Living permanently in a hostel or bed and breakfast
- Is in accommodation that is classed as not reasonable to continue living there.

Homeless people have rarely made themselves homeless intentionally. That is they are not a person who deliberately does something or fails to do something that results in them ceasing to occupy accommodation which is reasonable for them to occupy.

Possible homelessness priority groups

This will be influenced by the country, region or group the person resides in or is part of, for example:

- Those people with dependent children (those reasonably expected to be living with parents)
- Pregnancy
- Leaving armed forces
- Leaving prison
- Vulnerable due to ill health
- Aged 16–17 years
- Aged 18–20 years if at risk of financial or sexual exploitation, drug or alcohol misuse or previously looked after by social care
- Risk of violence or harassment based on discrimination (race, religion, sexuality, colour or ethnicity)
- Fire, flood or other disasters.

Homelessness and childbirth

The health and services issues that are important to recognise and the action needed for homeless women during the childbirth continuum are indicated in Figure 70.1.

Preconception

Some preconceptual health issues that need to be ascertained and addressed are:

- Sexual history including sexuality, partners and STIs
- Contraception history or need
- Diet/nutrition
- Alcohol, nicotine and drug use
- Hygiene
- Oral hygiene
- Folate and calcium supplements
- Risks of pregnancy
- Pap smear
- Human papilloma virus (HPV).

Antenatal

Some antenatal health issues that need to be ascertained and addressed are (Box 70.1):

- Pregnancy test
- Haemoglobin and other blood tests
- STIs
- Human immunodeficiency virus (HIV)
- Ultrasound scan
- Obstetric and medical history
- Antenatal appointments/walk-in
- Specific antenatal education
- Social service input
- Multiagency needs assessment.

Intranatal

Some intranatal health issues that need to be ascertained and addressed are (Box 70.2):

- Discuss services
- Antenatal care and advice
- Medical/obstetric history
- Blood test results
- Listen to woman's preferences
- Discuss birth plan.

Postnatal

Some postnatal health issues that need to be ascertained and addressed are (Box 70.3):

- Housing referral
- Family support
- Social support
- Services available
- GP service
- Regular midwifery visits
- Common assessment framework – multidisciplinary team.

Health services

Some areas may have specialist midwifery/obstetric services for homeless women. This is beneficial as many homeless women are not registered with a GP and the midwife can engage with the multiprofessional team to ensure cohesive maternity services are in place. These can include contraceptive/sexual health services, housing services and non-governmental organisations.

Asylum seekers and refugees

Table 71.1 Care and support for asylum seekers at present in the UK.

Asylum seeker – claim in process	Asylum seeker – claim refused (appealing)	Asylum seeker – claim failed	Refugee
Financial support	Supported (vouchers only, limited to certain goods and outlets)	Possible to apply for short-term support while you are preparing to return to your country. This is known as 'section 4 support'	Not supported
Housing	Housed	Housed for up to 3 weeks	Not housed, but some rights
Primary care access	Entitled to free prescriptions based on the individual country rules. On-going care or for conditions which deteriorate	Entitled to free prescriptions based on the individual country rules. On-going care or for conditions which deteriorate	Can use NHS free
Secondary care access	Different entitlements to free hospital treatment for refused asylum seekers exist in each of the UK nations. All emergency care and on-going care or for conditions which deteriorate	Different entitlements to free hospital treatment for refused asylum seekers exist in each of the UK nations. All emergency care and on-going care or for conditions which deteriorate	Can use NHS free
Right to work	Not permitted to work unless they have submitted further submissions for asylum and have waited for over 12 months for a decision	Not permitted to work	Eligible to work/obtain benefits

Box 71.1 Barriers to maternity care.

- Language and communication
- Engagement with maternity services
- Complexity of rights and entitlements
- Poverty and destitution
- Dispersal
- Housing
- Limited time and resources

Box 71.2 Best practice.

- Outreach services
- Translated materials
- Central website and national guidance
- Full-time specialists and specialist clinics
- Specifically trained practitioners
- Sufficient time to provide evidence-based, individualised care for these vulnerable women
- Need for specialist midwives
- Need for outreach workers

An asylum seeker is someone who has a well-founded fear of being persecuted for reasons of race, religion, nationality, membership of a particular social group or political opinion, is outside the country of his or her nationality, is unable or, owing to such fear, is unwilling to return to it and is applying for asylum in another country.

The system of seeking asylum and the status of a person can be complex and therefore a midwife needs to understand this system in their country to help all women during the childbirth continuum. In the UK, the UK Border Agency (UKBA) supply up-to-date information on asylum, refused or failed asylum and refugee status and Maternity Action supply up-to-date information that is specific to pregnant women who are accessing, refused and failed asylum seekers. This information often changes depending on government policy and country. Table 71.1 illustrates the different aspects of care and support at present in the UK.

Barriers to maternity care

There are certain barriers to the maternity services for asylum seekers that could be easily overcome with changes in practice and services (Box 71.1).

Best practice

There are certain practices that have been classified as best practice for asylum seekers within maternity care that could be easily be implemented (Box 71.2). The following discusses how some of the barriers identified in Box 71.1 can be alleviated.

Language and communication

A poor understanding of the language results in women's needs and the services available to the women not being well communicated. Communication could be enhanced with easily available professional translation services and translated materials.

Engagement with maternity services

This can be multifaceted and often is due to poor advertisement of what maternity services are available to women, especially when and where. Some women will be afraid of what they might consider to be government/official services which could be due to their past experiences of such services in their country of origin and their past histories. They may also think that maternity services are linked directly to UKBA and using this service might jeopardise their claim for asylum. Central websites and national guidance which is easily available as well as local maternity-related posters should be used to encourage early engagement with services.

Complexity of rights and entitlements

This is always a problem for health professionals due to the many changing statuses that exist (Table 71.1). It is important for the midwife that community and government agencies are known and easily available for the midwife to consult and for advice centres to be accessible for women. This could be enhanced by having specifically trained staff to help pregnant women and alleviate the stress that this situation causes.

Poverty and destitution

Most asylum seekers have lost most of their personal possessions and have little if any funds. This means that they rely on support from the government and charities for everything they need. This involves making sure that they have all the basic needs to live on such as food, warmth, hygiene, safety and housing as well as specialised needs they may have such as diet, psychological and legal support. This is especially relevant to issues involving the new baby and the needs of that baby.

Dispersal

The government has the right to locate asylum seekers in any area of the country where facilities are available. This may mean that communities or families can be separated. The unmarried partner of a pregnant woman could also be in another region. This can mean that the pregnant women may be isolated from any form of support apart from that given by the maternity and social services. Dispersal can also reduce continuity of care, cause important appointments to be missed and result in blood and screening reports being lost and therefore possibly being repeated unnecessarily.

Housing

It is important to discuss the housing situation for these women because some accommodation is inadequate because it lacks the facilities for hygienic and healthy living. This could be through damp, cold and limited living areas and poorly prepared food due to limited cooking facilities. The housing is often in deprived areas with high levels of poverty which can make the areas feel unsafe for these already vulnerable women. Midwives need to liaise with social services and other outreach groups to make sure that these women have all the support they can for housing, furnishings and cooking facilities applicable to their situation.

Limited time and resources

Midwives have limited time and resources made available to them and often many women to care for. It is important that the midwife acts as an advocate for this vulnerable group of women and tries to obtain more time and resources to make sure that their health and social needs are met. This can be achieved by utilising all members of the interdisciplinary team and co-ordinating available and accessible services for these women.

Need for specialist midwives and outreach workers

All health social care services need to educate and train specialised midwives and outreach workers as well as informing all health and social care practitioner of the needs of pregnant asylum seekers. This would help the midwife as the primary healthcare practitioner to be able to successfully co-ordinate the multidisciplinary teams that these women require at this special time in their lives. This will result in more successful, healthy mothers and infants.

72 Teenage mothers

Figure 72.1 Key points related to teenage mothers.

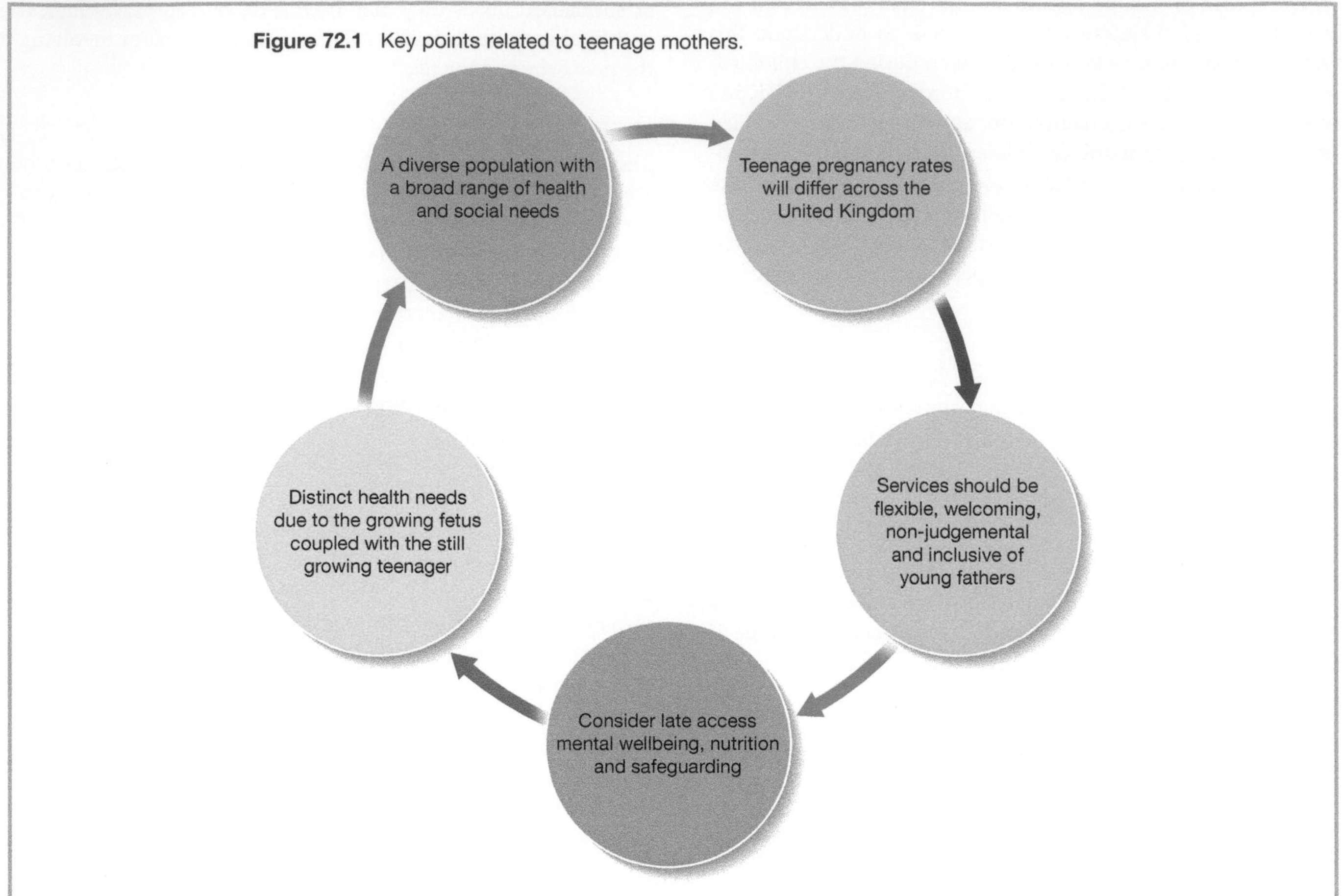

Midwifery at a Glance, First Edition. Edited by Eleanor Forrest © 2019 John Wiley & Sons, Ltd. Published 2019 by John Wiley & Sons, Ltd.
Companion website: www.wiley.com/go/forrest/midwifery

Teenage pregnancy continues to be prevalent throughout the UK with varying rates occurring across the country and strong associations existing between higher rates of teenage pregnancy and areas of deprivation. The service delivery and care planning within each locality will therefore depend on the number and needs of the pregnant teenagers within them.

Pregnant teenagers are a diverse population who bring with them a wide range of health and social needs. By definition a teenager spans the age range of between 13 and 19 years, and a pregnant teenager therefore may experience natural periods of transition coupled with pregnancy, which can be very challenging. Midwifery practice in relation to maternal age can differ, with some viewing the younger pregnant teenager (under 16 years of age) as being a higher risk pregnancy. Practitioners need to be mindful of their national and local guidance pertaining to age when planning and adopting appropriate maternity pathways of care for this client group.

Expectant teenage parents within the maternity setting should be supported with any social and health issues identified. Such issues can include support with maximising their financial capacity and support with honouring any educational, training and/or employment commitments. Maternity service providers should strive to be flexible, welcoming, non-judgemental and inclusive of the needs of expectant teenage fathers. Ideally teenage parents should have access to tailored antenatal educational information and materials that are age appropriate and that there should be clear signposting and referral pathways in place for all partner agencies applicable to the pregnancy.

Health needs

Pregnant teenagers have quite distinct and unique health needs due to the demands of the growing fetus, coupled with the pubertal demands of the still growing teenager. The expectant teenage mother should be informed of such unique demands at the earliest opportunity to maximise their health and wellbeing in pregnancy. Informing teenagers of their unique nutritional needs and the importance of maintaining a healthy diet in pregnancy is pivotal. If applicable, pregnant teenagers should be supported to access the national Healthy Start Voucher scheme and practitioners can facilitate the distribution of Healthy Start vitamins as soon as possible to maximise nutritional wellbeing and to reduce the risk of developing anaemia.

Support with health behaviours such as the cessation/reduction of smoking and the cessation/reduction of any drugs and/or alcohol use should be offered. Disclosure of experimental drug and/or alcohol use may occur in pregnancy as these types of risk-taking behaviours can be associated with this client group. Such disclosures, however, are not always indicative of an underlying addiction issue so sensitive and robust history taking from practitioners is paramount.

Later presentation into the maternity services is often associated with pregnant teenagers, thus hindering their access to the most timely uptake of maternal antenatal screening programmes. Barriers to accessing maternity services can include issues such as the fear of disclosure and being judged and a lack of trust. Such issues need to be considered when trying to maximise the earliest access into the maternity services for this group. Clear signposting, effective communication and pathway planning from partner agencies such as adolescent sexual health services providers and education providers can be beneficial and should be considered.

Psychological maturity will differ from person to person due to the wide age range of the teenage years. The impact of teenage pregnancy on the mental wellbeing for each mother may also differ depending on teenage transition and the broad range of social circumstances that pregnant teenagers may find themselves in. Poorer mental health outcomes in pregnancy are associated with this population, therefore emotional support and the monitoring of mental wellbeing should be continuous. Additionally, consideration should be given to using adolescent mental health service providers when maternity care planning as they are age appropriate and thus better suited to best meet the mental wellbeing needs of the expectant teenager.

Support with the planning of future pregnancies should begin at the earliest opportunity as there are strong associations between unplanned pregnancy and the teenage population. Practitioners need to be mindful that unplanned does not always mean unwanted and that any information sharing, such as the promotion of longer acting reversible contraception, which is currently being encouraged, should be discussed sensitively.

Safeguarding

Practitioners should be guided by local and national guidance and protocols pertaining to the safeguarding of children. Teenage pregnancy spans a broad age range therefore the issues of underage sexual activity, consent and confidentiality will occur and practitioners need to be mindful on how to sensitively and confidently address them. Pregnant teenagers can be quite fearful of disclosure and may withhold information in relation to the father of the baby or indeed in relation to the current partner who may or may not be the father. Transparency and honesty from practitioners around any safeguarding procedures that may apply to the teenage mother is encouraged as early as possible as it can engender trust and may assist the pregnant teenager with further disclosure throughout pregnancy.

Clear documentation, record keeping and timeous communication with other interagency partners such as GPs, health visitors and educational, social work and sexual health services should occur to ensure robust care planning that safeguards mothers and fetuses throughout the pregnancy journey.

Ultimately by recognising and supporting the health and social needs of teenage parents throughout the pregnancy and early postnatal period, it is hoped that they can achieve the potential of being the best parents possible (Figure 72.1).

73 Disability

Figure 73.1 Key points in law and guidance.

Generally, no adult can make decisions for another adult	The capacity to make decisions must be assumed unless otherwise assessed	Information for decision making must be in an understandable format
All adults with capacity may refuse treatment	The lead professional has responsibility to assess capacity & ability to communicate choices	A woman's capacity to consent must be evaluated in relation to every treatment decision

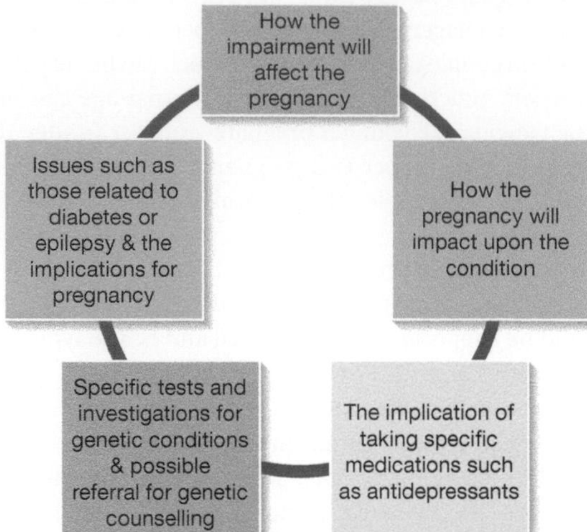

Figure 73.2 Knowledge of conditions and pregnancy.

Figure 73.3 Components of antenatal care.

Antental care

- 1st booking visit should be comprehensive & woman's preferred medium of communication identified. Perform a detailed assessment of needs from the woman's perspective, respecting the fact that she knows her disability & be guided her about service needs
- Offer antenatal care in the home; provides a non-threatening environment – some prefer to attend clinic as any other woman would do; home visits give midwives an opportunity to see the environment & discuss concerns for the future
- Agree frequency & location of antenatal visits with the woman; helpful for those who have more than 1 impairment or long-term medical conditions that need consideration, particularly those with earning disabilities
- Identify the woman's strengths, focusing on a social model & how needs can be met safely, rather than directly on the impairment; perform risk assessment if necessary; encourage the woman to bring aids & equipment into hospital
- Address complex needs by networking with the multiprofessional team to facilitate support & provide inclusive care; include those currently involved with the woman & her family

A plan of care should be discussed & written with the woman to include pregnancy, birth & postnatal care in hospital & home & communicated to the multi-disciplinary team

Figure 73.4 Components of care around birth.

Birth

- Home birth is possible because many impairments pose no increased risk
- Appropriate accommodation is needed for carers who sleep overnight during hospital admissions
- Identify appropriate sources of equipment, aids & other support for both parents & professionals

Figure 73.5 Components of postnatal care.

Postnatal

- Positive role models such as other disabled parents should be identified & women & their partners enabled to access them through support organisations
- Women have the right to access antenatal education but may require more specific information related to their impairment & pregnancy & birth
- Recognition of their long-term needs as parents

Box 73.1 Categories of impairment.

- Physical impairment:
  - Gross movements – Spina bifida, cerebral spinal cord injury, amputation & orthopaedic impairments, muscular dystrophy.
  - Gross & fine hand & finger movements – multiple sclerosis & rheumatoid arthritis
- Sensory impairment:
  - Sight & hearing problems
- Learning disability:
  - Significant impairment of intelligence & adaptive functioning
- Progressive disease:
  - HIV & AIDS, cancer, asthma, epilepsy, diabetes, sickle cell anaemia
- Chronic illness:
  - Heart disease, tuberculosis, neurological conditions & arthropathies
- Mental illness:
  - Schizophrenia, bipolar affective disorder, psychosis, severe postnatal depression, chronic depression, obsessive compulsive & eating disorders
- Speech & language impairment:
  - Disfigurements

Midwifery at a Glance, First Edition. Edited by Eleanor Forrest © 2019 John Wiley & Sons, Ltd. Published 2019 by John Wiley & Sons, Ltd.
Companion website: www.wiley.com/go/forrest/midwifery

Midwives need to be aware of the many disabilities that pregnant women may have: physical, mental, sensory, learning or other impairments that are less easy to classify (Box 73.1). All women with an impairment that fits the criteria of the Disability Discrimination Act 1995 and Equality Act 2010 are defined as disabled. The impairments from disability can be wide ranging and people often face barriers in society due to their disability.

Disabled people cite that a big barrier to receiving appropriate care is negative attitudes and behaviour of professional carers due to lack of disability awareness. Disabled childbearing women often experience poor understanding of their needs during childbearing from midwives, GPs, obstetricians and other professionals. Women are not asked directly about their needs and there may be no mention of the impairment and its implications on the pregnancy, birth and parenting. There can be an obvious lack of specialist knowledge. Midwives should seek support from the multiprofessional team in providing appropriate services to women. Specialists, the women's normal carers, for example partners, parents and siblings, are good sources of information. However, usually the individual is the expert in their own needs.

Disability awareness and duty of care

Decision making and consent for examination and treatment are key areas midwives need to understand. UK law on consent applies to who has the capacity to make decisions, including people with learning disabilities who benefit from equal rights. Key points in laws and guidance on decision making and consent are highlighted in Figure 73.1. Midwives need to ensure that women who have a disability have the same choices as other pregnant women. It is important not to overreact or ignore a person's disability but see the whole person. They need relevant and accessible information to remove barriers of communication and access.

Impact of pregnancy on disabled women

Concerns that are highly specific to women's individual circumstances and impairments include how their bodies will adjust to pregnancy, the effect of weight gain on mobility and independence and difficulties they may encounter with daily activities. There may be requirements for specific equipment, such as a special bed, cot, mobility aids or wheelchair. Women feel vulnerable for many reasons, such as having never been in hospital before, or may have memories of past negative experiences and barriers. First time expectant mothers may have concerns about the actual birth process such as choice of birth (vaginal or caesarean section), pain relief (an epidural analgesia if required) and postnatal mobility. Women with sensory impairments may have concerns relating to communicating their needs effectively and obtaining the information they need in appropriate formats. They should be given the opportunity to have support with communication and will need to familiarise themselves with the layout of facilities. Midwives need knowledge of basic awareness and guiding techniques.

The hormone changes of pregnancy can have a major impact on women with serious mental health difficulties or impaired mobility. Sleep patterns may change or be disturbed throughout childbearing and can affect women's wellbeing; these need to be explained to women.

Those who have progressive physical impairments (Box 73.1) may fear exacerbation of the condition following the birth. Women with significant mental health difficulties need to be aware of the risk that their mental health might deteriorate. With conditions such as epilepsy or diabetes, consultation with the wider health team involved in their management is important. Women may worry about their ability to look after a new baby – handling, bathing, lifting, changing and feeding, and locating and using specialist equipment to help with this.

Being dependent on others may give women more concerns, for example meeting personal needs such as eating, showering, toileting and mobilising. Women with learning disabilities may need information about pregnancy, birth and baby care presented in different ways and then repeated.

Effective care provision

Midwives need knowledge and awareness of conditions in order to ask specific and appropriate questions and provide information (Figure 73.2). The midwife needs to know about organisations that provide information for disabled parents and to contact them and use such resources. Information should be made available in accessible formats and media. A midwife should be familiar with the benefit system and disability allowances. There may be wider issues that require the midwife's assistance such as supportive letters. Midwives therefore need to listen and communicate directly with disabled parents. Although relevant information about a woman's impairment should be disclosed by the GP, the midwife is the front-line carer in pregnancy and a woman with a disability may arrive at hospital/clinic to discover barriers of access and communication and have to make adjustments to overcome these. Observing and asking appropriate questions when taking a history will identify any barriers to services and other healthcare professionals who may need to be involved in providing support to the woman.

Preconceptual care

Advice may be required when women take medication with possible harmful effects for the fetus, or by women who have hereditary conditions and want to be informed to make choices before becoming pregnant.

Antenatal care

Women with a disability should be identified early in pregnancy to ensure that they receive care that is tailored to their specific needs. As part of this, women should be referred to the specialist or named midwife with a responsibility for disability. For other key areas of antenatal care, see Figure 73.3.

Birth care

Individual needs must be assessed when considering labour and birth (Figure 73.4).

Postnatal care and parenting

It is important to remember that midwifery care can continue for as long as necessary following the birth. Joint working with other members of the multidisciplinary team is vital and devising a discharge plan with women would be helpful in this (Figure 73.5).

74 Health promotion education

Figure 74.1 Three main concepts of health.

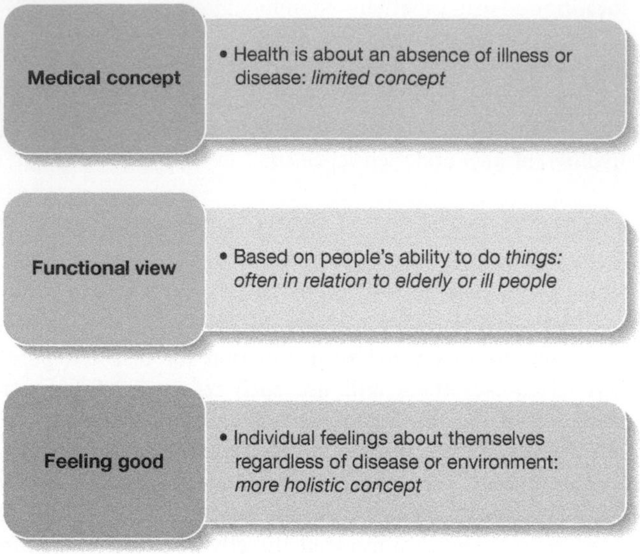

Medical concept	• Health is about an absence of illness or disease: *limited concept*
Functional view	• Based on people's ability to do *things: often in relation to elderly or ill people*
Feeling good	• Individual feelings about themselves regardless of disease or environment: *more holistic concept*

Figure 74.2 Salutogenisis.

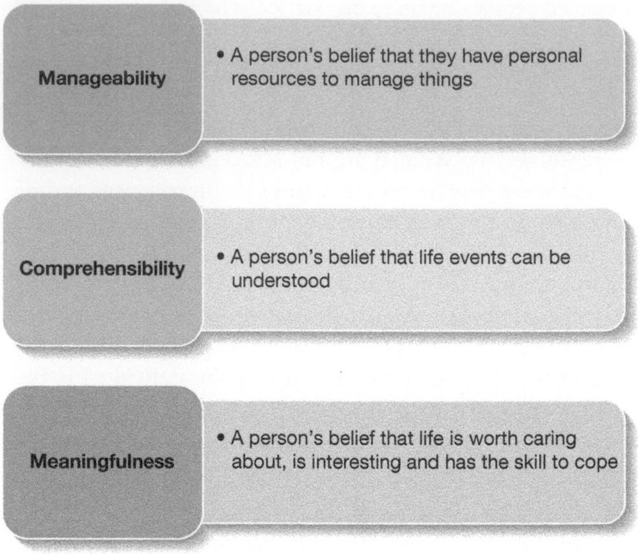

Manageability	• A person's belief that they have personal resources to manage things
Comprehensibility	• A person's belief that life events can be understood
Meaningfulness	• A person's belief that life is worth caring about, is interesting and has the skill to cope

Figure 74.3 Health promotion models.

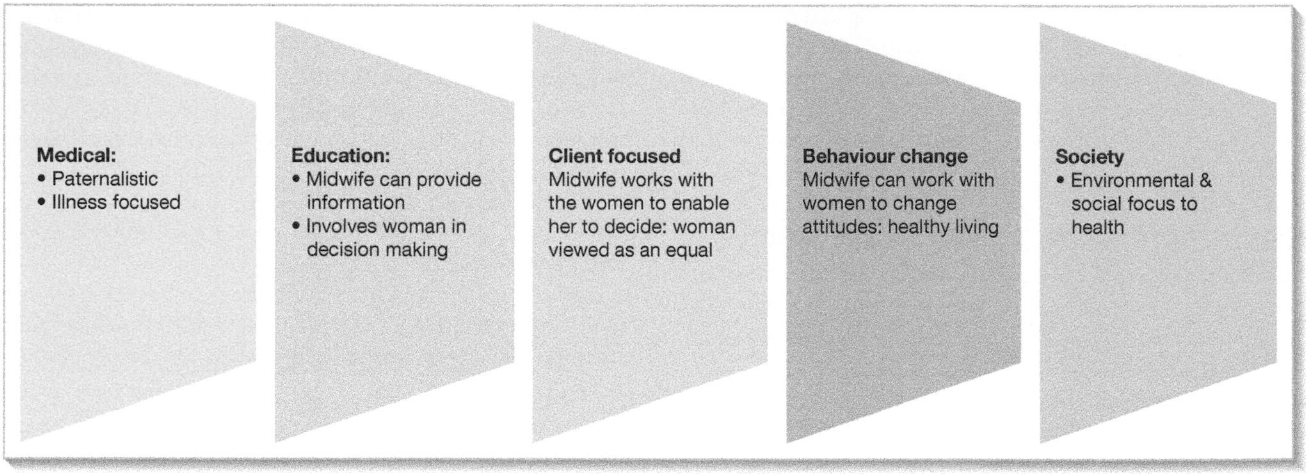

Medical:
- Paternalistic
- Illness focused

Education:
- Midwife can provide information
- Involves woman in decision making

Client focused
Midwife works with the women to enable her to decide: woman viewed as an equal

Behaviour change
Midwife can work with women to change attitudes: healthy living

Society
- Environmental & social focus to health

Figure 74.4 Health promotion by midwives.

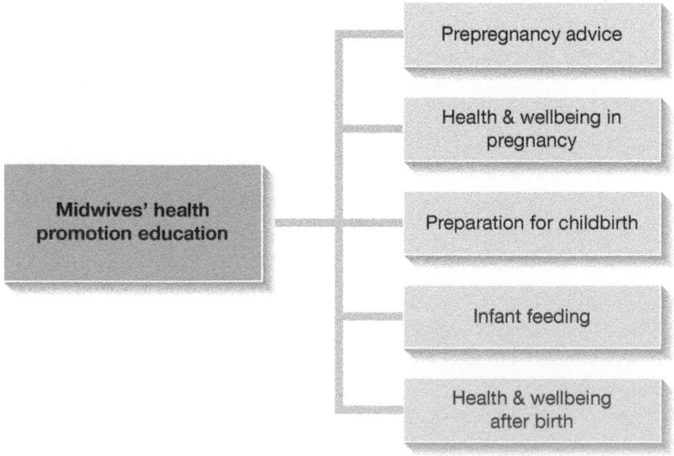

Midwives' health promotion education
- Prepregnancy advice
- Health & wellbeing in pregnancy
- Preparation for childbirth
- Infant feeding
- Health & wellbeing after birth

Health is 'a state of complete physical, mental and social wellbeing and not merely the absence of disease or infirmity' (WHO, 1946).

Health has a different meaning to different people, but its concept is embraced by the World Health Organisation quote above. The three main recognised concepts of health are provided in Figure 74.1. Health comprises many aspects, of which physical, emotional, social, spiritual and sexual wellbeing are interrelated; an imbalance in any aspect can affect the others.

Promoting health and wellbeing is an inherent part of the midwives' role; part of their day-to-day activities when working with women and their families at all times within the childbearing continuum. This aligns with midwives' public health role as they have knowledge of communities and can individualise care whilst implementing local and government policy. Midwives traditionally work in partnership with women to give and receive midwifery care. A salutogenic approach (Figure 74.2) considers the relationship between stress and coping and health and acknowledges that health fluctuates. By adopting salutogenesis, midwives are more likely to understand the health promotion needs of women and be able to provide the necessary information and support. However, there are many models to use within health promotion (Figure 74.3). Midwives are involved in providing health promotion education from preconception, through pregnancy and into the postnatal period. Preconception health advice can help women prepare for their pregnancy; this aids a healthier pregnancy and should be available to all women. Antenatal education should be on-going throughout the pregnancy and available at every visit, but is also commonly provided within organised classes as part of the preparation for childbirth and parenthood (Chapter 17). Health advice should also be given during labour and follow into the postnatal period (Figure 74.4).

Midwifery-related public health practices

Many of the following topics are discussed more fully as individual chapters within this book. However, the following sections address them in the context of health promotion education to promote awareness of the midwife's important role.

Diet

Although dietary advice is provided to women preconceptually and throughout pregnancy and the postnatal period, women may not change their dietary habits. Despite this, it is important that midwives inform women of their dietary requirements and the benefits of a balanced diet containing fruit and vegetables. This must be done in a way that takes account of women's ability to pay and source such items, if women are to be encouraged to make changes. Medical conditions such as diabetes, obesity, cardiac disease and hypertension which can be diet related are discussed in Part 7. Midwives require knowledge of current guidelines regarding certain foods to limit or restrict in pregnancy or when breastfeeding. Caffeine intake, for example, is a topic of much discussion worldwide. Midwives must be cognisant of current evidence to provide advice and support women's decisions about their caffeine intake in pregnancy.

Smoking

Although a preventable cause of death, smoking contributes greatly to morbidity and a reduced life expectancy. It also affects the developing fetus and newborn baby (Part 9). Midwives have an important role in providing information, support and smoking cessation advice. A client-centred approach (Figure 74.3) is the most likely to promote a trusting relationship and help women change their smoking behaviour. Normally ascertained at the booking visit, midwives can discuss a woman's smoking status and that of her household. Referral can then be made to a specialist smoke change midwife for on-going review and support. Current advice and information on nicotine, e-cigarettes and changing habits can be provided.

Alcohol

The safe measure of alcohol intake in pregnancy remains universally undecided. Current advice in the UK is that the safest approach is not to drink in pregnancy or if planning a pregnancy. Drinking in pregnancy can cause long-term harm to the baby (Chapters 55 and 68). However, although many women either do not drink alcohol or stop drinking during pregnancy, it is important for the midwife to discuss alcohol intake at the booking visit. Advice and support can then be given (Chapter 68).

Exercise

The benefits of exercise are well understood and women may wish to continue a level of fitness during pregnancy. With knowledge of how to exercise safely in pregnancy, the midwife can support women in their choice. Additionally, women can be encouraged to commence gentle exercise such as aquanatal whilst pregnant. Consultation with a maternity physiotherapist can provide further information and help support pelvic floor muscles in the postnatal period (Chapter 31).

Mental health

Maternal mental health and wellbeing are important aspects of a midwives' public health role and need to be addressed at all stages of the pregnancy continuum. Women with impaired mental health are less able to cope physically or emotionally with daily tasks (Chapter 65).

Points to note

- Midwives should be aware of their own attitudes and behaviours to health
- The concept and meaning of health promotion are key concepts of the midwife's role
- Midwives require up-to-date knowledge to meet the needs of childbearing women
- An appropriate approach to health promotion should be taken to ensure best outcomes of health for women.

75 Psychological changes

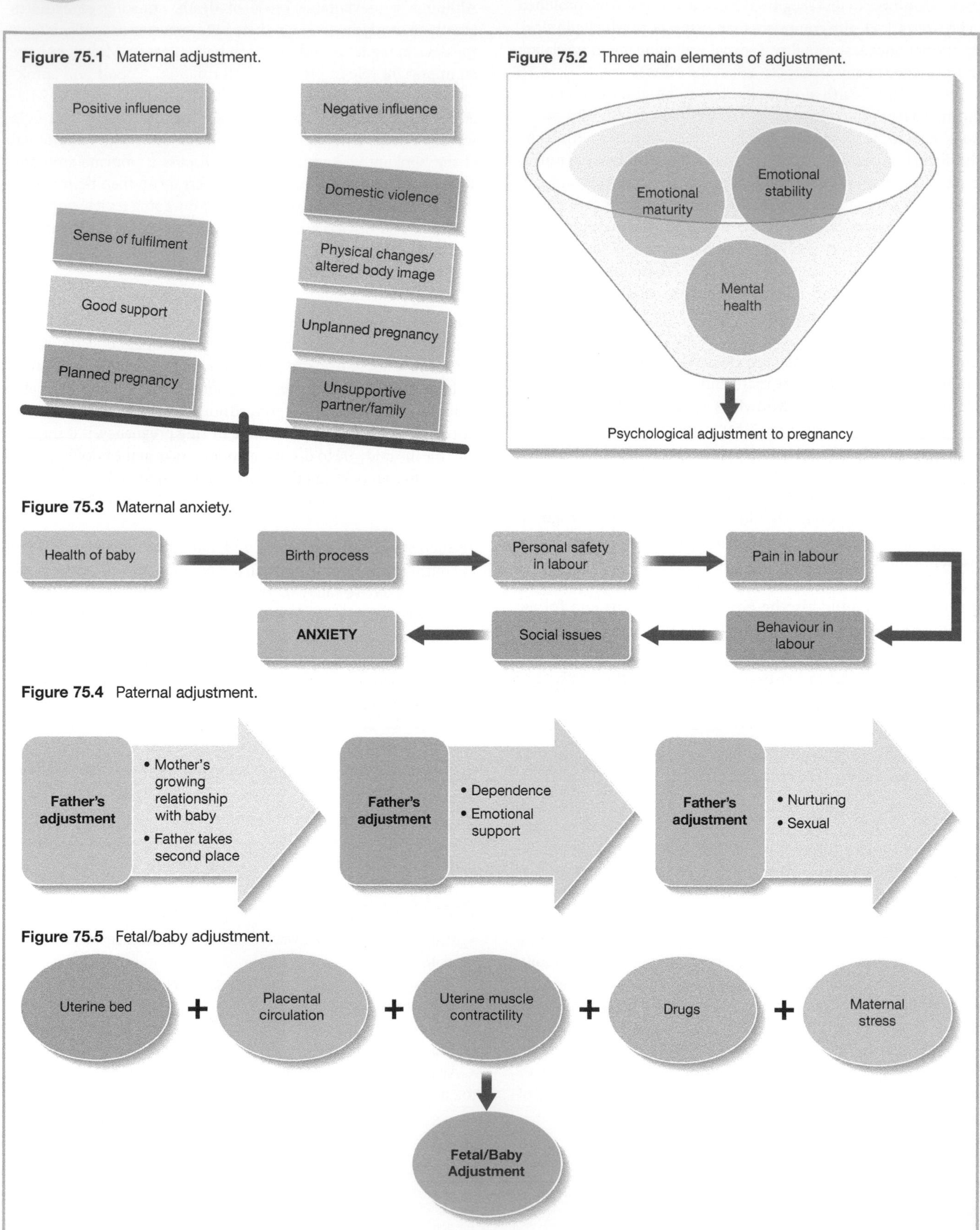

Figure 75.1 Maternal adjustment.

Figure 75.2 Three main elements of adjustment.

Figure 75.3 Maternal anxiety.

Figure 75.4 Paternal adjustment.

Figure 75.5 Fetal/baby adjustment.

There are many psychological changes that occur during pregnancy and the postnatal period. Many women embrace pregnancy and the postnatal period in a positive way, but as discussed in Chapter 64, pregnancy or childbirth is not always welcomed or enjoyed by women. There are many myths surrounding motherhood reflecting the expectations of society and this puts pressure on new parents to conform as they feel they should. Society can be very isolating and people are often presented by the media with a glamorous picture of mother and baby, which they feel they have to compete with. Most parents do adapt to becoming a family, but the reality is that it often takes time and there are many factors that can influence how positive this is (Figure 75.1). If a woman has strong support networks, views pregnancy and becoming a mother as a sense of fulfilment, she is more likely to adapt well to becoming a mother than a woman who has little or no support, did not plan the pregnancy or lives in an abusive relationship (Chapter 67). As such, there are three main elements that comprise psychological adjustment to pregnancy: emotional maturity, emotional stability and positive mental health (Figure 75.2).

Positive influences

- Planned pregnancy
- Thinking who the baby will look like
- Thinking of baby's name
- Sense of fulfilment and of being a 'real woman'
- Embrace impending motherhood
- At 'one' with peers.

Negative influences

- Unplanned pregnancy
- Unwilling father
- Unsupportive/resentful partner
- Altered body image/lack of control of body
- Physical effects.

Mother's adjustment

A mother's adjustment usually involves some degree of anxiety, such as the physical or mental health of baby, the birth process including her personal safety, pain, behaviour in labour, and financial, housing or employment issues (Figure 75.3). She may also experience emotional changes regarding her dependence versus independence. For example:

- Alone = grown up
- Pregnant = never alone; need for outside support.

There may even be a period of adjustment and grieving for her past role or image, part of letting go, previous lifestyle, body shape and relationships with partner or other children. Women have to adapt to their body image both during and after pregnancy. Some women view these changes in a positive way and embrace their pregnant or postnatal body, whilst others have a negative perception of how they look and this can affect how they feel.

Many women and their partners have sexual concerns during pregnancy and the postnatal period that they have to adjust to. For example:

- Damage to fetus
- Feelings of being watched
- Discomfort
- Dyspareunia
- Changes in libido
- Frustrated partner.

Parenthood often brings a realisation of adult responsibilities:

- Rite of passage: girl to woman
- Motherhood
- Thoughts of own childhood and relationship with own mother
- Financial.

Women often experience role conflict such as:

- Career
- Housewife
- Motherhood
- Lover
- 'Emancipation' and the need to be independent again.

Father's adjustment

Men have many psychological adjustments to make, but these often occur later than for women. It has been known for men to develop couvade syndrome, experiencing symptoms in sympathy with their partner. Men's adjustment and their needs often go unrecognised. Society's image of men also make it difficult for many men to discuss their psychological needs during this time. As such, many men often go unsupported; however the midwife can discuss this and offer support. Some men are fearful for their partner or baby's safety and wellbeing; they may feel helpless and powerless in the hospital environment and may be unsure of their role in a predominantly female environment. Role changes may occur as the mother becomes increasingly attached to her baby and there can be a realisation of responsibilities which can cause stress and anxiety (Figure 75.4). Attending preparation for childbirth and parenting sessions may help men understand their role and develop a sense of belonging in the maternity setting in addition to meeting other similar men.

Relationship changes

During pregnancy and following the birth of a baby, couples have to adapt to changes within their relationship (Figure 75.4). Often the baby becomes the centre of attention and parents often need encouragement to nurture their own relationship and spend together, on their own. Some relationship changes are:

- Mother's growing relationship with baby
- Father takes second place
- Dependence
- Emotional support
- Nurturing
- Sexual.

Fetal/baby adjustment

During pregnancy and the postnatal period, the baby also has adjustments to make as its environment is constantly changing. It is the midwife's role to ensure that parents are informed of the best possible environment to ensure optimal conditions for this adjustment. The developing fetus and newborn baby are sensitive to changes within the uterus and muscle contractility, placenta, drugs and maternal stress (Figure 75.5).

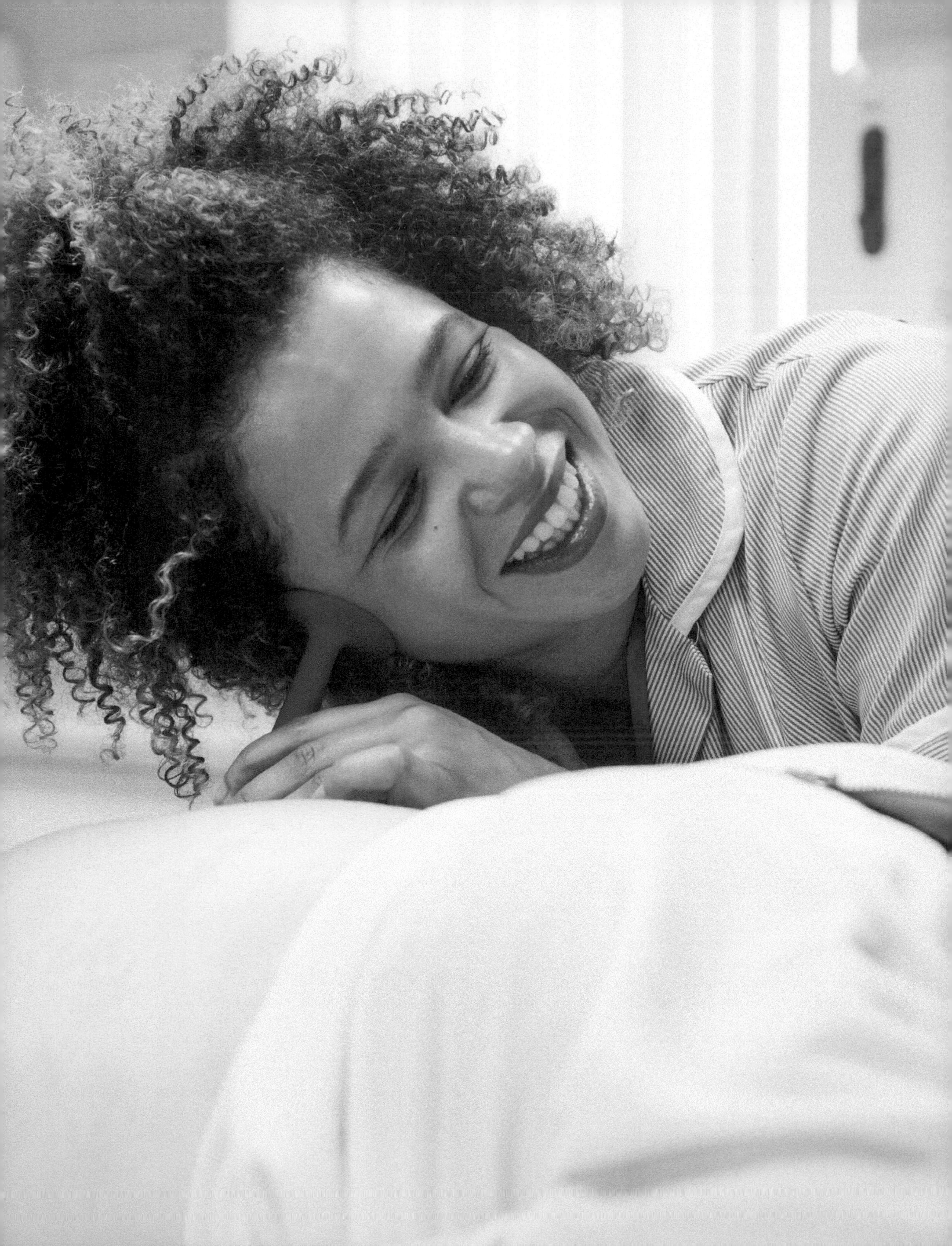

Midwifery skills

Chapters

76 Antenatal abdominal examination

Figure 76.1 Assessing fundal height.

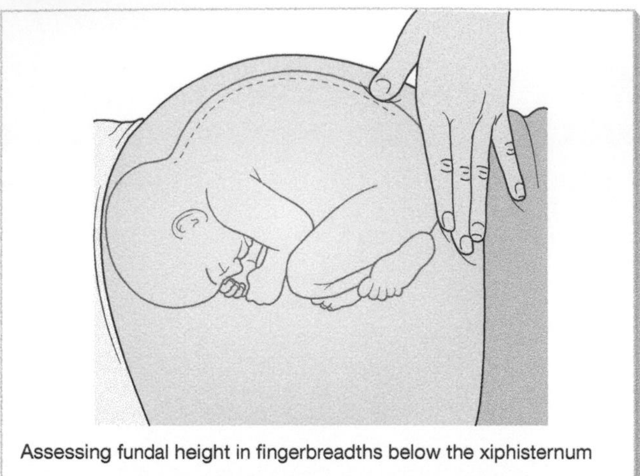

Assessing fundal height in fingerbreadths below the xiphisternum

Figure 76.2 Fundal palpation.

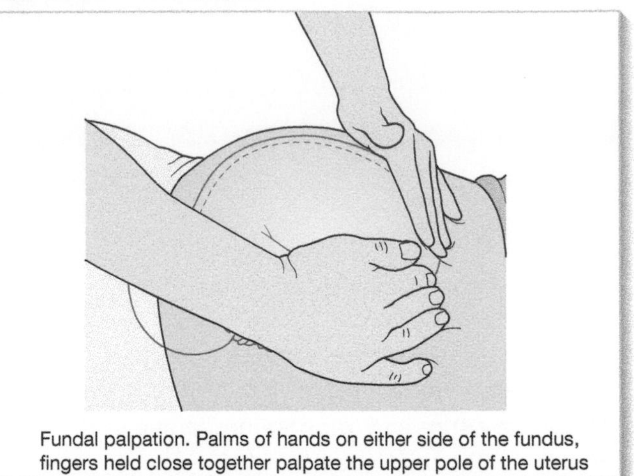

Fundal palpation. Palms of hands on either side of the fundus, fingers held close together palpate the upper pole of the uterus

Figure 76.3 Lateral palpation.

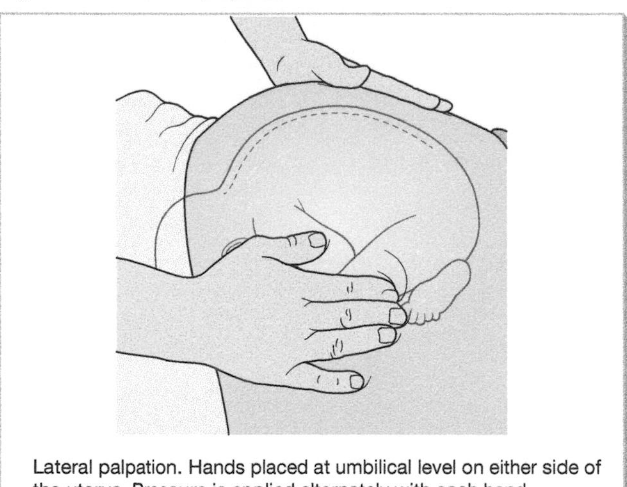

Lateral palpation. Hands placed at umbilical level on either side of the uterus. Pressure is applied alternately with each hand

Figure 76.4 Fairbairn's walk.

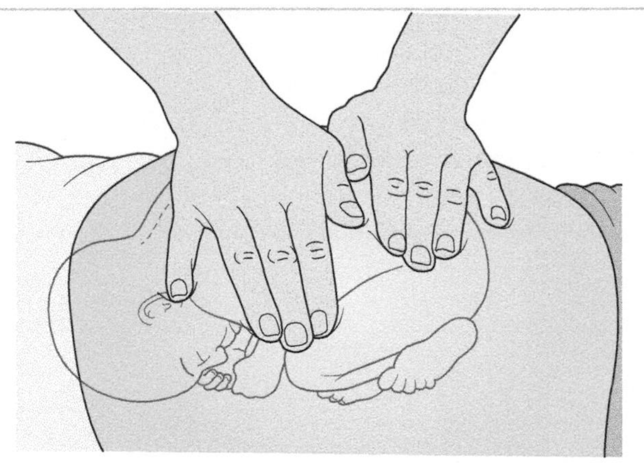

'Walking' the fingertips across the abdomen to locate the position of the foetal back

Figure 76.5 Pelvic palpation.

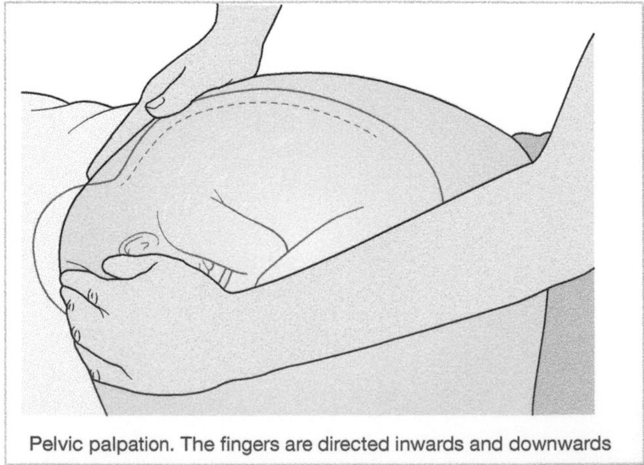

Pelvic palpation. The fingers are directed inwards and downwards

Figure 76.6 Pawlik's manoeuvre.

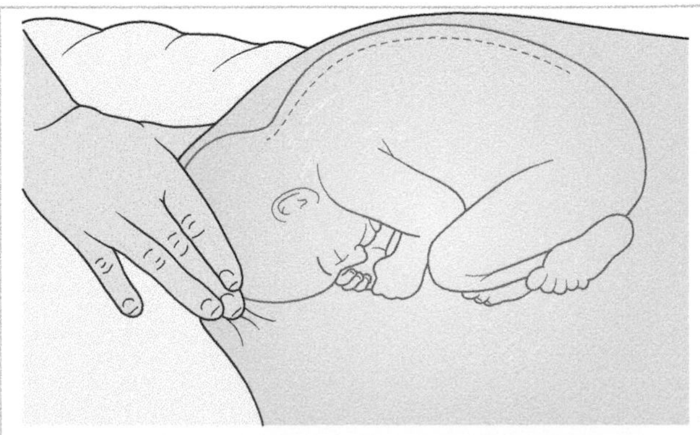

Pawlik's manoeuvre. The lower pole of the uterus is grasped with the right hand, the midwife facing the woman's head

The purpose for performing an antenatal abdominal examination is to:

- Assess fetal growth
- Ascertain lie, attitude, presentation and position of the fetus
- Auscultate the fetal heart rate, rhythm and volume.

Terminology relating to prenatal abdominal examination

Lie:

- The relationship of the long axis of the fetus to the long axis of the uterus
- Normal lie is longitudinal.

Attitude:

- The relationship of the fetal head and limbs to the fetal trunk
- Normal attitude is one of flexion.

Presentation:

- The part of the fetus that occupies the lower pole of the uterus
- Normal presentation is cephalic.

Position:

- The relationship of the denominator to one of six areas of the pelvic brim. These are:
  - Right posterior
  - Left posterior
  - Right lateral
  - Left lateral
  - Right anterior
  - Left anterior.

Engagement:

- The fetal head is engaged when the biparietal diameter has passed through the pelvic brim.

Preparation for examination

- The woman should be asked to empty her bladder
- The woman should lie comfortably with one or two pillows
- Privacy should be ensured
- The midwife should wash her hands in warm water.

Components of examination

Prenatal abdominal examination comprises three parts:

- Inspection
- Palpation
- Auscultation.

Inspection

- Size
- Shape
- Fetal movement
- Abdominal contours
- Skin changes such as pigmentation, scars and striae gravidarum.

Palpation

Prenatal abdominal palpation helps the examiner to estimate gestation. There are different stages to doing this:

- Fundal palpation (Figures 76.1 and 76.2) – xiphisternum, umbilicus and symphysis pubes
- Lateral palpation (Figure 76.3) – fetal back
- Fairbairn's walk (Figure 76.4)
- Pelvic palpation (Figure 76.5) – presenting part
- Pawliks' manoeuvre (Figure 76.6).

Auscultation

Use a Pinard's stethoscope placed appropriately on the woman's abdomen. With gentle pressure, remove your hands from the stethoscope and listen to the fetal heart whilst watching the woman's face for signs of discomfort. If the woman wishes to hear the baby's heartbeat, a doptone may then be used.

- Auscultate over the area where the anterior shoulder of the fetus is estimated to be
- Record for 1 minute taking note of the rate and regularity.

Vaginal examination

Figure 77.1 Information from vaginal examination.

Information

- **External genitalia** varicosities, bleeding, scars
- **Outlet of pelvis** feel for ischial spines
- **Vagina** soft, warm & moist
- **Cervix** position, consistency, effacement, dilatation
- **Presentation** landmarks of presenting part
- **Position** identification of sutures & fontanelles
- **Presenting Part** level to ischial spines
- **Membranes** intact or ruptured

Figure 77.2 Communication prior to examination per vaginam.

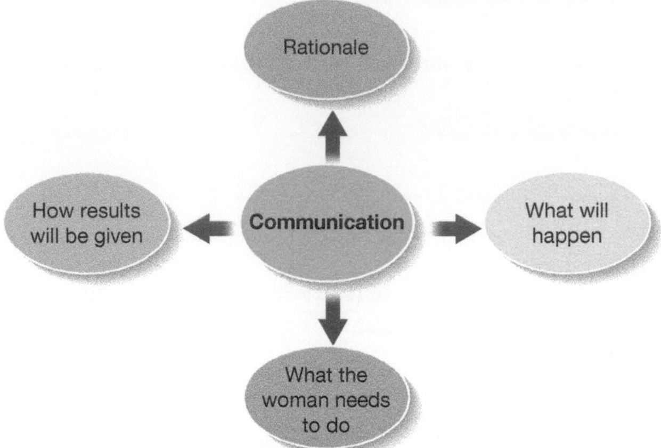

Figure 77.3 Contraindications to vaginal examination (VE).

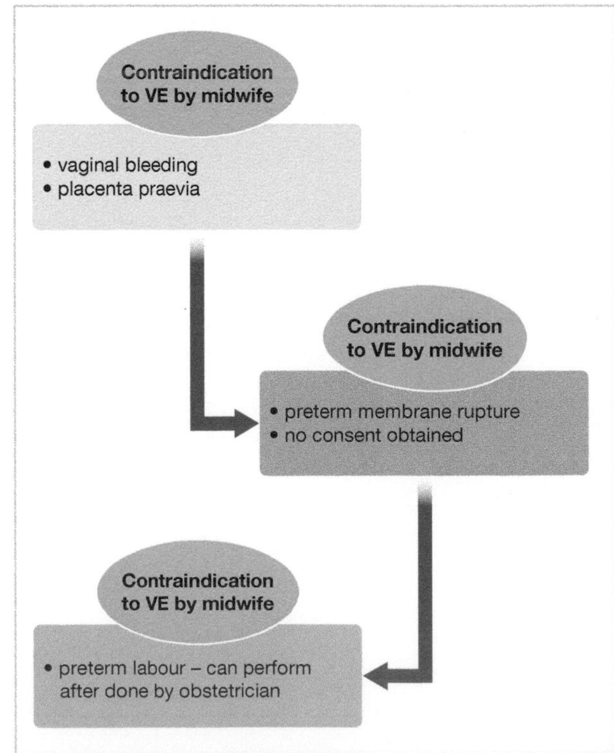

Figure 77.4 Vaginal examination to identify the saggital suture.
Source: Adapted from Mayes Midwifery 2012.

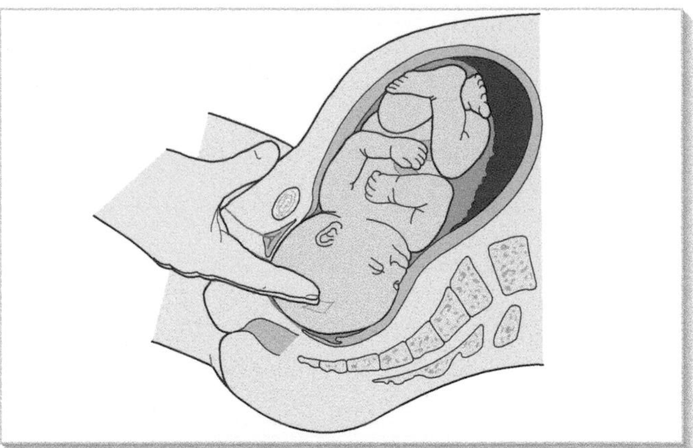

Table 77.1 Antenatal indications.

Sign	Findings
Hegar's sign	This is apparent when, during examination using two hands, the fingers in the anterior fornix almost meet those palpating the abdomen
Goodell's sign	The cervix and vagina are felt to be softer due to vascular increase; increased vaginal discharge is noted
Chadwick's sign	The mucous membranes of the vagina and cervix become a blueish, purple colour due to vascular increase
Osiander's sign	The uterine arteries can be felt to pulsate through the lateral fornices
Ballottement of the fetus	From approximately 16 weeks' gestation, the fetus can be balloted internally, using two fingers placed in the anterior fornix and giving the uterus a tap. This pushes the fetus up slightly and when it returns down, it can be felt
Uterine enlargement	The uterus is enlarged compared to a non-pregnant uterus and is consistent with the expected period of gestation

There are several reasons for conducting a vaginal examination and these will be discussed in this chapter. Due to the sensitive and intimate nature of an examination per vaginam, it should only be performed when deemed absolutely necessary and based on clear indications. As it is an invasive procedure, it can also introduce infection. Therefore consideration should be given to whether information obtained from conducting a vaginal examination will aid the decision-making process about the woman's care (Figure 77.1).

Many women are distressed by having a vaginal examination and may find it to be an uncomfortable procedure. Some women who have experienced post-traumatic stress disorder or sexual abuse have reported problems having vaginal examinations (Chapter 67). As such, communication with the woman should be a priority for the midwife to inform her of the rationale for conducting the examination, what the examination will entail, what the woman needs to do, how the results will be given to the woman and to obtain her consent prior to performing it (Figure 77.2). The information should be imparted in a way that allows the woman to ask questions and to refuse if she so wishes. Although the most common time in the perinatal period to perform an examination per vaginam is during labour, it is sometimes necessary to do this during pregnancy or the postnatal period. However, midwifery contraindications to performing a vaginal examination must be considered (Figure 77.3).

Antenatal examination

Although not common during the early antenatal period, a vaginal examination may still be performed in some situations to help with the diagnosis of pregnancy (Table 77.1):

- Hegar's, Goodell's, Chadwick's and Osiander's signs
- Ballottement of the fetus
- Uterine enlargement.

During pregnancy, woman can be prone to vaginal infections which require local medication. Later on in the pregnancy, if the woman is post-dates, a vaginal examination may be considered necessary to ascertain if the cervix is suitable for induction of labour to be commenced, with the use of drugs such as prostaglandin, or for the task of rupturing the membranes.

Intrapartum examination

Vaginal examinations are used as a guide to confirm labour onset and progress. However, it is only a tool and care should be taken when considering the need and frequency of performing them. Despite the discomfort women often feel, they may request a vaginal examination to reassure them and confirm their progress in labour and thereby help them make decisions about pain relief options. A vaginal examination may be performed if it is deemed necessary that the membranes be ruptured or if a fetal scalp electrode needs to be applied to monitor fetal wellbeing more closely.

Medicines per vaginam

Midwives have a role in administering medications per vaginam and as such they should be aware of their responsibilities. As women can be embarrassed by this route of drug administration, informed consent must be sought and given. An aseptic technique must be applied to reduce infection risk, especially if the membranes are not intact. Medication inserted vaginally ensures that it will have a local action. The most common reason for administering medication per vaginam is to insert prostaglandin to induce labour (Chapter 25); however, other drugs such as antifungals can also be administered vaginally. Care must be taken to use an appropriate lubricant, as required.

Procedure

An aseptic technique must be applied when performing a vaginal examination, including scrupulous hand hygiene and the use of sterile gloves. Local policy should be adhered to with regard to genital cleansing as evidence suggests that infection rates are not affected by the use of tap water alone.

The equipment required includes:

- Sterile gloves, apron and disposable sheet
- Lubricant (water soluble or obstetric cream – not if face presentation)
- Sonicaid or Pinard stethoscope, fetal scalp electrode or amnihook (as required).

The procedure should be discussed and agreed with the woman and privacy ensured.

- Ask the woman to empty her bladder, to ensure comfort
- Perform abdominal palpation to ascertain lie, presentation, position and engagement; auscultate fetal heart
- Place disposable sheet beneath the woman's buttocks and ask her to adopt a semi-recumbent position
- Wash and dry hands and apply apron
- Open equipment and put gloves on
- Using lubricant, apply to first two fingers of dominant hand, with other hand, part the labia and observe vulva
- Keeping the woman informed, insert two fingers gently in a downward and backward direction along the anterior vaginal wall (check no contraction present); avoid anus and clitoris
- Once the cervix has been located, feel for its position; consider effacement, dilatation, tone and the presenting part
- Once the fingers are through the cervical os, the forewaters should be felt. The position, presentation and level, flexion, any caput succedaneum or moulding can be ascertained (Figure 77.4)
- Depending on the reason for the vaginal examination, the membranes can be ruptured, a fetal scalp electrode can be applied or medications inserted
- Following the procedure, the fetal heart should be auscultated and the woman made comfortable
- Dispose of equipment, wash hands and document findings accurately; report as necessary.

78 Artificial rupture of membranes

Figure 78.1 Reasons for ARM.

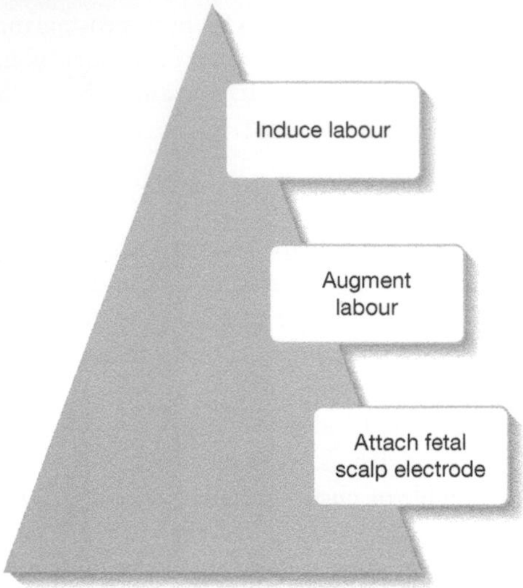

Induce labour
Augment labour
Attach fetal scalp electrode

Figure 78.2 Slow progress.

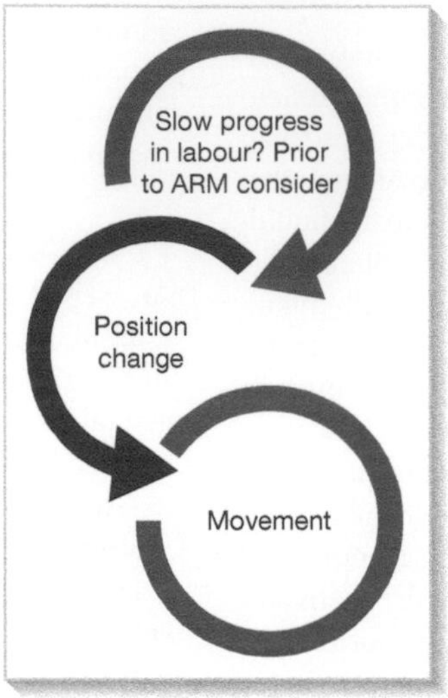

Slow progress in labour? Prior to ARM consider
Position change
Movement

Figure 78.3 Considerations prior to ARM.

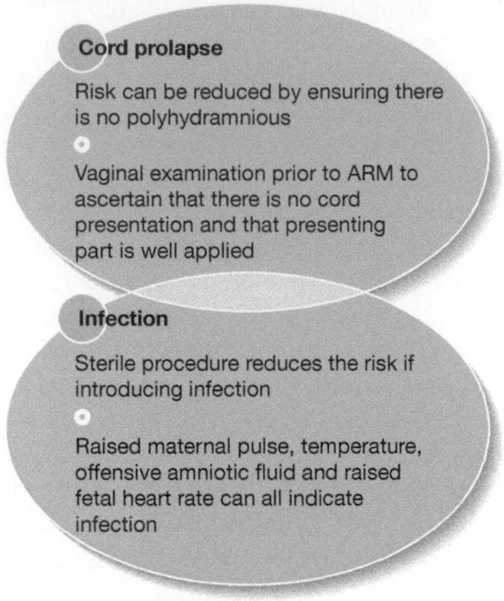

Cord prolapse
Risk can be reduced by ensuring there is no polyhydramnious
Vaginal examination prior to ARM to ascertain that there is no cord presentation and that presenting part is well applied
Infection
Sterile procedure reduces the risk if introducing infection
Raised maternal pulse, temperature, offensive amniotic fluid and raised fetal heart rate can all indicate infection

Figure 78.4 Contraindications to ARM.

Placenta praevia
Vasa praevia
Malpresentation
Active herpes lesions
Human Immunodeficiency virus (HIV) infection

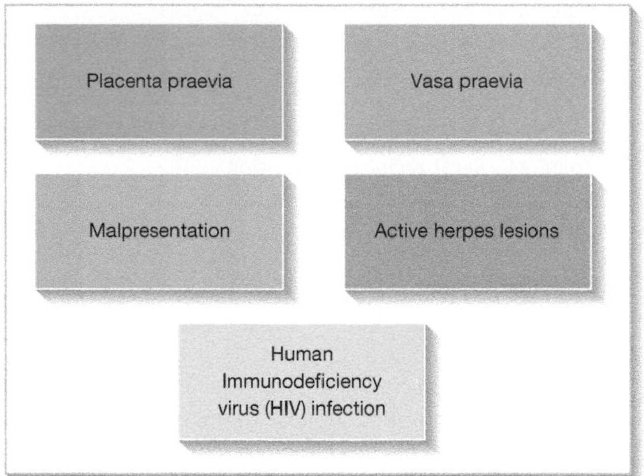

Figure 78.5 Vasa praevia.

Umbilical cord
Placenta
Fetal blood vessels
Internal os

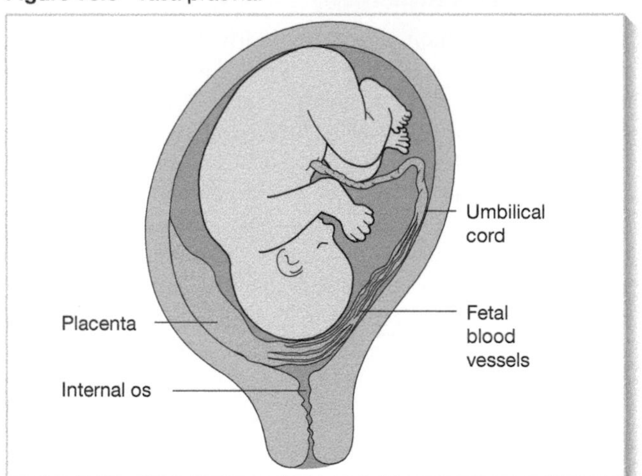

Figure 78.6 Position of amnihook.

Figure 78.7 Considerations post ARM.

Observe amniotic fluid for
Colour
Odour
Consistency
Assess FHR
FHR detects any changes which may indicate cord compression or prolapse
Maternal Observations
Temperature hourly
Pulse hourly
Liquor
Document all findings

Midwifery at a Glance, First Edition. Edited by Eleanor Forrest © 2019 John Wiley & Sons, Ltd. Published 2019 by John Wiley & Sons, Ltd.
Companion website: www.wiley.com/go/forrest/midwifery

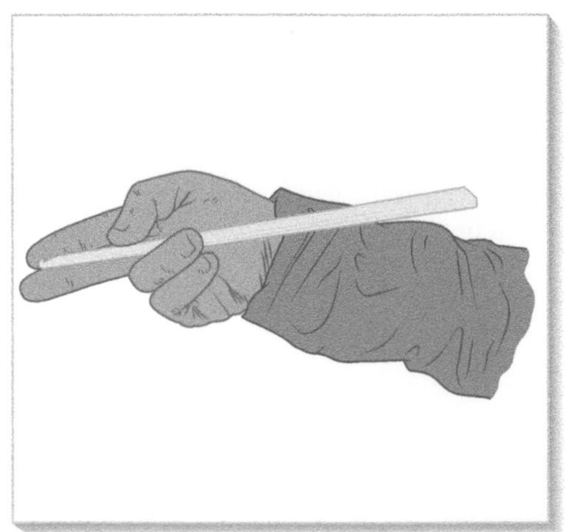

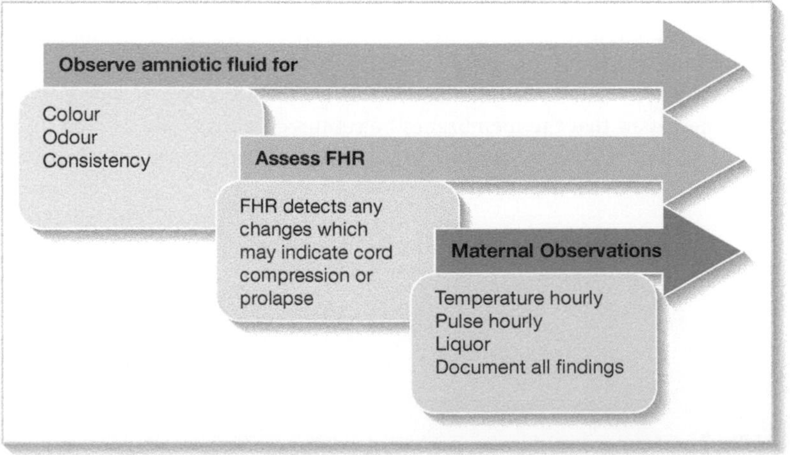

Amniotomy is the term used for the procedure to rupture the amniotic membranes. Artificial rupture of membranes (ARM) is the deliberate rupture of the amnion and chorion membranes to induce or augment labour or to introduce fetal monitoring tools such as the fetal scalp electrode. ARM is not part of the normal physiology of labour and should be considered only where there is a valid clinical reason or for women with slow labour progress when it may be the first intervention to consider following position change and mobilisation (Figures 78.1 and 78.2). It is believed that ARM speeds the process of labour because the production and release of prostaglandins and oxytocin increases, which leads to stronger contractions and faster cervical dilatation.

Note that this is limited evidence to support the use of ARM alone.

The majority of women report an increased strength and rate of contractions post ARM which was difficult to cope with and led to more analgesia and the feeling that the physiology of labour had been disturbed.

Timing of ARM

It is thought that ARM prior to 3 cm dilatation may slow the labour process. However, prolonged labour is associated with postpartum haemorrhage and infections, which are leading causes of maternal death, thus a well-timed ARM could reduce the risk of morbidity associated with long labour.

Considerations prior to ARM

Vaginal examination prior to ARM is essential to exclude cord presentation and to confirm that the presenting part is well applied to the cervix, thus eliminating the risk of the obstetric emergency that is cord prolapse (Figure 78.3).

ARM is carried out as a sterile procedure to reduce the risks of introducing infection. Regular observations of maternal pulse, temperature, amniotic fluid (colour and odour) and fetal heart rate are vital as changes can indicate maternal infection (Figure 78.3).

There are many contraindications to performing ARM and midwives must be aware of these prior to performing this procedure (Figure 78.4).

Placenta and vasa praevia

Placental position should be confirmed before vaginal examination. The midwife or doctor should exclude the presence of cord presentation and vasa praevia before considering or attempting ARM (Figure 78.5).

Presentation

Abdominal palpation and vaginal examination should determine the presentation and level of engagement. Ensuring the presenting part is well applied to the cervix minimises the risk of cord prolapse.

When is ARM performed by a doctor?

Where there is evidence of polyhydramnious, a high presenting part or a low lying placenta, ARM should only be performed by a senior doctor.

Equipment for ARM

- Dressing pack and sterile lotion
- Gloves
- Gel or obstetric cream
- Amnihook
- Incontinence pad
- Fetal scalp electrode if required
- Lithotomy poles only if deemed absolutely necessary.

Preparation for ARM

- Fully explain the procedure and gain informed consent
- Ensure the woman's bladder is empty
- Perform an abdominal palpation and auscultate the fetal heart
- Ensure the woman is comfortably positioned in a modified dorsal position (insert a wedge) or lithotomy position. Be aware that supine hypotension may occur if the woman has to lie on her back as the weight of the gravid uterus can occlude the aorta and vena cava.

Procedure

Perform a vaginal examination (Chapter 77) to confirm dilatation, effacement, fetal presentation, position, station and to exclude any contraindications to ARM (Figures 78.4 and 78.5). Be aware that although ARM is not painful as the membranes have no nerve endings, the vaginal examination can be uncomfortable for the woman.

Identify the cervical os and membranes, then gently slide the amnihook along the fingers with the hook facing towards your fingers, then rotate the hook towards the membranes and use the hook to tear the membranes (Figure 78.6).

Considerations following ARM (Figure 78.7)

1 Observe amniotic fluid – colour, odour and consistency. Inform the woman of findings or any abnormalities. Inform medical staff of any abnormalities in colour, odour or consistency of amniotic fluid.

2 Assess fetal heart rate (FHR) – assess FHR post ARM and according to local and national protocols thereafter.

3 Maternal observations – take the temperature hourly and pulse hourly or in accordance with protocols. Observe liquor levels.

4 Document –
- Vaginal examination findings
- Time of ARM
- Colour of amniotic fluid
- Maternal and fetal observations.

79 Urinary catheterisation

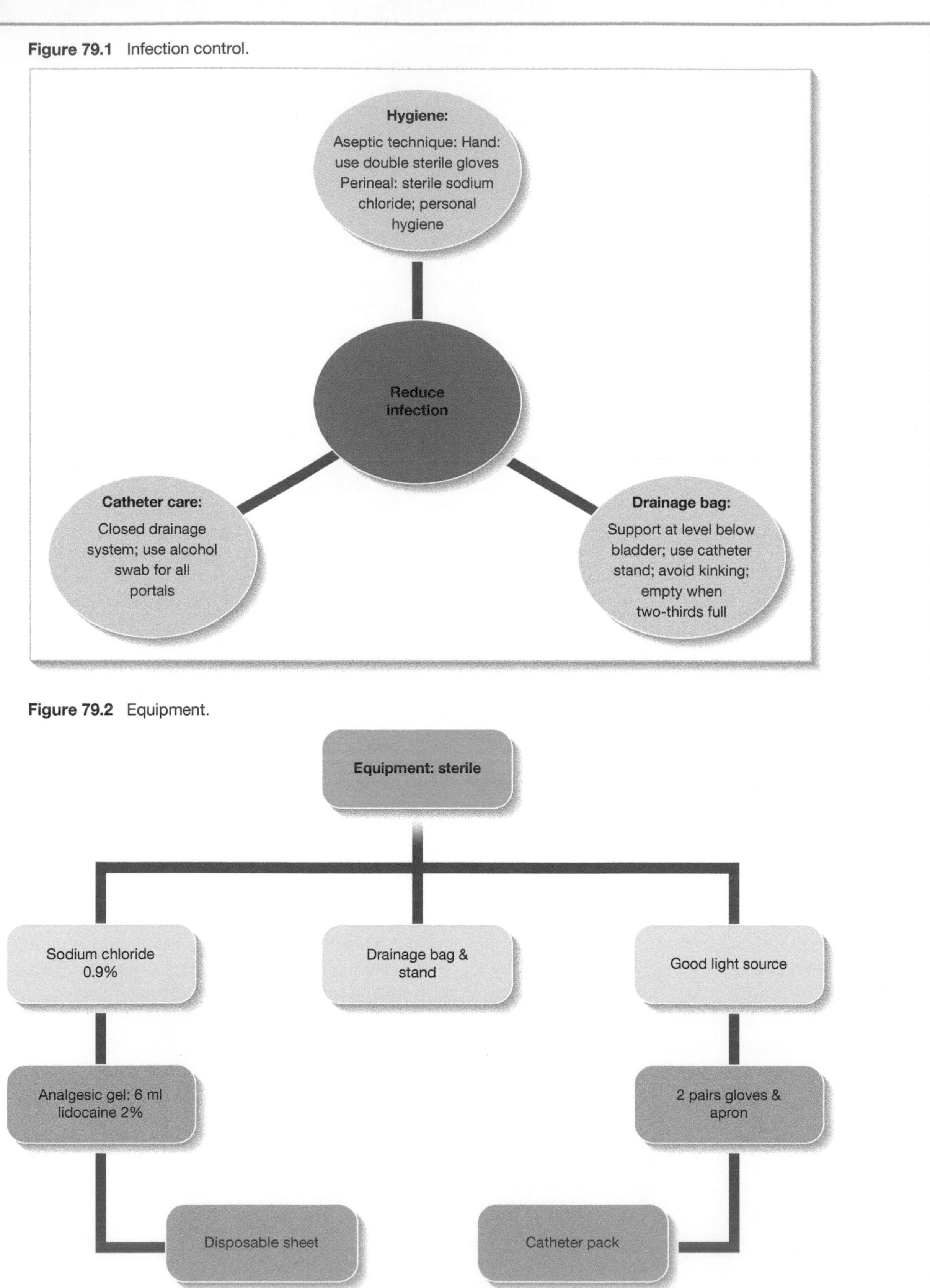

Figure 79.1 Infection control.

Figure 79.2 Equipment.

The aseptic procedure for urinary catheterisation involves the insertion of a sterile catheter into the bladder to subsequently drain urine. This is most commonly achieved via the urethra within maternity care, although suprapubic catheterisation via the abdominal wall is also possible, though much less likely.

Intermittent or indwelling

An intermittent catheter is inserted and removed following drainage of urine. The indwelling catheter is secured in the bladder. Urine can either drain freely into a catheter bag, or be emptied periodically, by use of a catheter valve.

Side effects

Catheterisation is a risk factor for infections such as the urinary tract (UTI) with about 2–6% of all women with a catheter being affected (Figure 79.1). More than 30% of all healthcare infections are UTIs which have detrimental effects on the woman and the health service. Blockage or bypass of the catheter can make the bladder spasm causing pain. Trauma or inflammation of the urinary tract can occur if due care is not taken during insertion or once indwelling; stones may form. Urinary catheterisation can lead to poor body image and impaired sexual function.

Indications

Although a fairly common procedure within maternity care, as mentioned, urinary catheterisation can have risks and side effects. Therefore, care must be taken to ensure that it is only performed when clinically indicated. The woman should also be fully informed as to the reasons and risks before consent is obtained. The decision about whether the catheter should be intermittent or indwelling will depend on each clinical indication.

During labour

If the woman is unable to pass urine during labour, urinary catheterisation should be considered. This is especially important in an instrumental delivery and the bladder must be emptied prior to this. If there is delay during the third stage of labour, a full bladder must be considered and catheterisation performed. This will help prevent a retained placenta or postpartum haemorrhage.

Postnatal or surgery

Postnatally, women can experience urinary incontinence and it may be necessary to have a catheter inserted to explore causes and aid diagnosis. Prior to abdominal surgery such as caesarean section, the bladder must be emptied to prevent damage. Women can experience urinary retention following surgery and may require having a catheter inserted.

Illness

During an episode of acute illness or shock, such as eclampsia or haemorrhage, accurate fluid balance monitoring is required; catheterisation will allow urinary output to be measured.

Procedure

Insertion of indwelling urinary catheter

Gather equipment (Figure 79.2) and following consent, ensure privacy throughout procedure. If possible, work with an assistant, but ensure hand hygiene at all times. Wash hands, put apron on, then apply an aseptic technique when opening equipment and performing the procedure.

- Woman's underwear should be removed; position her (semi-recumbent with ankles together, knees apart), on a disposable sheet and sterile drape
- Use opened pack as sterile field: place gloves, anaesthetic gel and catheter and drainage bag there
- Put on gloves (both pairs), expose tip of catheter and put gel on it; ask assistant to pour sodium chloride into the bowl
- Using swabs, separate the labia using the non-dominant hand, cleanse the vulva from front to back, swabbing once. Locate the urethra, and following insertion of anaesthetic gel wait 2–5 minutes. Remove top gloves and place receiver between the woman's thighs
- Holding the labia apart with a gauze swab in the non-dominant hand, gently insert the catheter with the dominant hand, upwards and backwards until urine flows. To ensure the balloon is in the bladder, insert a further 5 cm. Squeeze fluid from the external balloon or syringe to the inflate balloon; apply a clamp and remove the syringe
- Fully remove the plastic cover of the catheter and attach the drainage bag. Inform the woman that the procedure is complete; ensure her comfort and clear the area. Discuss care, mobility, infection and constipation prevention
- Ensure the catheter bag is secure at the side of the bed. Perform urinalysis as required. Document findings.

Insertion of intermittent urinary catheter

This is a similar aseptic technique, but the catheter is for single/residual use and is removed once the urine is drained.

Emptying/changing drainage bag

To promote drainage and reduce urethral pressure, empty the bag before it is two-thrids full. Using disposable gloves and an apron, wipe the tap with an alcohol swab before and after emptying. Measure urine and record if required. Drainage bags should be changed every 5 days or less.

Removal of indwelling urinary catheter

Removal should take place as soon as possible, depending on the woman's wellbeing. Local procedure may require a catheter specimen of urine to be obtained for culture. As for the insertion procedure, gain consent, ensure privacy and hygiene throughout and gather equipment as previously.

- Position the woman on a disposable sheet
- Wash hands and apply gloves and apron
- Deflate the balloon, remove the clamp and allow fluid to drain, either to an external balloon or by syringing off
- Ask the woman to take a deep breathe and whilst exhaling remove the catheter in a smooth but quick motion
- Cleanse the vulva and clear away the equipment
- Ensure the woman's comfort and provide advice regarding trauma, haematuria, retention, urgency or frequency of micturition, and the importance of drinking 2–3 litres of fluid and passing a good amount of urine within a 6–8-hour period
- Document findings of procedure.

Blood pressure and temperature, pulse and respiration: back to basics

Figure 80.1 MEOWS flowchart.

MEOWS $\leq$ 2 – continue as per plan of care

↓

MEOWS = 3
Inform Co-ordinator or Senior Midwife
Repeat observations
Senior Midwife to review
Consider medical review

↓

MEOWS $\geq$ 4
Inform Co-ordinator or Senior Midwife
Contact Obstetric Registrar to review
Think! ABC, increase frequency of observations, record oxygen saturations, ?i.v. access, ?urinary catheter, analgesia
Consider sepsis

↓

MEOWS $\geq$ 6
Inform Co-ordinator or Senior Midwife
Urgent Obstetric review by Specialist Registrar/Consultant
Contact Anaesthetic Registrar
Consider Critical Care Outreach Services

Box 80.1 Indications for performing and recording baseline observations.

- BP at each antenatal appointment (to exclude pre-eclampsia)
- On admission to hospital
- During labour (as per unit guidelines and not during a contraction)
- Immediately after delivery
- As the clinical condition changes (e.g. haemorrhage, shock/collapse, pre- and postoperative procedures)
- Blood transfusion (as per unit guidelines)
- Alongside auscultation of the fetal heart (maternal pulse)

Table 80.1 Normal values using a MEOWS score (NB these parameters do not apply to a normal labouring woman).

Score	3	2	1	0	1	2	3
Temperature		<35°C		35–37.4°C		37.5–39°C	>39°C
Systolic BP	≤70	71–79	81–89	90–139	140–149	150–159	≥160
Diastolic BP			≤45	46–89	90–99	100–109	≥110
Pulse		≤40	40–50	51–100	101–110	111–129	≥130
Respiratory rate		≤8		9–14	15–20	21–29	≥30

Blood pressure is measured in millimetres of mercury (mmHg) and usually reflects the arterial blood pressure – the pressure exerted on the arterial walls. Blood pressure is highest in the large arteries closest to the heart, decreasing gradually within the smaller arteries, arterioles and capillaries. Arterial blood pressure facilitates blood flow around the body to ensure optimal oxygenation to the vital organs and tissue. Blood pressure is measured using two parameters – systole (ventricular contraction) and diastole (when the ventricles relax) – therefore the pressure is not constant. It is important to measure both levels of pressure as these reflect different physiological responses.

Human core temperature is maintained at around 37°C and refers to the balance between heat gain and heat loss. The core temperature refers to the temperature within the brain, abdomen and chest, reflecting the warmest parts of the body housing the body's major organs. For optimal functioning it is critical that a constant, level body temperature is maintained to avoid cellular damage. Temperature is measured peripherally where it is generated by the skin and skeletal muscle, exposed to the external environment, and helping the body to regulate its core temperature. Peripheral temperatures reduce proportionally as the distance increases from the core.

As the left ventricle of the heart ejects blood into the circulatory system the arteries expand and recoil causing a 'pulse' which can be felt anywhere in the body where an artery can be palpated against something firm, such as against a bone. Typically, in an adult, the radial artery is used for monitoring a pulse as it is easily accessible. The pulse should be assessed for not only its rate, but also volume and regularity. A weak pulse or a full-bounding, rapid one may indicate changes in the amount of blood being pumped away from the heart and therefore the flow of oxygenated blood around the body.

The assessment of respiration involves the count of external breaths per minute. Respiration is the means by which the body gains oxygen through inhalation and excretes carbon dioxide through exhalation. It is important to observe associated signs of respiration such as colour, breath sounds, depth and regularity, especially when caring for a critically ill woman (Table 80.1).

Changes related to pregnancy, birth and the puerperium

Collectively, blood pressure (BP), temperature, pulse and respiration (TPR) are referred to as 'baseline observations'. The presence of progesterone in pregnancy and an increase in metabolic rate cause marked changes in baseline observations. Additional heat generated in pregnancy can be up to 35%, leading to a maternal increase in temperature of 0.5°C. Haemodynamic changes in pregnancy and anatomical adjustments, creating space for the growing uterus, result in an increase in blood volume, cardiac output and heart rate. Pregnancy is not normally associated with significant changes in arterial blood pressure, as progesterone relaxes blood vessel walls, decreasing peripheral resistance, counteracting the rise in blood pressure caused by increased cardiac output. However, when raised in pregnancy this is referred to as pregnancy-induced hypertension (PIH), which may also be a marker for pre-eclampsia and is therefore the only baseline observation to be recorded at each antenatal appointment. The woman's oxygen requirements are higher in pregnancy; breathing becomes largely diaphragmatic as the diaphragm is displaced upwards. Each breath is deeper as the smooth muscles are relaxed by progesterone; the respiratory rate may increase by 2 breaths per minute. The maternal heart rate increases in pregnancy by approximately 15–20 beats per minute (bpm), peaking at 28 weeks, corresponding with an increase in total blood volume.

During labour and birth each contraction returns 300–500 ml of blood to the circulation. TPR and BP can increase as a result of increased muscular activity and physical excursion but also in a psychosomatic response to pain and anxiety.

In the puerperium, physiological changes occur in the body, such as higher venous pressures. This results in increased blood pressure following birth and a transient rise in temperature in the first 24 hours (up to 38°C) and as milk production arrives on the second or third day.

Care must be taken when observing and recording all baseline observations, as early recognition of deterioration is essential for the on-going care and prognosis of a women who is severely compromised. Substandard care has been a frequent finding of confidential enquiries into maternal deaths. In many cases the early warning signs and symptoms of impending severe maternal illness or collapse go unrecognised; deterioration may be rapid, with catastrophic consequences. A balance must be sought between early identification of a woman requiring medical intervention and the avoidance of over-medicalising the normal physiological process.

Recognising pathology

See Box 80.1 for suggested indications for performing and recording baseline observations. However, as each woman is an individual, consent must be sought, and plans of care and the current situation must all be considered. Attention to detail is of most importance, observations should be timely, thorough, documented accurately and carefully, and with appropriate referral and escalation should an abnormality be detected.

A Confidential Enquiry into Maternal and Child Health report recommended the use of a modified early obstetric warning system (MEOWS) in all women admitted to an obstetric unit. It is universally agreed that all women, irrespective of risk, should be appropriately monitored and their observations documented. Having MEOWS in place at least ensures that women are clinically monitored whilst admitted. It is the response to an abnormal score that has the potential to alter an outcome, rather than merely the fact it was recorded (Figure 80.1).

81 Episiotomy

Figure 81.1 Layers of the pelvic floor.

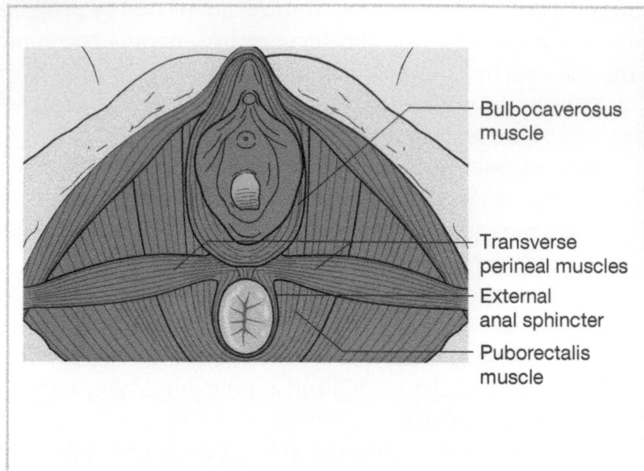

Figure 81.2 Distended perineum at crowning of the head.

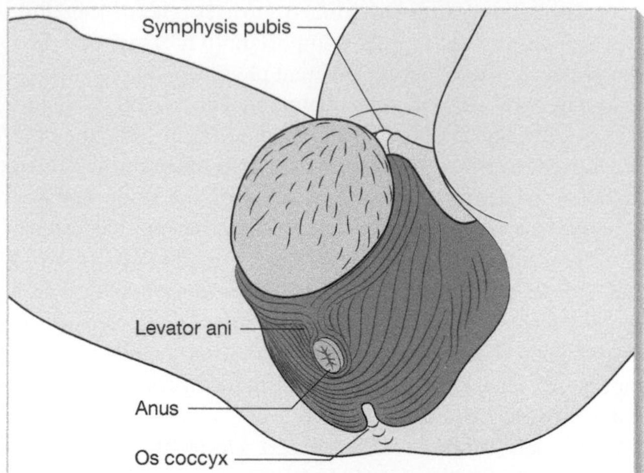

Figure 81.3 Infiltration of the perineum.

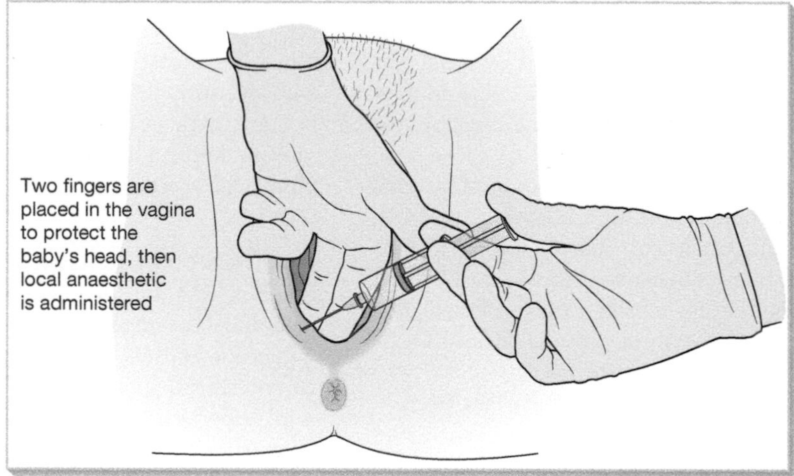

Figure 81.4 Performing the episiotomy.

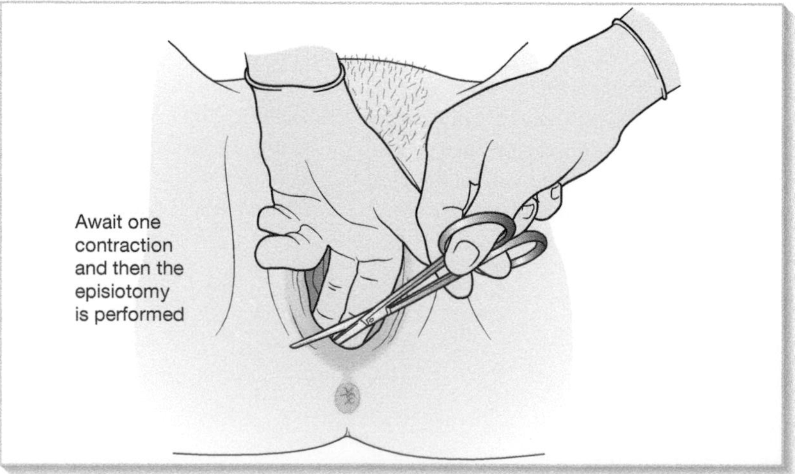

Within the UK around 85% of woman will have some degree of perineal trauma during childbirth, either spontaneously or as the result of an episiotomy. Episiotomy is a surgical incision made into the posterior aspect of the vagina to increase the vulval outlet and facilitate the birth of a baby. The UK has adopted restrictive episiotomies rather than routine episiotomy procedures. The recognised indications for restrictive episiotomy are to facilitate the birth of the baby if there is evidence of fetal distress; prior to an instrumental delivery (ventouse or forceps); and to minimise the risk of severe maternal trauma.

Evidence has demonstrated that midwives use a variety of practices and techniques when performing an episiotomy and some report that they have become deskilled and lack confidence in performing an episiotomy, even when it is required. The research reports that midwives are using differing angles, lengths and depths of incision, which may contribute to the increase risk and rates of obstetric anal sphincter injuries (OASIS). OASIS are injuries to the perineum involving the anal sphincter complexes and they are significant contributory factors in the development of anal incontinence. Traditionally in the UK the advised method for an episiotomy is mediolateral. However, definitions of a mediolateral episiotomy vary in textbooks and research studies. Most agree that an incision is made at the midline of the perineum at the fourchette, directed laterally at a 45° angle. However, due to the variation in midwives' techniques this angle is not always achieved.

The pelvic floor

The pelvic floor lies in the outlet of the bony pelvis and is a gutter-shaped structure, which is higher anteriorly than posteriorly. It consists of layers of tissue and supports the pelvic and abdominal organs (Figure 81.1). The levator ani muscle plays a crucial role in the preservation of urinary and bowel continence.

The pelvic floor has six layers. Starting externally and working internally the layers are as follows:

- Skin
- Subcutaneous fat
- Superficial muscles – bulbocavernosus, ischiocavernosus and transverse perineal
- Deep muscles (forming the levator ani) – pubococcygeus, iliococcygeus and ischiococcygeus
- Pelvic fascia thickened to form pelvic ligaments
- Peritoneum.

Functions of the pelvic floor

- Supports the abdominal and pelvic organs
- Maintains intra-abdominal pressure
- Controls voluntary function of micturition and defecation
- Facilitates the mechanisms of labour during birth
- Allows flexion and extension of the sacrum and coccyx.

The perineal body

This is a triangular-shaped structure that lies between the vagina and rectum and consists of the superficial muscles and the deep pelvic floor muscle.

Assessment of the perineum

The perineal body can be overstretched and damaged during childbirth. During the birth, as the fetal head crowns, the maternal perineum and the anal sphincter complexes stretch and distend (Figure 81.2). Following the birth the perineal tissues will then shrink. This distortion of the perineum means that an incision made as the head is crowning at a presumed 45° angle will then be approximately at a 25° angle or less following birth when the perineum is at rest.

Incisions that are performed very close to the fourchette, short episiotomies and angles of less than 45° are all associated with increased OASIS rates. Large studies show that true 45° mediolateral and 60° lateral episiotomies have a protective effect against OASIS.

To ensure that a 45° angle is achieved when the perineum is at rest post birth the incision should be made using a 60° angle when the fetal head is crowning. Making the incision laterally to the midline at 7 o'clock may also have a protective effect. Traditionally, the length of the episiotomy is 2.5 cm, and with the stretched perineum a median of 3 cm may prevent OASIS.

Infiltration of anaesthetic

An explanation of the procedure should be given and consent obtained. The perineum should be adequately anaesthetised using 5–10 ml of lidocaine hydrochloride 1%. Two fingers are inserted into the vagina along the line of the proposed incision protecting the fetal head.

1 The needle is inserted beneath the skin for 4–5 cm following the line of your fingers (Figure 81.3).

2 The piston of the syringe should be withdrawn prior to injecting the lidocaine hydrochloride 1%. If blood is aspirated then reposition needle, aspirate again until no blood is withdrawn.

3 Lidocaine hydrochloride 1% is continuously injected as the needle is slowly withdrawn.

Do not remove the needle completely from the skin, but redirect needle to either side of first line and repeat steps 1–3.

The anaesthetic takes about 3–5 minutes to take effect. For adequate analgesia, wait for the following contraction before performing the episiotomy.

Performing the episiotomy

To perform the episiotomy two fingers are inserted into the vagina along the line of the proposed incision protecting the fetal head. The scissors are inserted into the vagina at 7 o'clock around 1 cm laterally to the midline and then angled at 60°. The incision should be 3 cm in length (Figure 81.4). This should be performed at the peak of a contraction when the head is crowning as the perineal body tissues are at their thinnest. The scissors should then be removed and delivery of the head should be supported.

The tissues that are involved in an episiotomy are the same as a second degree tear and comprise the skin of the fourchette, perineum and perineal body (superficial muscles: bulbocavernosus and transverse perineal; deep pelvic floor muscles: pubococcygeus).

82 Perineal repair

Figure 82.1 Structures of the pelvic floor.

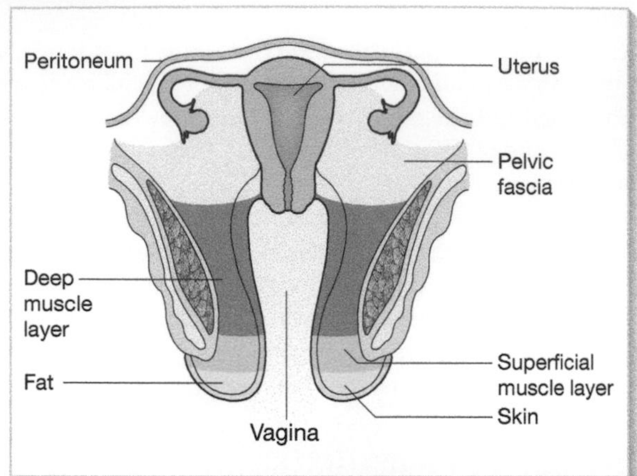

Figure 82.2 The perineal body.

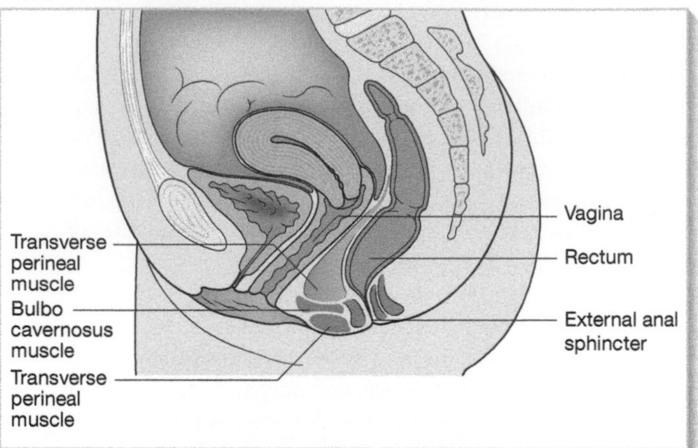

Figure 82.3 Second degree laceration.

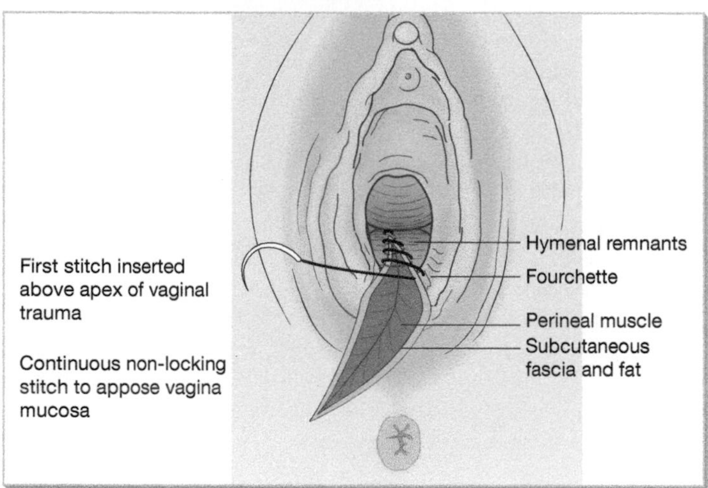

Figure 82.4 Infiltration of the perineum.

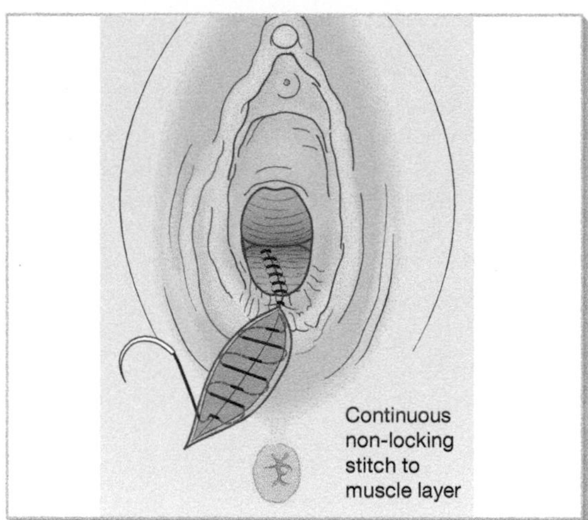

Figure 82.5 Perineal repair – continuous non-locking technique.

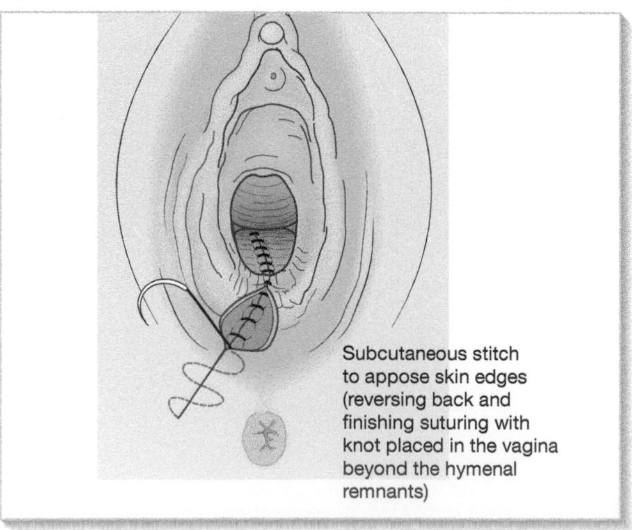

In childbirth 85% of women with a vaginal birth will experience some degree of perineal trauma. Identification of perineal trauma and its subsequent repair must be conducted efficiently to prevent future morbidity to the woman. The different degrees of perineal trauma that can occur and a detailed account of how to repair a second degree perineal laceration will follow. Third and fourth degree lacerations must be referred for medical management.

Anatomical structures

The structures of the pelvic floor are skin and superficial and deep pelvic floor muscles (Figure 82.1). The anal sphincter and urethral sphincter also form part of the muscle structures. The perineal body (Figure 82.2) is the main area associated with perineal trauma in childbirth.

Degrees of perineal trauma

Perineal trauma is defined as the following:

1 **First degree laceration** – skin of the fourchette only.

2 **Second degree laceration** (resulting from perineal tear or episiotomy) – skin of the fourchette, bulbocavernosus (superficial muscle), transverse perineal and pubococcygeus (deep pelvic floor muscles) (Figure 82.3).

3 **Third degree laceration** – skin of the fourchette, bulbocavernosus, transverse perineal and pubococcygeus muscles and internal and external anal sphincter muscle(s):

3a: less than 50% of the external anal sphincter torn
3b: more than 50% of the external anal sphincter torn
3c: internal anal sphincter torn.

4 **Fourth degree laceration** – skin of the fourchette, bulbocavernosus, transverse perineal and pubococcygeus muscles; laceration has transcended through both the internal and external anal sphincters muscles and anal epithelium.

Identification of perineal trauma

Following birth the midwife must identify the correct anatomical structures involved in the perineal trauma to ensure appropriate management. Inspect the perineal region and vagina under a good light source. A digital rectal examination must also be performed to exclude any occult lacerations even if the perineum is intact. Informed consent must be obtained from the woman; then gently insert a lubricated finger into the rectum to examine the rectum and sphincters. Once a first or second degree laceration is confirmed the midwife can commence perineal repair.

Preparation prior to perineal repair

Following explanation, informed consent must be obtained to conduct the perineal repair. Place the woman in the lithotomy position. Cleanse the perineal area with sterile solution from top to bottom and from the centre outwards. Place sterile drapes appropriately. The midwife must wear an apron, gown, face/mouth shield and sterile gloves. Count sterile swabs, cotton wool balls, tampons, instruments and suture needles prior to the repair and recheck immediately following the repair. Rapid absorbable polyglactin 910 is the preferred suture material; it dissolves within 42 days with less perineal pain, dehiscence and suture removal compared with a standard polyglycolic acid/polyglactin 910, which takes 60–90 days to dissolve.

Infiltration of anaesthetic

Ensure adequate analgesia prior to suturing the perineum. An epidural top-up can be administered if the woman has had no epidural, then up to 15–20 ml of local anaesthetic (lidocaine hydrochloride 1%) is administered via injection. If 5 ml of lidocaine hydrochloride 1% has already been given prior to an episiotomy then only 15 ml would now be administered. In Figure 82.4, the needle is inserted at point A and moved towards point B. Once the needle is at point C the syringe piston is withdrawn to ensure the needle is not in a blood vessel. The needle is withdrawn down towards A whilst simultaneously inserting the local anaesthetic. Without removing the needle the same process is repeated for A to D. The perineum is then infiltrated from point C to B and C to D using the same process. Leave for 3–5 minutes to ensure effectiveness of the anaesthetic. Entonox gas can be self-administered by the woman during infiltration to reduce pain. A tampon might be gently inserted into the vagina to help prevent blood occluding the view of the laceration. This must be securely attached to the sterile drapes and removed post repair.

Perineal repair

This is conducted using an aseptic technique. A continuous non-locking suture throughout (the vaginal wall, muscle and skin) is the preferred method (Figure 82.5). The apex of the perineal laceration is identified and an anchoring knot is inserted 5–10 mm above the apex. This knot should be tied three times to prevent slippage and to lie flat. To do this (i) put the suture material over the needle holder and round it for two throws, then pull the suture taught; (ii) do one throw in the opposite direction and pull taught; (iii) repeat one throw in the first direction and pull taught. A loose continuous non-locking suture is then performed down the posterior aspect of the vaginal wall where the laceration has occurred. The needle should then exit the vagina at the hymenal remnants and come out into the muscle layer on the same side of the laceration just exited. The muscle layer is also done using a continuous non-locking method. Start at the top of the muscle layer nearest to the fourchette. Depending on the depth of the laceration this layer might have to be sutured in two layers; then use a continuous non-locking subcuticular stitch to close the skin layer. Start at the area of the skin nearest to the anus and suture up towards the fourchette, then continue up into the vagina to the hymenal remnants. The repair ends with a non-slip knot (Aberdeen knot). Conduct a small stich to the left or right of the sutured laceration to move the knot to the side of the repair, leaving it visible.

Post-perineal repair

Once completed, another rectal examination is conducted to ensure the rectum is patent with no sutures through it. Count all instruments and swabs/needles to ensure none have been left in situ. Ensure the woman is comfortable and restore dignity. Document the procedure as per professional regulations. Offer advice on perineal wound care, and provide appropriate analgesia and follow-up.

Feeding support and breast expression

Box 83.1 Reasons to express breast milk.

- To encourage baby to feed, by expressing a little colostrum/milk onto the nipple
- To relieve engorgement and assist a baby to attach at the breast by softening the breast
- To maximise milk production
- If a baby or mother is unable to breastfeed (Chapter 61)
- Manage a blocked duct and prevent or reduce symptoms of mastitis
- If a mother and baby are separated
- If a mother wishes to offer her baby a bottle or to facilitate someone else giving the baby a bottle

Box 83.2 Expressing milk for sick and preterm babies.

- Mothers who are expressing to provide milk for sick or preterm babies should express 8–10 times in 24 hours, at least one of these expressions should be during the night

Figure 83.1 Hand expression of breast milk.

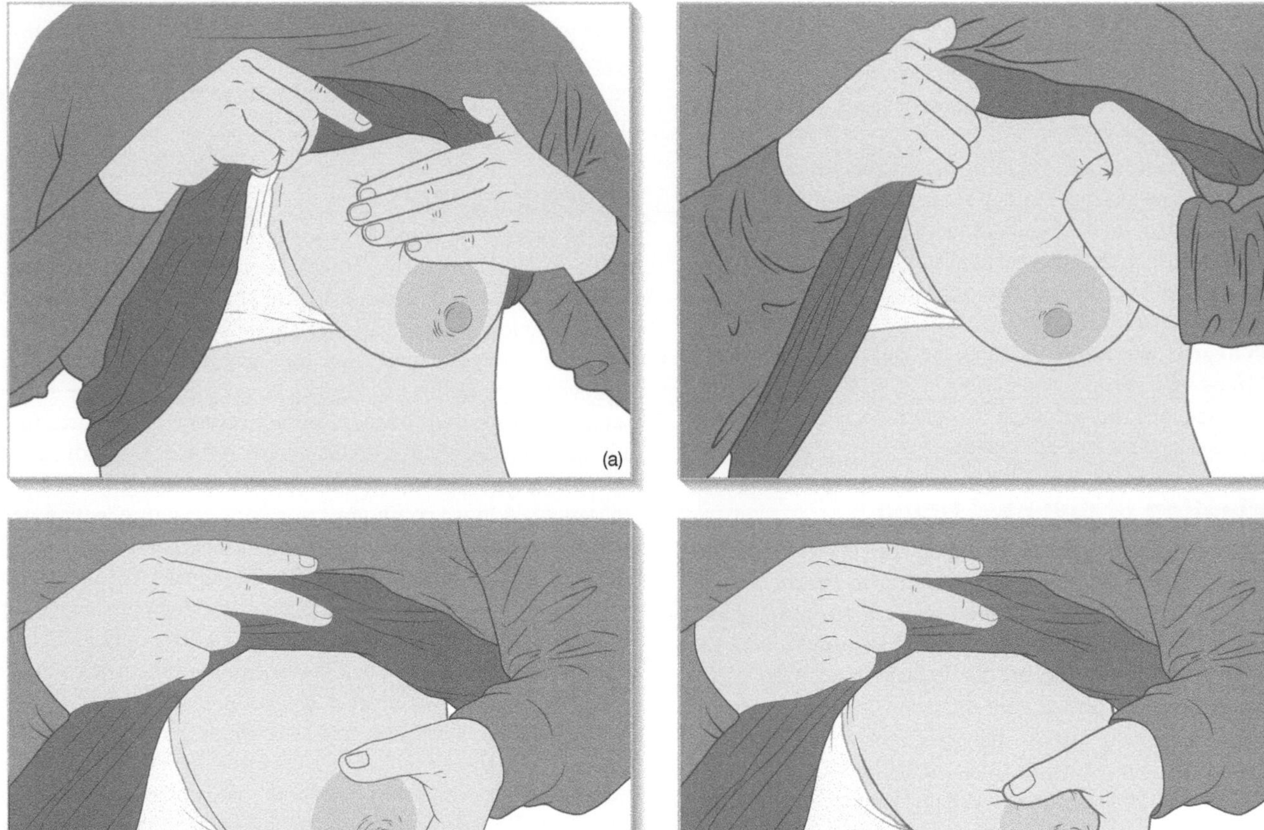

Box 83.3 Additional support for a mother's learning.

- http://www.feedgoodfactor.org.uk/breastfeeding-worries/expressing-your-milk/
- http://www.unicef.org.uk/babyfriendly
- https://www.bestbeginnings.org.uk/
- www.healthscotland.com/documents/120.aspx
- Minekawa R. et al. 2014. Human breast milk suppresses the transcriptional regulation of IL-1beta-induced NF-kappaB signaling in human intestinal cells. Am J Physiol Cell Physiol. 287(5):C1404–11

The World Health Organisation (WHO) International Code of the Marketing of Breast Milk Substitutes (WHO, 1981) seeks to:

- Protect and promote breastfeeding as the best way to feed babies
- Ensure the provision of appropriate information regarding infant feeding
- Regulate the advertising of breast milk substitutes/infant formula, bottles, teats and dummies
- Ensure that health services do not promote breast milk substitutes and that free samples of breast milk substitutes are not provided to pregnant women, new mothers or families.

The WHO code includes infant formula, milk products, foods and drinks used in place of breast milk. Product information to health professionals must contain scientific and factual information only and be free from advertising. Further, the WHO code indicates that promotional material from infant formula manufacturers such as pens, tape measures, weight conversion charts and calendars that advertise breast milk substitutes, bottles, teats and dummies should not be accepted or used by health professionals. Health professionals should not accept equipment or sponsorship from infant formula manufacturers to undertake study or attend study days.

In addition nurses and midwives are required to adhere to the Nursing and Midwifery Council (NMC)'s *The Code* (NMC, 2015) which states that as a health professional you must 'refuse all but the most trivial gifts, favours or hospitality. . .'.

Further information for woman needing support in breast feeding can be found from the sources listed in Box 83.3.

The law

In Scotland the Breastfeeding Scotland Act 2005 states that it is against the law to prevent a woman from breast or bottle feeding a child under the age of 2 years in a public place. In addition, the Equality Act of 2010 affords further protection throughout the UK by making it unlawful to discriminate against a woman because she is breastfeeding. Breastfeeding employees are also afforded protection by the Equality Act 2010 as employers must not prevent a woman from breastfeeding in the course of her employment.

Expressing breast milk

Breast milk can be expressed by hand or by using a breast pump. The choice of expression method can be dependent on the reason for expressing (Box 83.1). Hand expressing is a useful skill for breastfeeding women to have as it gives them a method of solving many breastfeeding challenges just using their fingertips! Even if a woman chooses to use a breast pump to express her milk, she will improve the yield by stimulating her lactation hormones by hand expressing some milk first.

Preterm and ill babies

For all babies breast milk is important in helping them get the best start in life. However, it is imperative that preterm babies benefit from the protection from infection and support for growth and development that breast milk provides. There is evidence to suggest that the use of breast milk decreases the incidence and severity of the life-threatening disease necrotising enterocolitis. Expressing breast milk for a sick or preterm baby can provide a mother with a sense of satisfaction that her unique milk is making a difference to the wellbeing of her baby (Box 83.1). However, skilled and sensitive support is imperative for such mothers as expressing breast milk over a long period of time is demanding (Box 83.2).

Teaching hand expression

Use a diagram or model of a breast to illustrate the anatomy of the breast and relevant structures. Show the mother how to stimulate her lactation hormones by having her baby close by, using gentle massage and, if she cannot be close to her baby, having something that reminds her of her baby, for example, a photo or vest. The woman should locate the area in her breast for her to put her fingers on and express milk (Figure 83.1b). Placing her fingers 2–3 cm back from the base of the nipple should work for most women (Figure 83.1a).

Now describe and allow mother to practice the technique for expressing:

- Place the index finger and thumb in a C shape, opposite each other at either side of the nipple (Figure 83.1c)
- Compress and release bringing the finger and thumb together in a steady rhythm (mimicking the baby's sucking pattern) (Figure 83.1d)
- Avoid sliding the fingers on the skin
- Move round the breast once flow slows
- Once flow slows/ceases move to the other breast.

Storing expressed milk

Expressed breast milk (EBM) can be stored in the body of the fridge for up to 5 days, in the freezer compartment of the fridge for up to 2 weeks or in the freezer for up to 6 months. The fridge and/or freezer being used should be clean and able to maintain a reliable temperature of 4°C or lower for the fridge and −18°C or lower for the freezer. Any stored EBM should be labeled, dated and used sequentially.

If freezing breast milk it is less wasteful to freeze EBM in small quantities in ice cube trays or freezer bags. Milk should be defrosted slowly, ideally in the fridge overnight. This reduces the degradation of the living cells within the milk. EBM can be gently warmed prior to offering it to a baby but should *never* be warmed in a microwave due to the high risk of scalding.

Blood and blood products

Box 84.1 Positive patient identification.

Ask person or use official hospital identification (band) for following details:

- Last name
- First name
- Date of birth
- Unique identification number (NHS, CHI, HSC)

Box 84.2 Incompatible intravenous fluids.

Solutions containing:

- Calcium: Ringer's lactate, Haemaccel, Gelofusine
- Hypotonic i.v. solutions: 5% dextrose

Box 84.3 Administration.

- Use blood administration set with integral mesh filter (170–200 microns)
- Complete within 4 hours after leaving temperature-controlled environment
- Change administration set 12 hourly

Box 84.4 Infusion devices.

- Gravity or electronic infusion device
- Rapid infusion devices (6–30 litres per hour)
- Blood warming device (if necessary)
- All equipment needs to have manufacturer safety approval for use with blood

Box 84.5 Monitoring.

- Pre-transfusion observations
- Visual observation during process
- Observations every 15 minutes
- Observe for reaction
- Post-transfusion observations after 60 minutes
- Observe closely for 24 hours
- Inform patient of sign and symptoms of possible late reactions
- Give patient contact details for 24-hour clinical advice

According to the British Committee for Standards in Haematology (BSCH, 2012) the following guidelines should be adhered to when administering blood components. Staff involved in the blood transfusion process should receive regular (minimum 2 yearly) training and be assessed as competent.

Patient identification and documentation

A patient identification band (or risk assessed equivalent) must be worn by all patients receiving a blood transfusion. The minimum patient identifiers must be legible and accurate. This is best done by printing the identification band directly from the organisation's computerised patient administration system (PAS). Positive patient identification is essential at all stages of the blood transfusion process; key identifiers are shown in (Box 84.1). The patient or their legal carers must consent to receive blood or blood products. Full and complete documentation, governed by local policies and guidelines, is required at every stage of the blood transfusion process to provide an unambiguous audit trail. All paperwork relating to the patient must include, and be identical in, every detail with the minimum identifiers contained on the patient's identification band.

Pre-transfusion

Requests must include patient core identifiers, gender, current diagnosis and any relevant significant comorbidities, a clear unambiguous reason for the request, type of component and volume/number of units required, any clinical special requirements, time needed, the location of the patient (and location where transfusion will occur if known to be different), and name and contact number of the requester. The minimum dataset to be recorded in the patient's clinical records should contain documentation of the reason for transfusion (clinical and laboratory data), details of the information provided to the patient (risks, benefits and alternatives to transfusion) and consent to proceed.

Prescription

Must contain the patient's core identifiers and must as a minimum specify what components are to be transfused, date of transfusion, the volume/number of units to be transfused, the rate of transfusion and any other clinical special instructions or requirements – for example irradiated, cytomegalovirus-seronegative, blood warmer or any concomitant drugs needed.

Communication and collection of blood products

Clear and unambiguous communications between all staff involved in the transfusion process, including all clinical and laboratory staff and any other support staff, is essential. Organisations should have local policies and guidelines to minimise the risk of misinterpretation or transcription errors in all communications relating to transfusion, whether written, verbal or electronic. Blood samples for pretransfusion testing requires the same stringent identifications as all other blood component processes.

Administration equipment and infusion devices

A peripheral or central venous catheter can be used as can multilumen catheters. Umbilical venous or arterial catheters should not be used. Generally no other i.v. fluid should be administrated via the same infusion line as the blood/blood components because some i.v. fluids are incompatible with blood (Box 84.2). However, other i.v. fluids can go via a separate lumen if the catheter has multiple lumens.

When blood components are being administered the correct administration sets need to be used. These require an integral mesh filter of 170–200 microns. Each unit of blood needs to be completed within 4 hours after leaving the temperature-controlled environment. If several blood components are being administrated then the administration set needs to be changed at least 12 hourly (or in accordance with manufacturer instructions) to reduce risk of bacterial growth (Box 84.3). Platelets should not be administered through a set previously used for other blood components.

Staff must be competent in use of the device and should only use devices that are compatible with blood component administration sets. Gravity or an electronic devise for precise infusion rates can be used. Rapid infusion devises can be used as well as pressure devices that exert even pressure over the blood component bag. These latter devices need a pressure gauge which does not exceed 300 mmHg. Blood warmers can also be used to administer red cells to prevent hypothermia (Box 84.4).

Monitoring

Observations should be undertaken for every unit transfused. Minimum monitoring of the patient should include (Box 84.5):

- Regular visual observation throughout the transfusion episode
- Pre-transfusion pulse (P), blood pressure (BP), temperature (T) and respiratory rate (RR) measurements. These should be taken and recorded no more than 60 minutes before starting the transfusion.
- P, BP and T (Chapter 80) should be taken 15 minutes after the start of each component transfusion. If these measurements have changed from the baseline values, then RR should also be taken. More frequent observations may be required, for example in rapid transfusion, or in patients who are unable to complain of symptoms that would raise suspicion of a developing transfusion reaction
- If the patient shows signs or symptoms of a possible transfusion reaction, P, BP, T and RR should be monitored and recorded and appropriate action taken
- Post-transfusion P, BP and T should be taken and recorded not more than 60 minutes after the end of the component transfusion
- Patients should be observed during the subsequent 24 hours for (or, if discharged, counselled about the possibility of) late adverse reactions
- Organisations should ensure that systems are in place to ensure patients have 24-hour access to clinical advice.

Administration of drugs with blood products

This is not considered good practice and should be avoided due to the preservative and additive nature of these drugs. There has been some research on the use of opioid infusions at the same time for those who have limited i.v. access, but the evidence is controversial. However, there may be an organisational policy permitting this for those with limited i.v. access due to the differences of opinion on the evidence.

85 Maternal resuscitation

Table 85.1 Causes of cardiac arrest during childbirth.

Thromboembolism	Sepsis/infection
Amniotic fluid embolism (anaphylactoid syndrome of pregnancy)	Trauma
Pregnancy-induced hypertension (pre-eclampsia and eclampsia)	Haemorrhage (including disseminated intravascular coagulation)
Latrogenic • Medication allergy/error • Anaesthetic complication • Hypermagnesemia	Asthma
Pre-existing heart disease • Congenital • Acquired	Cerebral vascular accident

Table 85.2 Physiologic changes and their effect on CPR.

Physiological difference	Resuscitation modification
Cardiac output increased (maternal & fetal demand)	Caesarean section within 5 minutes & replace any blood loss immediately
Aortocaval compression when supine	Lateral uterine displacement – wedge or manual
Increased oxygen requirements	Resuscitation with 100% oxygen immediately
Splinting of diaphragm	May be harder to ventilate lungs
Relaxation of cardiac sphincter	Application of cricoid pressure & use cuffed endotracheal tube when intubated
Oedema of glottis, neck obesity, large breasts	More difficult to intubate; smaller tube possibly needed

Figure 85.1 Two procedures for manual lateral uterine displacement.

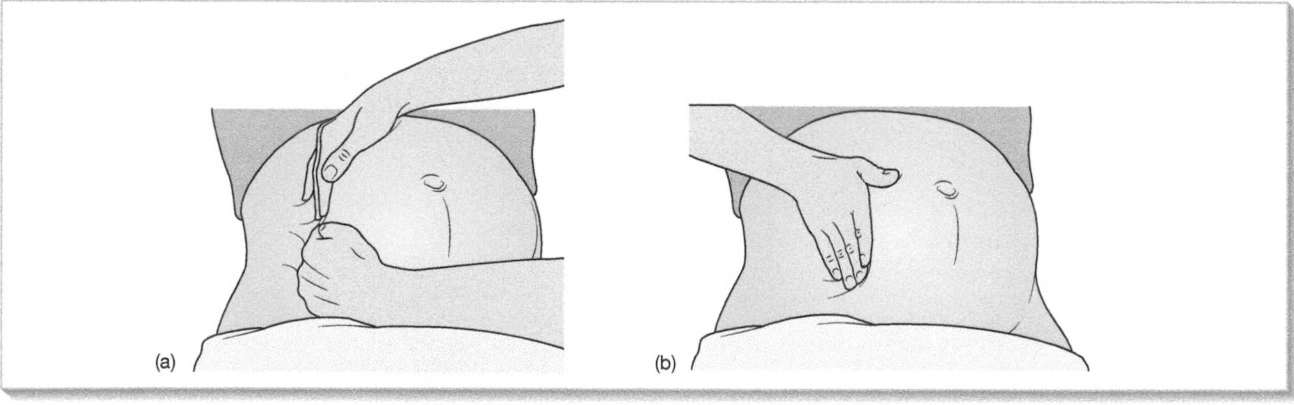

Figure 85.2 Cricoid pressure.

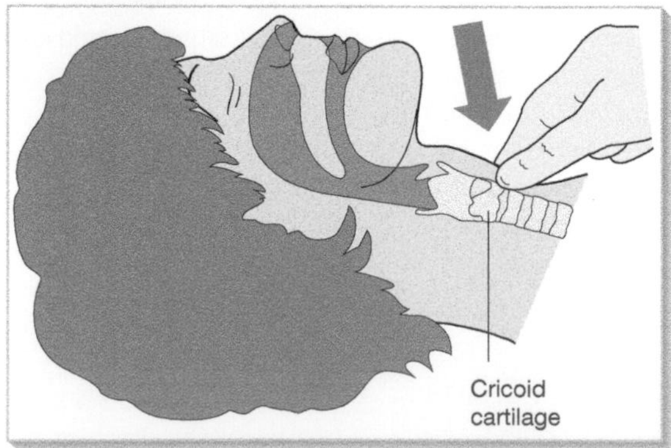

Cardiac arrest in pregnancy affects around 1:30 000 women in the UK. The incidence is thought to be rising due to the increasing age and morbidity of the antenatal population in the UK. Figures quoted from the USA indicate a rate of 1:20 000 and this is attributed to pregnancy occurring at a later age – 35 years or over – and more women with serious underlying medical conditions undertaking pregnancies.

Cardiac arrest during late pregnancy or birth is quite rare. However, when it does occur, maternal and fetal survival rates are low. Maternal survival is around 40%, partly due to the fact that the events leading to cardiac arrest tend to be overwhelming and incurable, but another factor of major importance is the physiological changes of pregnancy which hamper resuscitative efforts (Table 85.1).

Outcome is more successful when there is a good knowledge of:

- The risk factors of cardiac arrest
- The physiologic alterations of pregnancy
- Basic life support and advanced life support protocols
- Cardiopulmonary resuscitation (CPR) adaptions during pregnancy.

Resuscitation in pregnancy

When a maternal cardiorespiratory arrest occurs, resuscitation should begin immediately and should follow the special basic and advanced life support guidelines. The physiological changes of pregnancy and the presence of the fetus require some additions to the normal algorithms (Table 85.2).

The 30° left lateral tilt of the mother is controversial, with the latest guidelines advocating manual lateral uterine displacement (Figure 85.1). This has better results and complies with the resuscitation science that advocates high-quality chest compression which are not possible when tilted.

Basic life support

Airway

Initially establish that cardiorespiratory arrest has occurred by first trying to rouse the collapsed woman by calling her name. Help needs to be obtained immediately. She then needs to be laid on a firm surface and the uterus displaced. A clear airway should be established as quickly possible using the head tilt–jaw thrust or head tilt–chin lift manoeuvre. This should then be maintained throughout. Suctioning should be used to aspirate any vomit. Badly fitting dentures or any other foreign bodies should be removed from the mouth.

Breathing

To ascertain if the woman is independently breathing, look at the chest, listen for breathing and feel for breath against the side of your face for 10 seconds. If not breathing then ask for an ambulance with an automated external defibrillator (AED) and start cardiac compressions with intermittent positive pressure ventilation at a ratio of 30 compressions to 2 breaths. Each breath should be 1 second and be carried out by mouth to mouth, mouth to nose or mouth to airway ventilation until a self-inflating bag mask and reservoir bag are available. Ventilation should then be continued with 100% oxygen. Due to the increased risk of regurgitation and pulmonary aspiration of gastric contents in late pregnancy and early postnatal period, cricoid pressure (Figure 85.2) should be applied until the airway has been protected by a cuffed tracheal tube.

Ventilation is made more difficult by the increased oxygen requirements and reduced chest compliance in pregnancy. The reduced compliance is due to rib spread and splinting of the diaphragm by the pregnancy. Observing chest movement in pregnant patients is also more difficult. However, if the chest does not appear to inflate then reposition the head before the second breath or insert an oropharyngeal airway if available.

Chest compressions

Commence chest compressions if there is an absence of a palpable pulse in a large artery (carotid or femoral). Chest compressions should be given at the standard rate and ratio of 30 compressions to 2 breaths. Chest compression should be given at a rate of 100–120 per minute. Chest compression on a pregnant woman is made difficult by the ribs, raised diaphragm, obesity and breast hypertrophy. The diaphragm is pushed upwards by the pregnancy therefore the hand position for chest compressions should be moved up the sternum, although currently no guidelines suggest exactly how far.

CPR should continue until the women starts to show signs of regaining consciousness.

Advanced life support

Intubation

Intubation should be carried out as soon as a skilled attender is available because difficulty in tracheal intubation is common in pregnant women and specialised equipment may be needed.

Mouth to mouth or bag and mask ventilation is best done without pillows under the head and with the head and neck fully extended. The position for intubation, however, requires at least one pillow to flex the neck and extend the head. In the event of failure to intubate the trachea or ventilate the woman's lungs with a bag and mask, insertion of a laryngeal mask airway should be attempted. Cricoid pressure must be temporarily removed in order to place the laryngeal mask airway successfully. Once the airway is in place, cricoid pressure should be reapplied.

Defibrillation and drugs

Defibrillation and drug administration should be in accordance with advanced life support recommendations.

Caesarean section

Caesarean section is not performed merely to save the life of the fetus but is an important part in the resuscitation of the mother. Prompt surgical interventions have resulted in many successful resuscitation attempts. The probable mechanism for a favourable outcome is that occlusion of the inferior vena cava is relieved completely by emptying the uterus, whereas it is only partially relieved by manual uterine displacement. Removal of the baby will also improve thoracic compliance, which will improve the chest compressions and the ability to ventilate the lungs.

CPR must be continued throughout the operation and afterwards because this improves the prognosis for mother and child.

86 Neonatal resuscitation

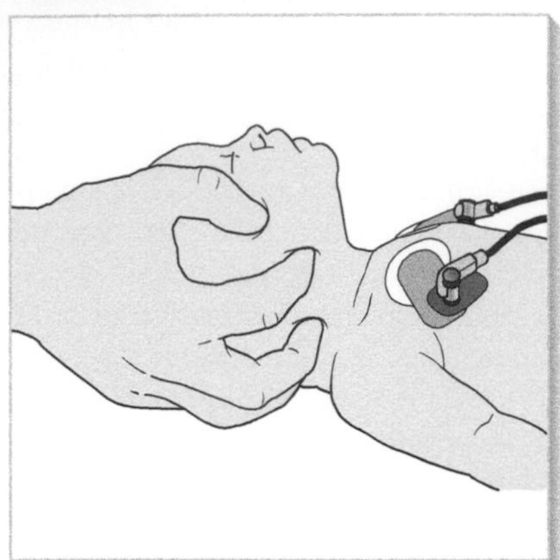
Figure 86.1 Neutral position.

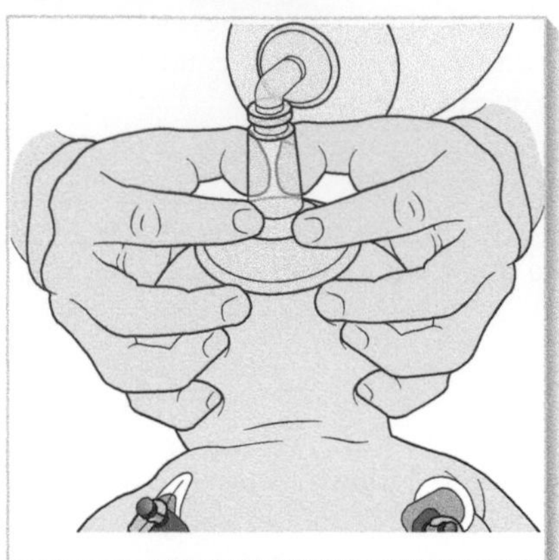
Figure 86.2 Jaw thrust.

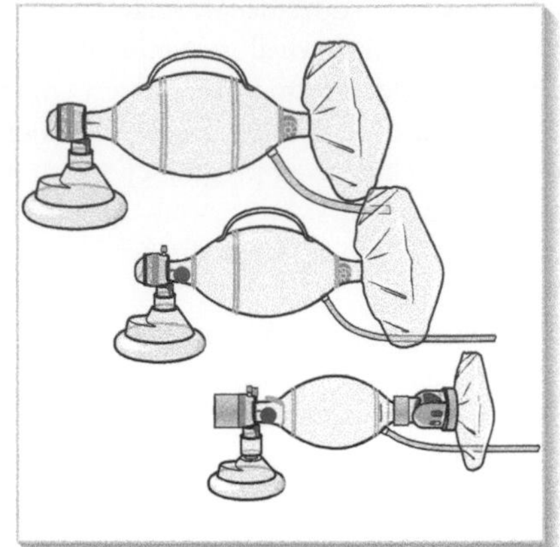
Figure 86.3 Ambubag.

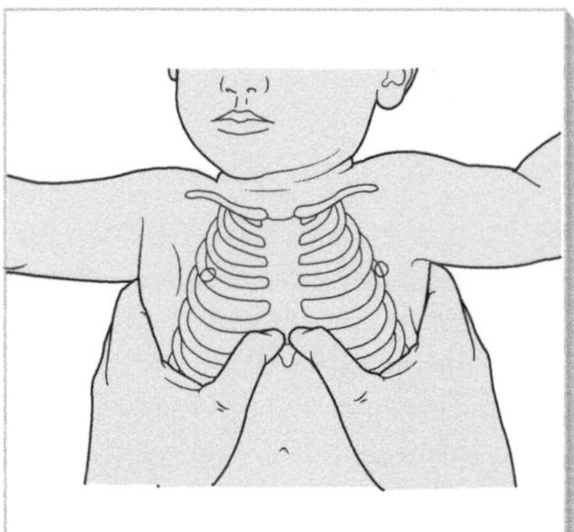
Figure 86.4 Position of thumbs for cardiac compression.

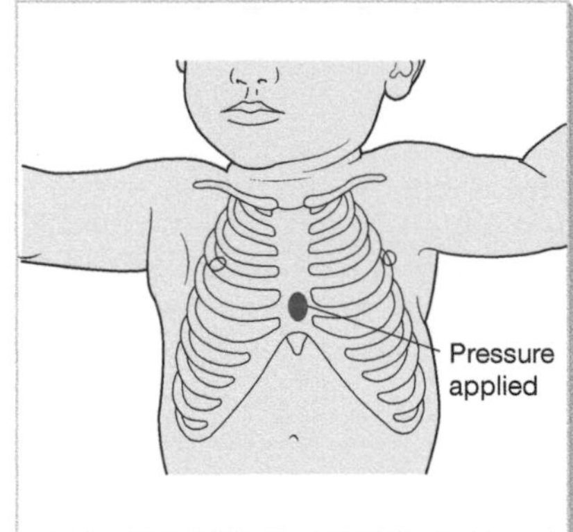

Figure 86.5 Position on sternum for cardiac compression.

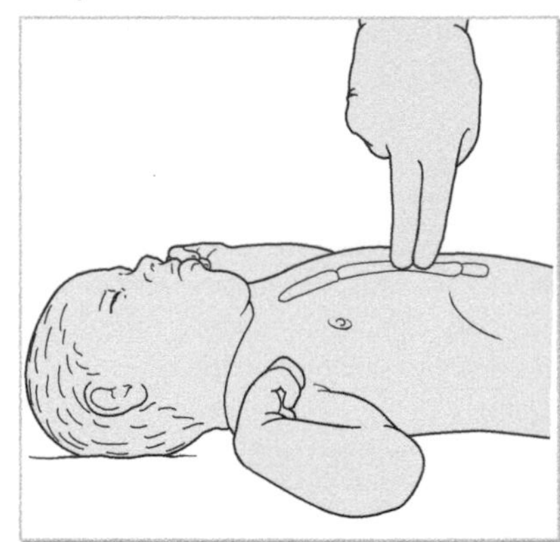
Figure 86.6 Two finger cardiac compression.

Figure 86.7 Drugs via umbilical venous catheter.

Drugs given via umbilical venous catheter

- Epinephrine Adrenaline 1:10 000 dose 10 μg/kg (0.1 ml/kg) if not successful then and other dose of 30 μg/kg (0.3 ml/kg)
- Sodium bicarbonate 4.2% 1 to 2 mmol per kg (2 to 4 ml)
- (i) 10% dextrose 250 milligrams/kg (2.5 ml/kg). If hypovolaemia is present then a bolus of 10 ml/kg of 0.9% (ii) sodium chloride given over 10–20 seconds

Table 86.1 Apgar score.

Sign	0	1	2
Appearance (colour)	Blue, pale	Body pink, limbs blue	All pink
Pulse (heart rate)	Absent	<100	>100
Grimace (response to stimuli)	None	Grimace	Cry
Activity (muscle tone)	Limp	Some flexion of limbs	Active movements, limbs well flexed
Respiratory effort	None	Slow, irregular	Good strong cry

Midwifery at a Glance, First Edition. Edited by Eleanor Forrest © 2019 John Wiley & Sons, Ltd. Published 2019 by John Wiley & Sons, Ltd.
Companion website: www.wiley.com/go/forrest/midwifery

During labour and the passage through the birth canal a fetus will have a hypoxic experience or lack of respiratory exchange during the 50–70-second average contraction. Few require assistance with normal breathing at birth, however if life support is needed a specific process of events should be followed. This process can be halted at any stage if breathing is established. The process for resuscitation should have the following steps:

- Drying and covering to conserve heat
- Assessing the need for any intervention
- Airway opening
- Lung inflation
- Rescue breathing
- Chest compressions
- Drugs.

Drying and covering

Babies are born wet and get cold easily, especially if they remain wet and in a draught. Being wet will impede their ability to recover from any hypoxic experience. Therefore it is imperative that the baby is dried and that the wet towels are removed and they are covered with dry towels (Chapter 60). This process provides good stimulation which encourages the baby to breathe and also allows the midwife to assess the baby's colour, tone, breathing and heart rate.

Assessing condition

To assess the baby's condition at birth the Apgar scoring system is used to assess the following signs: appearance (colour), pulse (heart rate), grimace (response to stimuli), activity (muscle tone) and respiratory effort and to give a score of 0, 1 or 2 at 1 minute, 5 minutes and possibly 10 minutes (Table 86.1) (Chapter 60).

A healthy baby at 1 minute is likely to have the following signs: blue extremities that become pink during the first 90 seconds from birth, a heart rate of 120–150 beats/min, will cry within few seconds from birth, have good tone, and be breathing regularly by 90–120 seconds from birth. A less healthy baby at 1 minute will be blue, have a heart rate <100 beats/min, have made only a weak cry at birth, have a tone that is not good and will not establish regular breathing by 90–120 seconds from birth. An ill baby at 1 minute will be born pale, have a very slow heart rate judged by stethoscope or pulsation of cord, no peripheral pulse, will not cry, will be floppy and will have no breathing.

Airway

If a baby is not breathing or is having difficulty breathing, after drying and covering, as assessed by looking, listening and feeling for 5 seconds, you need to check for any obstruction in the nose or mouth. You then need to open the airway by lying the baby flat on its back on a hard surface with the head in a neutral position (Figure 86.1) or apply a chin–jaw thrust (Figure 86.2), and check for breathing again.

Suctioning

Suctioning should not be routine as it can cause vagal stimulation which leads to an autonomic nervous system reaction. This leads to bradycardia and apnoea. If an obstruction is present then suction should only be done under direct vision using a laryngoscope.

If meconium is present and the baby is crying no suctioning is needed. If meconium is present without the baby breathing, suction under direct vision.

Breathing

To assist a baby with breathing you need the appropriate equipment. A Laerdal/ambu bag with a pressure release valve (Figure 86.3) is needed and possibly a Guedel airway. If the baby is not breathing adequately by 90 seconds give five inflation breaths. An inflation breath requires sustained pressures of 30 cmH_2O for 2–3 seconds using air only. It is important that you watch for chest movement to make sure that the air is getting into the lungs. If effective ventilation occurs the heart rate should increase. If the heart rate responds but the baby fails to begin breathing itself, it will be necessary to give ventilation breaths using the Laerdal/ambu bag with a pressure release valve of 20 cmH_2O at a rate of 30–40 breaths per minute until the baby breathes independently.

Lack of response to inflation breaths

If the heart rate does not respond to the inflation breaths it is most likely caused by a failure to inflate the chest. Therefore you need to:

- Check head and neck are in a neutral position
- Check pressure of 30 cmH_2O is given
- Check correct length of breath of 2–3 seconds
- Check chest movement
- If no movement ask for help
- Two people are required for chin–jaw thrust
- Consider obstruction
- Suction under direct vision
- Use oropharyngeal airway (Guedel).

Chest compressions

After the five inflation breaths, if the heart rate remains less than 60 per minute or is absent despite good chest movement, then chest compressions need to be started. Almost all babies needing help at birth will respond to successful lung inflation, with an increased heart rate and spontaneous breathing.

Chest compressions should only occur after inflation of the lungs. Grip the chest in both hands with the thumbs of both hands pressed on the sternum (Figure 86.4) at the point of the imaginary line joining the nipples (Figure 86.5).The fingers are over the spine at the back or use two fingers on the sternum (Figure 86.6).

When compressing the chest it should be done quickly and firmly, reducing the anterior posterior diameter by about one-third. The rate of compression to inflation should be 3:1.

Drugs

Drug use is very rare and only really needed if lung inflation and chest compressions are not sufficient for effective circulation. Drugs should be given via an umbilical venous catheter:

- Adrenaline 1:10 000, dose 10 μg/kg (0.1 ml/kg); if not successful then another dose of 30 μg/kg (0.3 ml/kg)
- Sodium bicarbonate 4.2%, 1–2 mmol/kg (2–4 ml)
- 10% dextrose, 250 mg/kg (2.5 ml/kg)
- If hypovolaemia is present then a bolus of 10 ml/kg of 0.9% sodium chloride should be given over 10–20 seconds (Figure 86.7).

87 Examination of the newborn

Figure 87.1 Antenatal history.

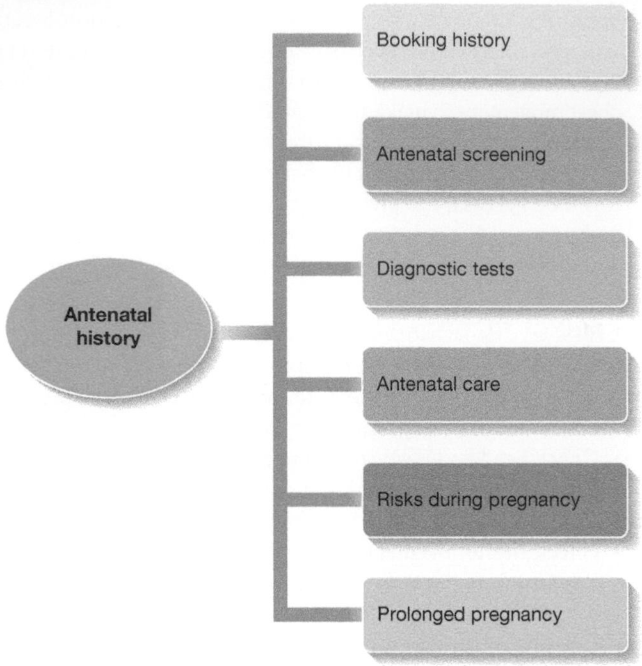

- Antenatal history
  - Booking history
  - Antenatal screening
  - Diagnostic tests
  - Antenatal care
  - Risks during pregnancy
  - Prolonged pregnancy

Figure 87.2 Intranatal events.

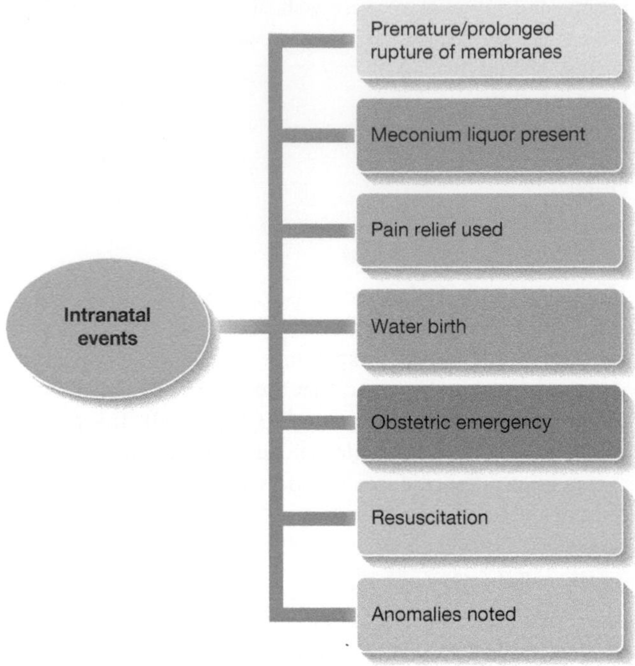

- Intranatal events
  - Premature/prolonged rupture of membranes
  - Meconium liquor present
  - Pain relief used
  - Water birth
  - Obstetric emergency
  - Resuscitation
  - Anomalies noted

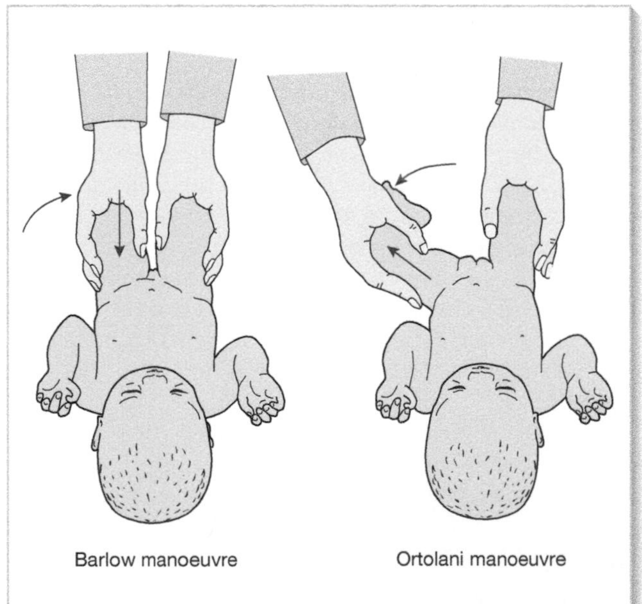

Figure 87.3 Testing for hip dysplasia.

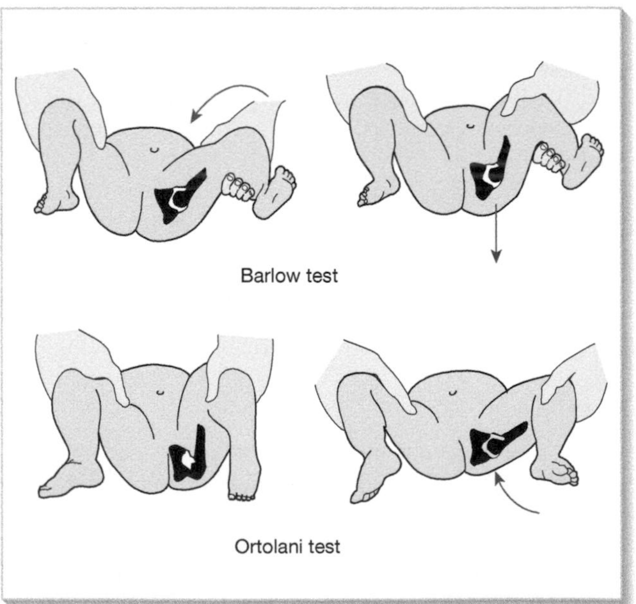

Figure 87.4 Barlow and Ortolani tests. Source: Adapted from http://www.cssd.us/body.cfm?id=512.

Box 87.1 Barlow's manoeuvre.

- Adduct the hip (bringing the thigh towards the midline)
- Apply light pressure on the knee, directing the force posteriorly
- If the hip is dislocatable, the hip can be popped out of socket (positive)

Box 87.2 Ortolani's manoeuvre.

- Flex the hips and knees of a supine infant to 90°
- Apply anterior pressure on the greater trochanter
- Apply gentle and smooth abduction of the infant's legs using the examiner's thumbs
- A positive sign is a 'clunk' which can be heard and felt as the femoral head relocates anteriorly into the acetabulum

Midwifery at a Glance, First Edition. Edited by Eleanor Forrest © 2019 John Wiley & Sons, Ltd. Published 2019 by John Wiley & Sons, Ltd.
Companion website: www.wiley.com/go/forrest/midwifery

The clinical examination is a top to toe physical examination of a newborn baby usually carried out as an examination prior to discharge. The examination will allow major congenital abnormalities to be excluded and provides information and reassurance to the parents of the health of their baby at that moment in time, thus addressing any concerns. The examination should also be the time to educate the parents on what to observe about their baby's health and when they should seek medical advice. The examination is part of the post birth screening of all babies which also includes: an immediate check after birth (Chapter 60); hearing testing; neonatal blood spot (Chapter 88); and a physical examination at 8 weeks of age. Examination of the newborn requires detailed knowledge of fetal development and neonatal systems and an understanding of theory with regard to screening these systems for abnormities in the newborn infant. The examination involves auscultation of the lungs and heart and examination of the eyes, including the use of an ophthalmoscope to look at the back of the eye. The abdomen should be palpated and the hips assessed.

The content of the neonatal examination should include three main elements: (i) preparation, which involves acquiring information and knowledge of antenatal history and intranatal events; (ii) observation of the baby; and (iii) the physical and clinical examination of the newborn.

Preparation

Antenatal history

Before commencing examination of the neonate, the practitioner should take the essential step of reading the mother's case notes and thus becoming familiar with the antenatal history (Figure 87.1). Details of the mother's general health, family health and social habits, screening tests and care need to be reviewed. This information and knowledge of fetal development will alert the practitioner to whether the baby has been compromised as a result of hazardous exposure during pregnancy. For example, if exposed to rubella during pregnancy, or to sources of potential fetal compromise such as smoking, alcohol, drug abuse, infection and environmental hazards. The practitioner will need to consider the implications of these antenatal events for the mother and baby so that they can be anticipated during the examination.

Intranatal events

There are many aspects of the intranatal history that it is important to know before examining the new born (Figure 87.2). Being aware of these issues will allow the practitioner to understand and rationalise certain aspects of their observations and physical and clinical examination and to look for sequelae of any risk factors that occurred during this time, for example maternal pyrexia in labour.

Observation before examination

Checking the baby should start with a general observation of their appearance, including colour, breathing, behaviour, activity and posture. This can be done prior to disturbing the newborn.

Physical and clinical examination

Examine the exposed parts of the baby first; again this will not disturb the baby too much and will not expose it to a cooler environment. These areas are the head (including fontanelles), scalp, face, nose, mouth (including palate), ears, neck and general symmetry of head and facial features. The rest of the examination covers the following:

- Measure and plot the head circumference
- The eyes should be checked for opacities and red reflex using an ophthalmoscope
- If exposed, the limbs, hands, fingers, feet and toes could be examined at this time for proportion and symmetry
- The newborn then needs to be undressed, so make sure the environment is warm
- The heart needs to be checked for position, heart rate, rhythm, sounds and murmurs and the femoral pulse needs to be palpated for volume
- The lungs need to be checked with a stethoscope for effort, and rate of breathing and lung sounds
- The abdomen needs to be checked in relation to shape and be palpated to identify any organomegaly. The condition of the umbilical cord should be noted. The renal area should also be palpated
- The genitalia and anus need to be examined for completeness and patency and in males the testes are examined to ensure they are descended
- The spine is inspected and palpated for bony structures and to check the integrity of the skin
- The clavicles should be observed and palpated to identify any abnormalities such as fractures
- The skin's colour and texture needs to be observed, also noting any birthmarks or rashes
- The central nervous system is examined by observing the baby's tone, behaviour, movements and posture, and reflexes can be elicited
- The hips are checked for symmetry of the limbs and skin folds and the Barlow and Ortolani manoeuvres performed (Boxes 87.1 and 87.2 and Figures 87.3 and 87.4)
- The baby's cry should be noted, considering both sound and pitch
- A check of the baby's weight should be made and plotted on the growth chart.

Following the examination

The baby should be redressed as soon as possible and made comfortable, either in the cot or in the arms of a parent. The findings need to be discussed with the parents and any questions answered. It is important that the parents are aware that the examination is for that moment in time and are given information on how to look for possible problems in the future in their newborn. Parents need to be treated as individuals and their need for reassurance will be based on their experiences of pregnancy and childbirth. All findings of the examination need to be appropriately and accurately recorded.

If a referral is deemed necessary, this should be made in accordance with the policies, routes and systems of the specific health board. For example, babies with a cardiac murmur will usually be referred for immediate review and investigation. Babies with a high risk of hip problems should be referred for secondary screening regardless of clinical finding. Babies with a family history of hereditary eye conditions should be referred to a specialist.

88 Newborn bloodspot screening

Figure 88.1 Newborn conditions screened.

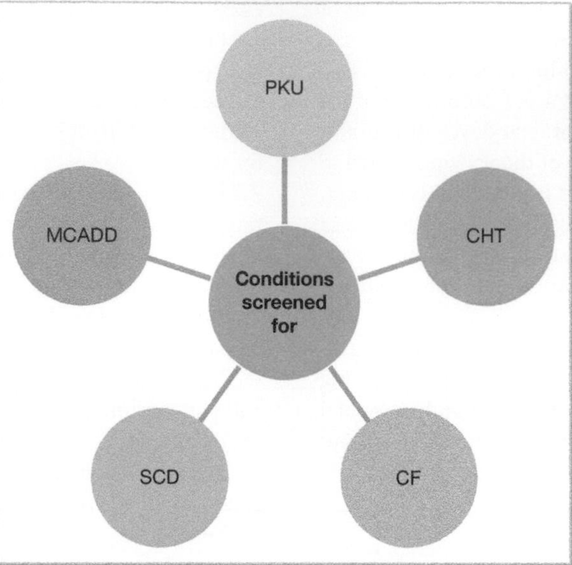

Figure 88.2 Puncture site for bloodspot.

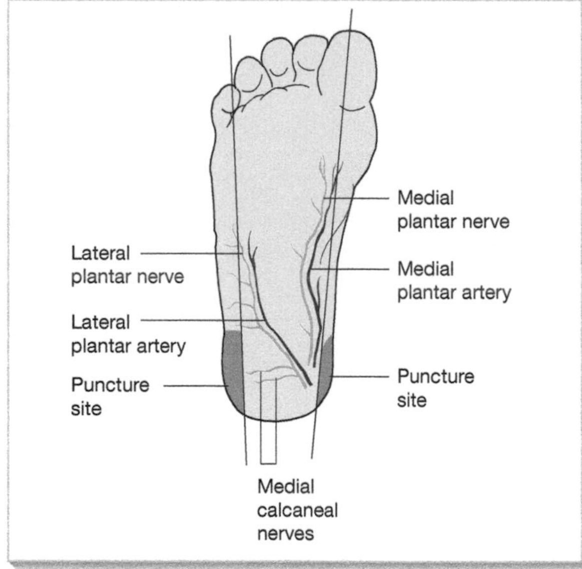

Newborn bloodspot screening is a recommended test in the UK for all newborn babies to identify those who may have rare but serious conditions. The aim of screening is to ensure early detection, referral and treatment of babies thought to be affected by the following conditions (Figure 88.1):

- Phenylketonuria (PKU)
- Congenital hypothyroidism (CHT)
- Cystic fibrosis (CF)
- Sickle dell disorders (SCD)
- Medium chain acyl CoA dehydrogenase deficiency (MCADD).

The NHS Newborn Blood Spot Screening Programme in England has offered expanded screening for a total of nine disorders, which include the following inherited metabolic diseases in addition to the above list: maple syrup urine disease (MSUD), isovaleric acidaemia (IVA), glutaric aciduria type 1 (GA1) and homocystinuria (pyridoxine unresponsive) (HCU). Due to the importance of newborn bloodspot screening, such as the health implications for a baby if any of the above conditions are not detected, and to prevent any newborn not being followed up, there should be a very comprehensive process in place.

Maternity services

The first stage of this process is providing the parents with information about all the tests to be undertaken so that they can give informed consent, or decline the test/s. If they decline some or all the tests, the GP needs to be informed. Additionally, the parents need information about the fact that the benefits of screening may be lost by delay, what to do if they change their minds, or if the baby develops signs and symptoms of the conditions that would have been screened for. Parents' understanding of this information needs to be established. If they decide at a later stage to have the tests they need to ask their GP or health visitor to organise it and they will liaise with the screening laboratory.

If parents have given consent then the blood sample needs to be taken on day 5, or in exceptional circumstances between days 5 and 8, after birth (day of birth counted as day 0), using the approved card (Figure 88.2). The process should be explained to the parents so they can choose if they are present or not. If they choose to be present one of them can hold the baby whilst the blood is taken. The mother could breastfeed or either parent could hold the wrapped baby. A good quality bloodspot sample is necessary to ensure that babies with rare but serious conditions are identified and treated early. Poor-quality samples can cause inaccurate results and can give false negative (underfilled circles or compression of the sample) or false positive (layering the blood or applying the blood to the front and back of the card) results.

- To obtain capillary blood from the baby, usually the heel is used
- The heel should be cleansed with either alcohol or water and should be dried carefully to prevent contamination of the specimen
- It is important to use the lateral and medial parts of the heel as puncture sites (Figure 88.2). Imagine a line from between the fourth and fifth toe and the middle of the big toe
- Capillary blood taking is done by the heel pricking process using a lancet or automated blood-letting device process; allow a few seconds for the blood to flow so that a large drop can collect
- When you have finished, apply pressure to the site with gauze or cotton wool and when bleeding has stopped a small plaster should be applied
- Each circle on the card needs to be filled with one drop of blood so that it soaks through the absorbable paper; do not layer the blood
- The specimen card should be filled in with all the relevant details: baby's CHI number or bar code label and gestational age (weeks and days) and then sent to the specific laboratory in the correct envelope
- Document that the bloodspot has been taken in the mother's maternity notes and the baby's health record.

Newborn screening laboratory

The newborn screening laboratory will check the sample for quality and if necessary they will request a repeat sample from the maternity services. If the sample is accepted it will then be tested and the results sent to the child health record team. If an abnormality is found it is sent to a specialist team. The specialist team will request an appointment with the baby to make a confirmatory diagnostic test. If the diagnosis is confirmed they will instigate the intervention/treatment.

Child health record team

The child health team will generally consist of the GP and health visitor and other professionals such as a paediatrician. The GP is notified of the birth of the baby and informed of the acceptance or not of the bloodspot testing. They are also notified of the receipt of the sample in the laboratory and the results. They are also informed if the screening is incomplete. Subsequently:

- Primary care child health record team will notify the health visitor of any missing results
- The primary care team will take samples in older babies
- The health visitor ensures that the parents receive the results and records these in the baby's records by 8 weeks
- If these results are normal this notification will sent be by letter to the parents
- If a problem is detected, the health visitor and/or a counsellor will inform the parents of the results and inform the newborn screening laboratory of this notification
- This process may differ slightly depending on health board area.

Care of women having surgery

Box 89.1 Possible surgical procedures.

- Caesarean section
- Perineal repair
- Manual removal of placenta
- Abscess drainage
- Cervical suture removal (cervical cerclage)
- General surgery (e.g. appendicectomy, cholecystectomy)

Box 89.2 Rationale for identification.

- Personal identification of the woman is necessary as she may be compromised or unconscious

Box 89.3 Rationale for psychological preparation.

- The midwife can ensure that the woman (and her partner) are fully informed of what is happening and give an explanation of the procedure where possible. It can also be useful to allow parents to meet theatre staff

Box 89.4 Rationale for fasting.

To ensure that there are no gastric contents which could be regurgitated, and subsequently inhaled, fasting is recommended

- Stomach empties of food in 6–8 hours and fluids in 2–3 hours
- Pregnancy, labour, anxiety and drugs such as pethidine can delay gastric emptying
- Women having elective surgery should fast for 6 hours prior

Box 89.5 Preoperative blood tests.

- The most recent haemoglobin must be noted
- The availability of saved serum in the laboratory must be established in case urgent cross-matching is required

Box 89.6 Principles of asepsis.

To provide an area free from infectious agents all staff should wear:

- Clean scrub outfit, face mask, hat and protective footwear

If directly involved in surgery:

- 5-minute hand scrub with antiseptic soap or detergent
- Sterile gown
- Sterile gloves

i.v. antibiotics should be offered routinely to prevent postoperative infection

Box 89.7 Positioning in theatre.

The anaesthetist will help position the woman for the anaesthetic.
For spinal anaesthesia:

- Tilt theatre table to 15°
- Woman should be supported upright, in a seated position, bending forward. Place a pillow on her lap to support the abdomen and provide reassurance

Box 89.8 Airway maintenance.

For a general anaesthetic this includes:

- Use of preoxygenation
- Cuffed endotracheal tube
- Cricoid pressure
- Rapid sequence induction
- Mechanical ventilation

Should ventilation fail, refer to local protocol

Box 89.9 Recording vital signs postoperatively.

- Every 5 minutes for 20 minutes…then
- Every 15 minutes for the first hour…then
- Half hourly if woman remains stable…then
- Hourly until the woman leaves the recovery area
- Use pulse oximetry to record oxygen saturation and assessment of colour

Midwifery at a Glance, First Edition. Edited by Eleanor Forrest © 2019 John Wiley & Sons, Ltd. Published 2019 by John Wiley & Sons, Ltd.
Companion website: www.wiley.com/go/forrest/midwifery

Many childbearing women will require surgery for a variety of reasons (Box 89.1) and it is therefore not uncommon for midwives to be involved in their pre-, peri- and postoperative care. Careful preparation can reduce complications and midwives have an important role as part of the multidisciplinary team caring safely for women at this time. Women are likely to have anxieties about surgery and the safety of their baby and the midwife should be sensitive to their particular concerns. Whether surgery is elective or emergency, involves local or general anaesthesia, surgical care should be holistic and include midwifery skills from pre- through to the postoperative period. *At all stages, check local protocols and guidelines which may have a care pathway outlining management requirements and ensure concise documentation.* These should include the following components.

Preoperative care

This relates to the care provided before the surgical procedure and should include psychological, physical and pre-anaesthetic assessment and checklist.

Identification

Correct identification of the woman must be written on an identification (ID) band and placed on her wrist: name, date of birth and hospital ID number (Box 89.2).

Written consent

A woman's decision to consent to surgery should be based on full information being provided and her understanding that information, including eventualities. The discussion should help the woman prepare psychologically for surgery (Box 89.3). A consent form signed by the woman and the obstetrician should be placed in the woman's notes. Prior to surgery this should be checked again against her ID band.

Drugs and fasting

Premedication drugs may be prescribed according to need as relaxant, antiemetic and analgesic. This should be given at the prescribed time in order to take effect prior to surgery. Antacids are prescribed to reduce the risk of aspiration and aspiration pneumonitis (Mendelson's syndrome). An H_2 antagonist (such as ranitidine 50 mg), given i.v. 1 hour prior to surgery can reduce gastric secretions, in conjunction with medication to reduce stomach pH (such as citric acid 30 ml). Fasting is indicated to also reduce the risk of aspiration (Box 89.4).

Other preparations

There is no conclusive evidence about the best preoperative skin preparation. It is recommended that, at the least, women should shower prior to surgery and remove all make-up and nail varnish to ensure visible nail bed colour. No deodorants or powder should be used as these may be flammable and jewellery should be removed or taped if a wedding ring. Hair removal from the operative site is not obligatory but, if required, clipping is preferred shaving. A gown should then be provided and underwear removed. Recent blood test results should be checked (Box 89.5). Baseline observations of temperature, pulse (P), respiration (R), blood pressure (BP) (Chapter 80) and fetal heart rate (Chapter 76) should all be recorded.

Perioperative care

Depending on the role assumed by the midwife in theatre, duties will vary. This may range from assisting in the operation to receiving the baby in a caesarean section. The principles of asepsis should be adhered to throughout (Box 89.6). The primary focus should always be the woman and maintenance of her safety and dignity, whether awake or anaesthetised. On transfer to theatre, check the woman's identity again and discuss any wishes she has regarding the baby and give time for both parents to prepare (if having an epidural). Check resuscitaire if preparing for the birth of the baby. A drape is generally placed over the woman to prevent her seeing the operation site, but if she requests to immediately see her baby a low screen should be put in place.

Positioning

The theatre table should be tilted to 15° to prevent aortocaval occlusion (Box 89.7).

Monitoring, airway maintenance and fluid management

Pulse oximetry is used to detect hypoxia, and BP is monitored and i.v. fluid volume adjusted to maintain BP as necessary. Record the woman's temperature every 30 minutes; use fluid warming device if required. For respirations and airway maintenance see Box 89.8. Depending on local protocol, an indwelling Foley catheter should be inserted into the woman's bladder (Chapter 79) either prior to or following the anaesthetic, and then attached to a drainage bag. An empty bladder during surgery reduces the risk of bladder trauma.

Postoperative care

Following the birth of the baby, the cord should be clamped and cut and the baby handed to the receiving midwife to take to the prepared resuscitaire. Dry, assess and wrap the baby to ensure warmth is maintained and then give the baby to the parents to hold for skin-to-skin contact and feeding (Chapter 60).

Following transfer from theatre to a recovery area, the woman should receive individual skilled midwifery care. A handover from the anaesthetist should provide the midwife with information regarding the procedure, medications and intravenous infusion regimen. If the woman had a general anaesthetic, remove the airway which the anaesthetist will have inserted following extubation; oxygen therapy may be required. Regardless of type of anaesthetic, assessment of BP, P and R should be recorded regularly (Box 89.9). Ensure correct positioning to care for numb and pressure areas. The following should also be cared for:

- Check for vaginal blood loss
- Care of wound and drain if applicable
- Care of urinary catheter and urinary output.

Pain relief and medication

Administer analgesia as appropriate following pain assessment. Ensure the woman has access to her patient-controlled analgesia (PCA). Administer subcutaneous heparin as prescribed.

References and further reading

Andrees M, Rankin J (2007) Amniotomy in spontaneous, uncomplicated labour at term. *British Journal of Midwifery*, 15(10), 612–616.

Andrews V, Sultan AH, Thakar R, Jones PW (2006) Risk factors for obstetric anal sphincter injury: a prospective study. *Birth*, 33, 117–122.

Arai L (2009) *Teenage Pregnancy: The Making and Unmaking of a Problem*. Policy Press, Cambridge.

ASH (Action on Smoking and Health) (2017) Home page. Available at: http://ash.org.uk/home/ (accessed August 2018).

Baghurst M, Antoniou G (2012) Risk models for benchmarking severe perineal tears during vaginal childbirth: a cross-sectional study of public hospitals in South Australia, 2002–08. *Paediatric and Perinatal Epidemiology*, 26, 430–437.

Ball HL, Howel, D, Bryant A, et al. (2016) Bed-sharing by breastfeeding mothers: who bed-shares and what is the relationship with breastfeeding duration? *Acta Paediatrica*, 105, 628–634.

Barlow J, Davis H, McIntosh E, et al. (2008) *The Oxfordshire Home Visiting Study: Three Year Follow Up*. University of Oxford, Oxford.

Baston H (2014) Antenatal care. In: Marshall J, Raynor M (eds) *Myles Textbook for Midwives*, 16th edn. Elsevier, Edinburgh, pp. 127–287.

BCSH (British Committee for Standards in Haematology) (2012) *Guideline on the Administration of Blood Components*. Available at: www.bcshguidelines.com (accessed August 2018).

Bentham K (2003) Maternity care for asylum seekers. *British Journal of Midwifery*, 11(2), 73–77.

Bick D, Ismail KMK, MacDonald S, et al. (2012) How good are we at implementing evidence to support the management of birth related perineal trauma? A UK wide survey of midwifery practice. *BMC Pregnancy and Childbirth*, 12, 57.

Bick D, Kettle C, MacDonald S, et al. (2010) Perineal Assessment and Repair Longitudinal Study (PEARLS): protocol for a matched pair cluster trial. *BMC Pregnancy and Childbirth*, 10(10), 1–8.

Billington M, Stevenson, M (2007) *Critical Care in Childbearing for Midwives*. Blackwell Publishing, Oxford.

Blackburn ST (2013) *Maternal, Fetal and Neonatal Physiology: A Clinical Perspective*, 4th edn. Saunders, St Louis.

Blake D (2008) Midwives: all things to all women? *British Journal of Midwifery*, 16(5), 292–294.

Bornstein MH (ed.) (2001) *Handbook of Parenting: Vol. 1 Children and Parenting*. Lawrence Erlbaum, Mahwah, NJ.

Bothamley J, Boyle M (2009) *Medical Conditions Affecting Pregnancy and Childbirth*. Radcliffe Publishing, Oxford.

Bowlby J (1982) *Attachment, Vol. 1 Attachment and Loss*. Basic Books, New York.

Briscoe L, Lavender T (2009) Exploring maternity care for asylum seekers and refugees. *British Journal of Midwifery*, 17(1), 17–24.

Burke N (2012) Clinical risk management of obstetric anal sphincter injury. *Clinical Risk*, 18, 19–22.

Caveretto P, Serafini A, Valsecchi L, et al. (2009) Early diagnosis, follow-up, and prenatal treatment of a case of TRAP sequence occurring in a dichorionic triamniotic triplet pregnancy. *Journal of Clinical Ultrasound*, 37(6), 350–354.

Children in Scotland (2011) *Working for Inclusion: the Role of the Early Years Workforce in Addressing Poverty and Promoting Social Inclusion*. Available at: https://childreninscotland.org.uk/working-for-inclusion/ (accessed August 2018).

CMACE (Centre for Maternal and Child Enquiries) (2011) Saving Mothers' Lives: Reviewing Maternal Deaths to Make Motherhood Safer: 2006–08. The Eighth Report on Confidential Enquiries into Maternal Deaths in the United Kingdom. *British Journal of Obstetrics and Gynaecology*, 118(Suppl. 1), 1–203.

Coad J, Dunstall M (2011) *Anatomy and Physiology for Midwives*, 3rd edn. Churchill Livingston Elsevier, Edinburgh.

Collins CH, Zimmerman C, Howard LM (2011) Refugee, asylum seeker, immigrant women and postnatal depression: rates and risk factors. *Archives of Women's Mental Health*, 14(1), 3–11.

Cooper AP (2005) *Structure of the Breast in the Human Female. On the Anatomy of the Breast, by Sir Astley Paston Cooper, 1840*. Paper 6. Available at: http://jdc.jefferson.edu/cooper/6 (accessed August 2018).

Department for Children, Schools and Families (2010) *Teenage Pregnancy Strategy: Beyond 2010*. Available at: http://dera.ioe.ac.uk/11277/1/4287_Teenage%20pregnancy%20strategy_aw8.pdf (accessed August 2018).

Department of Health (2007) *Maternity Matters: Choice, Access and Continuity of Care in a Safe Service*. HMSO, London.

Department of Health (2012) *Healthy Start. Retailer Research Summary*. Available at: https://assets.publishing.service.gov.uk/government/uploads/system/uploads/attachment_data/file/216866/DH-template-retailer-research-FINAL1.pdf (accessed August 2018).

Dobbing J, Kaiser AM, Sullivan J, et al. (1994) Warm chain for breastfeeding. *Lancet*, 344(8938), 1700–1702.

Downe S (2013) Physiology and care during transition and second stage phases of labour. In: Marshall J, Raynor M (eds) *Myles Textbook for Midwives*, 16th edn. Elsevier, Edinburgh, p. 367.

Dunn P (1994) Perinatal lessons from the past: Dr Grantly Dick-Read (1890–1959) of Norfolk and natural childbirth. *Archives of Disease in Childhood*, 71, F145–F146.

Edwards NP (2004) Why can't women just say no? And does it really matter? In: Kirkham M (ed.) *Informed Choice in Maternity Care*. Palgrave Macmillan, Basingstoke, pp. 1–22.

Elharmeel S, Chaudhary Y, Tan S, et al. (2011) Surgical repair of spontaneous perineal tears that occur during childbirth versus no intervention. *Cochrane Database of Systematic Reviews*, 8, Article No. CD008534.

Fernando RJ, Sultan AH, Freeman RM, et al. (2007) *Green-top Guideline No. 29. The Management of Third and Fourth-Degree Perineal Tears*. RCOG, London.

Freeman R (2013) Can we prevent childbirth-related pelvic floor dysfunction? *British Journal of Obstetrics and Gynaecology*, 120, 137–140.

Godfrey KM, Gluckman PD, Hanson MA (2010) Developmental origins of metabolic disease: life course and intergenerational perspectives. *Science Direct*, 21(4), 199–205.

Hanley J (2009) *Perinatal Mental Health.* Wiley, Chichester.

Hedayati H, Parsons J, Crowther CA (2003) Rectal analgesia for pain from perineal trauma following childbirth. *Cochrane Database of Systematic Reviews,* 3, Article No. CD003931.

Henley-Einion A (2009) The medicalisation of childbirth. In: Squire C (ed.) *The Social Context of Birth,* 2nd edn. Radcliffe, Oxford, pp. 180–190.

Hoekstra C, Zhao Z, Lambalk C, et al. (2008) Dizygotic twinning. *Human Reproduction Update,* 14(1), 37–47.

Howie L, Watson J (2017) The second stage of labour. In: Rankin J (ed.) *Physiology in Childbearing with Anatomy and Related Biosciences,* 4th edn. Elsevier, Edinburgh, pp. 411–427.

ICM (International Confederation of Midwives) (2011) ICM International definition of the midwife. Available at: https://internationalmidwives.org/who-we-are/policy-and-practice/icm-international-definition-of-the-midwife/ (accessed August 2018).

Inskip H, Crozier S, Godfrey K, et al. (2009) Women's compliance with nutrition and lifestyle recommendations before pregnancy: general population cohort study. *British Medical Journal,* 12, 338:b481.

Jentsch B, Durham R, Hundley V, Hussein J (2007) Creating consumer satisfaction in maternity care: the neglected needs of migrants, asylum seekers and refugees. *International Journal of Consumer Studies,* 31(2), 128–134.

Johnson R & Taylor W (2010) *Skills for Midwifery Practice,* 3rd edn. Elsevier, Edinburgh.

Jones RL, Jewsbury SM (2007) *Teenage Pregnancy and Reproductive Health.* Royal College of Obstetricians and Gynaecologists/Dorchester Press, Dorchester.

Kalis V, Laine K, De Leeuw JW, et al. (2012) Classification of episiotomy: towards a standardisation of terminology. *British Journal of Obstetrics and Gynaecology,* 119, 522–526.

Kalis V, Landsmanova J, Bednarova B, et al. (2011) Evaluation of the incision angle of mediolateral episiotomy at 60 degrees. *International Journal of Gynaecology and Obstetrics,* 112, 220–224.

Kennedy P, Harris M, Humphries K, Nabb J (2006) Delivering care for women seeking refuge. *RCM Midwives Journal,* 9(5), 190–192.

Kettle C (2012) The pelvic floor. In: Macdonald S, Magill-Cuerden J (eds) *Mayes' Midwifery: A Textbook for Midwifery,* 14th edn. Baillière Tindall, London.

Kettle C, Dowswell T, Ismail K (2010) Absorbable suture materials for primary repair of episiotomy and second degree tears. *Cochrane Database of Systematic Reviews,* 6. Article No. CD000006.

Kettle C, Dowswell T, Ismail K (2012) Continuous and interrupted suturing techniques for repair of episiotomy or second-degree tears. *Cochrane Database of Systematic Reviews,* 11, Article No. CD000947.

Kettle C & Raynor MD (2010) Perineal management and repair. In: Marshall J, Raynor M (eds) *Advancing Skills in Midwifery Practice.* Churchill Livingstone, Edinburgh, pp. 103–121.

Khaled M, Ismail K, Kettle C, et al. (2013) Perineal Assessment and Repair Longitudinal Study (PEARLS): a matched-pair cluster randomized trial. *BMC Medicine,* 11, 209.

King R, Glover P, Byrt K, Porter-Nocella L (2011) Oral nutrition in labour: 'Whose choice is it anyway?' A review of the literature. *Midwifery,* 27, 674–686.

Kitzinger S (2005) *The Politics of Birth.* Elsevier, Edinburgh.

Knight M, Tuffnell D, Kenyon S, et al. (eds) on behalf of MBRRACE-UK Saving Lives, Improving Mothers' Care (2015) *Surveillance of Maternal Deaths in the UK 2011–13 and Lessons Learned to Inform Maternity Care from the UK and Ireland Confidential Enquiries into Maternal Deaths and Morbidity 2009–13.* National Perinatal Epidemiology Unit, University of Oxford, Oxford.

Kurth E, Jaeger FN, Zemp E, et al. (2010) Reproductive health care for asylum-seeking women – a challenge for health professionals. *BMC Public Health,* 10, 659.

Laine K, Glisser M, Pirhonen J (2009) Changing incidence of anal sphincter tears in four Nordic countries through the last decades. *European Journal of Obstetrics, Gynecology and Reproductive Biology,* 146(1), 75.

Laine K, Stedenfeldt FE, Sandvik L, et al. (2012) Incidence of obstetric anal sphincter injuries after training to protect the perineum: cohort study. *BMJ Open,* 2, e001649

Lawrence A, Lewis L, Hofmeyr GJ, et al. (2009) Maternal positions and mobility during first stage of labour. *Cochrane Database of Systematic Reviews,* 15, Article No. CD003934.

Leeman L, Spearman M, Rogers R (2003) Repair of obstetric perineal lacerations. *American Family Physician,* 68(8), 1585–1590.

Lenders C, McElrath T, Scholl T (2000) Nutrition in adolescent pregnancy. *Current Opinions in Pediatrics,* 12(3), 291–296.

Lewis G (ed.) (2007) *The Confidential Enquiry into Maternal and Child Health (CEMACH). Saving Mothers' Lives: Reviewing Maternal Deaths to Make Motherhood Safer – 2003–2005. The Seventh Report on Confidential Enquiries into Maternal Deaths in the United Kingdom.* CEMACH, London.

MacDonald S, Magill-Cuerden J (2012) *Mayes Midwifery,* 14th edn. Elsevier, Edinburgh.

Magill-Cuerden J (2012) Choosing homebirth. In: Steen M (ed.) *Supporting Women to Give Birth at Home.* Routledge, London, pp. 15–44.

Marieb EN, Hoehn K (2013) *Human Anatomy and Physiology,* 9th edn. Pearson, Boston.

Marshall J, Raynor M (eds) (2014) *Myles Textbook for Midwives,* 16th edn. Elsevier, Edinburgh.

Martin EA (ed.) (2010) *Oxford Concise Colour Medical Dictionary,* 3rd edn. Oxford University Press, Oxford.

Maslow AH (1988) *Motivation and Personality,* 3rd edn. Harper & Row, New York.

Matthews L, Rankin J (2017) Muscle – the pelvic floor and the uterus. In: Rankin J (ed.) *Physiology in Childbearing with Anatomy and Related Biosciences,* 4th edn. Elsevier, Edinburgh, pp. 263–275.

McAndrew F, Thompson J, Fellows L, et al. (2012) *Infant Feeding Survey 2010.* NHS Health and Social Care Information Centre. Available at: http://www.greenwichbreastfeeding.com/media/1634/infant-feeding-survey-2010-consolidated-report.pdf (accessed August 2018).

McLeish J (2005) Maternity experiences of asylum seekers in England. *British Journal of Midwifery,* 13(12), 782–785.

Mendelson L (1946) Aspiration of gastric contents into lungs during obstetric anaesthesia. *American Journal of Obstetrics and Gynaecology,* 52, 191–205.

Meetoo D (2010) In too deep: understanding, detecting and managing DVT. *British Journal of Nursing,* 19(16), 1021–1027.

Midwifery 2020 (2010) *Delivering Expectations.* Available at: https://assets.publishing.service.gov.uk/government/uploads/system/uploads/attachment_data/file/216029/dh_119470.pdf (accessed August 2018).

Moatti Z, Gupta M, Yadava R, Thambian S (2014) A review of stroke and pregnancy: incidence, management and prevention. *European Journal of Obstetrics and Gynecology and Reproductive Biology,* 181, 20–27.

Moore ER, Bergman N, Anderson GC, Medley N (2012) Early skin-to-skin contact for mothers and their healthy newborn infants. *Cochrane Database of Systematic Reviews,* 16(5), Article No. CD003519.

Moran VH (2007) A systematic review of dietary assessments of pregnant adolescents in industrialised countries. *British Journal of Nutrition,* 97(3), 411–425.

Murphy-Lawless J (2003) The maternity care needs of refugee and asylum seeking women in Ireland. *Feminist Review*, 73, 39–53.

Nelson-Piercy C (2015) *Handbook of Obstetric Medicine*, 5th edn. CRC Press, Boca Raton, FL.

NHS Choices (2018) *Drinking Alcohol While Pregnant*. Available at: http://www.nhs.uk/conditions/pregnancy-and-baby/pages/alcohol-medicines-drugs-pregnant.aspx#close (accessed August 2018).

NHS Smokefree (2018) Home page. Available at: http://www.nhs.uk/smokefree (accessed August 2018).

NICE (National Institute for Health and Care Excellence) (2005) *Clinical Guideline 30. Long-Acting Reversible Contraception*. NICE, London. Available at: https://www.nice.org.uk/guidance/cg30/resources/longacting-reversible-contraception-pdf-975379839685 (accessed August 2018).

NICE (National Institute for Health and Care Excellence) (2006) *Clinical Guideline 37. Postnatal Care up to 8 Weeks After Birth*. Available at: https://www.nice.org.uk/guidance/cg37 (accessed August 2018).

NICE (National Institute for Health and Care Excellence) (2008a) *Clinical Guideline 62. Antenatal Care for Uncomplicated Pregnancies*. Available at: https://www.nice.org.uk/guidance/cg62 (accessed August 2018).

NICE (National Institute For Health and Care Excellence) (2008b) *Clinical Guideline 70. Inducing Labour*. Available at: https://www.nice.org.uk/guidance/cg70 (accessed August 2018).

NICE (National Institute for Health and Care Excellence) (2010a) *Weight Management Before, During and After Pregnancy*. NICE, London.

NICE (National Institute for Health and Care Excellence) (2010b) *Hypertension in Pregnancy: Diagnosis and Management*. NICE, Manchester.

NICE (National Institute for Health and Care Excellence) (2011a) *Public Health Guidance 11 Update. Maternal and Child Nutrition*. Available from: http://www.nice.org.uk/nicemedia/live/11943/40097/40097.pdf (accessed August 2018).

NICE (National Institute for Health and Care Excellence) (2011b) *Clinical Guideline 129. Multiple Pregnancy: Antenatal Care for Twin and Triplet Pregnancies*. NICE, London.

NICE (National Institute for Health and Care Excellence) (2012a) *Venous Thromboembolic Diseases: the Management of Venous Thromboembolic Diseases and the Role af Thrombophilia Testing*. NICE, London.

NICE (National Institute for Health and Care Excellence) (2012b) *Pre-Conception – Advice and Management*. Available at: http://cks.nice.org.uk/pre-conception-advice-and-management (accessed August 2018).

NICE (National Institute for Health and Care Excellence) (2014a) *Clinical Guideline 192. Antenatal and Postnatal Mental Health: Clinical Management and Service Guidance*. Available at: https://www.nice.org.uk/guidance/cg192 (accessed August 2018).

NICE (National Institute for Health and Care Excellence) (2014b) *Clinical Guideline 190. Intrapartum Care for Healthy Women and Babies*. Available at: https://www.nice.org.uk/guidance/cg190 (accessed August 2018).

NICE (National Institute for Health and Care Excellence) (2015) *Quality Statement 4. Infant Health – Safer Infant Sleeping*. Available at: http://www.nice.org.uk/postnatal-care-qs37/quality-statement-4-infant-health-safer-infant-sleeping#quality-statement-4 (accessed August 2018).

NMC (Nursing and Midwifery Council) (2012) *Midwives Rules and Standards*. NMC, London.

NMC (Nursing and Midwifery Council) (2015) *The Code: Professional Standards of Practice and Behaviour for Nurses and Midwives*. NMC, London.

Oates J (ed.) (2007) *Attachment Relationships: Quality of Care for Young Children. Early Childhood in Focus, 1*. Open University, Milton Keynes.

O'luanaigh P, Carlson C (2005) *Midwifery and Public Health*. Elsevier, Edinburgh.

ONS (Office for National Statistics) (2013) *General Lifestyle Survey: 2011*. Available at: https://www.ons.gov.uk/peoplepopulationandcommunity/personalandhouseholdfinances/incomeandwealth/compendium/generallifestylesurvey/2013-03-07 (accessed August 2018).

Page L, McCandlish R (2006) *The New Midwifery*, 2nd edn. Elsevier, Amsterdam.

Parenting Across Scotland (2018) Home page. Available at: http://www.parentingacrossscotland.org/about-us.aspx (accessed August 2018).

Ramsay DT, Kent JC, Hartman RA, Hartman PE (2005) Anatomy of the lactating breast redefined with ultrasound imaging. *Journal of Anatomy*, 206(6), 525–534.

Raynor M & England C (2010) *Psychology for Midwives*. Open University Press, Maidenhead.

RCM (Royal College of Midwives) (2004) *Teenage Parents: Who Cares? A Guide to Commissioning and Delivering Maternity Services for Young Parents*. Teenage Pregnancy Unit, DH Nursing and Midwifery Policy, Royal College of Midwives/Department of Health, London.

RCOG (Royal College of Obstetricians and Gynaecologists) (2004) *Guideline No. 23. Methods and Materials Used in Perineal Repair*. RCOG, London.

RCOG (Royal College of Obstetricians and Gynaecologists) (2007) *Guideline No. 29. The Management of Third- and Fourth-Degree Perineal Tears*. RCOG, London.

RCOG (Royal College of Obstetricians and Gynaecologists) (2008) *Clinical Governance Advice No. 6. Obtaining Valid Consent*. RCOG, London.

RCOG (Royal College of Obstetricians and Gynaecologists) (2010) *Consent Advice No. 9. Repair of Third- and Fourth-Degree Perineal Tears Following Childbirth*. RCOG, London.

RCOG (Royal College of Obstetricians and Gynaecologists) (2011) *Green-top Guideline No. 57. Reduced Fetal Movements*. Available at: https://www.rcog.org.uk/globalassets/documents/guidelines/gtg_57.pdf (accessed August 2018).

RCOG (Royal College of Obstetricians and Gynaecologists) (2015) *Green-top Guideline No. 37b. Thromboembolic Disease in Pregnancy and the Puerperium: Acute Management*. Available at: https://www.rcog.org.uk/globalassets/documents/guidelines/gtg-37b.pdf (accessed August 2018).

RCOG (Royal College of Obstetricians and Gynaecologists) (2016) *Alcohol and Pregnancy*. Available at: https://www.rcog.org.uk/en/patients/patient-leaflets/alcohol-and-pregnancy/ (accessed August 2018).

Reynolds B & White J (2010) Seeking asylum and motherhood: health and wellbeing needs. *Community Practitioner*, 83(3), 20–23.

Robson E, Marshall J, Doughty R, McLean M (2014) Medical conditions of significance to midwifery practice. In: Marshall J, Raynor M (eds) *Myles Textbook for Midwives*, 16th edn. Churchill Livingston, Edinburgh, pp. 244–253.

Robson Se, Waugh J (2013) *Medical Disorders in Pregnancy: A Manual for Midwives*, 2nd edn. Wiley-Blackwell, Oxford.

Scottish Government (2011) *A Refreshed Framework for Maternity Care in Scotland*. Scottish Government, Edinburgh. Available at: https://www.gov.scot/Resource/Doc/341632/0113609.pdf (accessed August 2018).

Seu BI (2003) The woman with the baby: exploring narratives of female refugees. *Feminist Review*, 73, 158–165.

SIGN (Scottish Intercollegiate Guidelines Network), HIS (Healthcare Improvement Scotland) (2012) SIGN 127. *Management of Perinatal Mood Disorders*. Available at: https://www.sign.ac.uk/assets/sign127_update.pdf (accessed August 2018).

Simkin P (2010) The fetal occiput position: state of the science and a new perspective. *Birth*, 37(1), 61–71.

Smyth R, Aldred S, Markham C, Dowswell T (2007) Amniotomy for shortening spontaneous labour. *Cochrane Database of Systematic Reviews*, 6, Article No. CD006167.

Snowden A, Martin C, Jomeen J, Hollins Martin C (2011) Concurrent analysis of choice and control in childbirth. *BMC Pregnancy and Childbirth*, 11(40), 1–11.

Stables D & Rankin J (2010) *Physiology in Childbearing*. 3rd edn. Elsevier, Edinburgh.

Start 4 Life (2018) *Can I drink alcohol when pregnant?* Available at: https://www.nhs.uk/start4life/pregnancy/alcohol/ (accessed August 2018).

Stedenfeldt M, Pirhonen J, Blix E, et al. (2012) Episiotomy characteristics and risks for obstetric anal sphincter injuries: a case-control study. *British Journal of Obstetrics and Gynaecology*, 119, 724–730.

Steegers E, Van Dadelszen P, Duvekot J, Pijenborg R (2010) Pre-eclampsia. *Lancet*, 376, 631–644.

Symon A (2008) Third degree tears: the three-stage negligence test. *British Journal of Midwifery*, 16(3), 192–193.

Thakar R, Sultan A (2014) The female pelvis and reproductive organs. In: Marshall J, Raynor M (eds) *Myles Textbook for Midwives*, 16th edn. Churchill Livingston, Edinburgh, pp. 64–69.

Trochez R, Waterfield M, Freeman R (2011) Hands-on or hands-off the perineum: a survey of care of the perineum in labour (HOOPS). *International Urogynecology Journal*, 22(10), 1279–1285.

Thorell SE, Parry-Jones A, Punter M, et al. (2015) Cerebral venous thrombosis – a primer for the haematologist. *Blood Reviews*, 29, 45–50.

Ukoko F (2005) Sure Start midwife: giving a voice to the voiceless. *British Journal of Midwifery*, 13(12), 776–780.

UNICEF (2001) *A League Table of Teenage Birth of Rich Nations. Innocenti Report Card, Vol. 3*. UNICEF Innocenti Research Centre, Florence.

UNICEF (2013) *The Evidence and Rationale for the UNICEF UK Baby Friendly Initiative Standards*. Available at: https://www.unicef.org.uk/babyfriendly/wp-content/uploads/sites/2/2013/09/baby_friendly_evidence_rationale.pdf (accessed August 2018).

United Nations (2011) *The Millennium Development Goals Report*. Available at: http://www.un.org/millenniumgoals/pdf/(2011_E)%20MDG%20Report%202011_Book%20LR.pdf (accessed August 2018).

Verralls S (1980) *Anatomy and Physiology Applied to Obstetrics*, 2nd edn. Churchill Livingstone, Edinburgh.

White Ribbon Alliance, The (2011) *Respectful Maternity Care: The Universal Rights of Childbearing Women*. Available at: https://www.whiteribbonalliance.org/wp-content/uploads/2017/11/RMC_Brochure.pdf (accessed August 2018).

Wickham A (2012) Management of obstetric anal sphincter injury. *British Journal of Midwifery*, 20(8), 540–543.

Widstrom Am, Lilja G, Aaltomaa-Michalias P, et al. (2011) Newborn behaviour to locate the breast when skin-to-skin: a possible method for enabling early self-regulation. *Acta Paediatrica*, 100(1), 79–85.

WHO (World Health Organisation) (1981) *International Code of Marketing of Breast-milk Substitutes*. Available at: http://www.who.int/nutrition/publications/code_english.pdf (accessed August 2018).

WHO (World Health Organisation) (2003) *The World Health Report 2003 – Shaping the Future*. Available at: http://www.who.int/whr/2003/en/ (accessed August 2018).

WHO (World Health Organisation) (2006) *Pregnant Adolescents: Delivering on Global Promises of Hope*. WHO, Geneva.

WHO (World Health Organisation) (2013) *Meeting to Develop a Global Consensus on Preconception Care to Reduce Maternal and Childhood Mortality and Morbidity*. Available at: http://apps.who.int/iris/bitstream/10665/78067/1/9789241505000_eng.pdf?ua=1 (accessed August 2018).

Index

Page numbers in *italics* refer to illustrations or tables

Midwifery at a Glance, First Edition. Edited by Eleanor Forrest © 2019 John Wiley & Sons, Ltd. Published 2019 by John Wiley & Sons, Ltd.
Companion website: www.wiley.com/go/forrest/midwifery